Thinking in Circles About Obesity

Thinking in Circles About Obesity

Applying Systems Thinking to Weight Management

Tarek K.A. Hamid

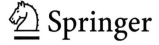 Springer

Tarek K.A. Hamid
Department of Operations Research
Naval Postgraduate School
Monterey CA 93943
USA
tkabdelh@nps.edu

ISBN 978-0-387-09468-7   e-ISBN 978-0-387-09469-4
DOI 10.1007/978-0-387-09469-4
Springer New York Dordrecht Heidelberg London

Library of Congress Control Number: 2009931951

Printed on acid-free paper

Springer is part of Springer Science+Business Media (www.springer.com)

To Nadia: My wife and best friend.

Preface

Today's children may well become the first generation of Americans whose life expectancy will be shorter than that of their parents. The culprit, public health experts agree, is obesity and its associated health problems.

Heretofore, the strategy to slow obesity's galloping pace has been driven by what the philosopher Karl Popper calls "the bucket theory of the mind." When minds are seen as containers and public understanding is viewed as being a function of how many scientific facts are known, the focus is naturally on how many scientific facts public minds contain. But the strategy has not worked. Despite all the diet books, the wide availability of reduced-calorie and reduced-fat foods, and the broad publicity about the obesity problem, America's waistline continues to expand. It will take more than food pyramid images or a new nutritional guideline to stem obesity's escalation.

Albert Einstein once observed that the significant problems we face cannot be solved at the same level of thinking we were at when we created them, and that we would have to shift to a new level, a deeper level of thinking, to solve them. This book argues for, and presents, a different perspective for thinking about and addressing the obesity problem: a *systems thinking* perspective. While already commonplace in engineering and in business, the use of systems thinking in personal health is less widely adopted. Yet this is precisely the setting where complexities are most problematic and where the stakes are highest. Though the tools and concepts associated with systems thinking are new and advanced, the underlying worldview is extremely intuitive. Even young children can learn systems thinking very quickly.

This book aims to apply systems thinking to personal health in a form that is accessible to the general reader, with the hope that it will have a profound influence on how ordinary people think about and manage their health and well-being. The book is written to help the following readers:

- Individuals seeking to better understand how to control/manage their bodies and their well-being.
- Parents who need to address the systemic, long-term risks of this complex but slowly developing threat before children get trapped in lifestyles that ultimately result in chronic obesity.
- Public policy makers who need to move beyond the *infomercial* model to prevention, that is, aiming to stuff people's "mental buckets" with nutritional guidelines and food pyramid images, to a customized knowledge *restructuring* model—one that challenges people's deeply ingrained assumptions about health risk and well-being.

The Book's Outline

The book has five parts. Part I is an introductory discussion of the problem's scope and its burden (on people and society), and the argument for a *different* way of thinking.

Part II traces the development of the epidemic and delineates its multiple causes. One of the few reasonably reliable facts about the obesity epidemic is that it started in the early 1980s. We need to understand why. The trigger that induced obesity's escalation was not a single factor (e.g., a sudden upsurge in moral failure), but rather the confluence of multiple socioeconomic and technological factors.

Parts III and IV focus on the solution. Reducing the national waistline will require a major shift in thinking about managing our instincts and our environment; motivation alone is not going to be enough. Effective self-regulation of health behavior, as with the regulation of any dynamic system (whether it is the energy regulation of our bodies or the energy regulation of an atomic reactor), requires two essential skills: understanding and prediction. Part III focuses on understanding—helping people think systematically about the inner workings of human weight/energy regulation so that they can better manage their own bodies and health.

Part IV discusses prediction. While understanding helps us look *backward* to make sense of the past (e.g., explaining weight gain), we need prediction to look *forward* (e.g., to devise treatment strategies and assessing treatment outcomes). The ability to infer a system's behavior is essential if we are to know how actions influence the system, and thus is essential in devising appropriate interventions for change. Perfect understanding without a capability to predict the system's behavior is of little practical utility. The two skills—understanding and prediction—are needed together.

Part V discusses prevention. While the attention to the treatment of obesity has heretofore overwhelmed that given to prevention, interest in obesity prevention is attracting increasing attention because of the growing realization that it may be easier, less expensive, and more effective to change behavior, so as to prevent weight gain or to reverse small gains, than to treat obesity after it has fully developed.

The great advances in systems sciences, medicine, and communication technology are converging with another powerful trend: the increase in public initiative, so that people take greater responsibility for their well-being. This is opening enormous possibilities for empowering people with the tools they need for disease prevention and personal health management. Part V discusses the possibilities.

The Story of the Book

The series of events that ultimately led to writing this book are a bit unusual. In the mid-1990s I became extremely interested in the confluence of information and medical technologies, and saw it as one of the most promising new frontiers for system dynamics research and public policy. But I had a lot to learn. So, in 1997, I took an open-ended leave-of-absence and enrolled in the master's program at Stanford University's Engineering Economic Systems and Operations Research Department, where I focused on decision analysis and medical decision making. (Returning to become a master's student while already holding a PhD was certainly a weird experience, for me and for my professors, but it was a lot of fun.) It was during my studies at Stanford that I began to see the natural fit between the obesity problem (as a dynamic system of energy regulation) and system dynamics. (Research was revealing that human bioenergetics belongs to the class of multiloop nonlinear feedback systems, the same class of system that system dynamics aims to study.)

Upon graduation, I spent a year (1999–2000) as an affiliate at Stanford's Medical Informatics Department (part of Stanford's Medical School), where I worked on developing system dynamics models of human physiology and metabolism. In December 2001, I returned to my faculty position at the Naval Postgraduate School where I continued to conduct research on medical decision making and modeling of human metabolism and energy regulation.

I started writing this book in the winter of 2003.

Acknowledgments

Many authors, sitting with keyboard at the ready, must have thought, as I did, of the first few phrases of *Don Quixote*: "Idle reader, you may believe me without any oath that I would want this [work], the child of my brain, to be the most beautiful, the happiest, the most brilliant imaginable. But I could not contravene that law of nature according to which like begets like." If such can be said of Cervantes's brainchild, what can one possibly say about one's own[1]? Only that one has done one's best. And yet, if the truth be told, that "best" may prove to belong as much to certain others as to one's self.

This book is a product of the stimulating environments at three institutions. For twenty years, the Naval Postgraduate School has provided a hospitable environment for my research and writing. I am especially indebted to Dan C. Boger, chairman of the Department of Information Sciences, who fosters camaraderie and an intellectual climate that celebrates bold original thinking that I believe I could not have found elsewhere. My students are not only the country's "fittest" but also our finest. They make going to work every day a lot of fun and have been a source of pride and inspiration. (My only complaint: they are all so "Navy fit" that they proved to be very poor research subjects.)

I have been blessed to have attended two great learning institutions: MIT and Stanford. Among the many people who have contributed to my work and thinking at MIT, I am particularly indebted to Professors Stuart E. Madnick, John Sterman, and John Morecroft.

I have also been fortunate to have had the opportunity to learn from Professor Elizabeth Paté-Cornell at Stanford. She taught me everything I know about risk management, and she is the one who sparked my interest in health prevention.

---

[1] Konner, M. J. (1982). *The Tangled Wing: Biological Constraints on the Human Spirit*. New York: Holt, Rinehart and Winston.

At Springer I am grateful for the excellent support, genuine enthusiasm, and good cheer of my editor Janice Stern and her tireless assistant Ian Marvinney.

Special thanks to Rena Henderson and David Kaplan, whose editorial suggestions have been invaluable and for teaching me a thing or two about style and clarity.

But there is only one person who has made every single aspect of this book possible—my wife, Nadia. Others have contributed greatly, but nobody could possibly match her encouragement, guidance, commitment, and sacrifices.

Contents

I   Mismanaging the Obesity Threat   1

1   Like Boiled Frogs   3
    How the Problem Sneaked Up on Us   3
    The Temperature Is Rising   5
    The Heavy Burden of Obesity   7
    For Older Americans, The Future Is Now.   9
    The Sociocultural Burden   10
    "Globesity"   11
    A Bucket Half-Empty?   12
    The Leverage (or the Impediment) Is with the People.   13
    It Is Not Easy Becoming a *Top Gun*   14
    States *In* Mind   16
    Emotions Play a Role   20
    Failure to Learn from Failure   22
    Single-Loop vs. Double-Loop Learning   22
    Barriers to Learning   27
    What Is to Be Done?   28
    Metanoia   28
    Synthesis, Not Analysis   28
    What Is Feedback?   32
    Circles, Not Straight Lines   32
    Dynamic, Not Static   36
    Obliterating, Not Automating   38
    Notes   41

II   How We Changed Our Environment, and Now Our Environment
    Is Changing Us   51

2   Unbalanced Act   53
    Moving Beyond Individual-Centric Explanations   56
    Evolved Asymmetry of Our Physiology   58

How Asymmetry Is Achieved by Our Physiology 60
Asymmetry in Energy Intake............................... 60
Asymmetry in Energy Expenditure......................... 63
Asymmetry in Energy Storage............................. 65
Conclusion 66

3   Human–Environment Interactions: Not One Way ... and
    Not One-Way 69
Human Behavior Is Not Expressed in a Vacuum.................. 71
It Is Not Just *Physical*....................................... 72
A Symphony Out of Tune?...................................... 75

4   Tilting the Energy Balance: More Energy In 77
The Quantity of Food We Eat 78
The Causes Behind the Cause 80
How America's Eating Habits Started to Change................. 80
The First Mechanism: The *Time* We Eat........................ 86
Soft Drinks: The Liquid Snack............................. 88
The Second Mechanism: *Where* We Eat 90
Fast Food: Eat Anywhere, Everywhere 91
The Qualitative Dimension 92
The *Quantity* Dimension 95
Events Give Birth to Trends, But What Escalates Them
Are Self-Reinforcing Processes 100
Demand–Pull 103
Supply–Push... 105
Putting It All Together....................................... 108
Hurricane Obesa... 109

5   Tilting the Energy Balance: Less Energy Out. 111
The Water Is Boiling!... 111
Work: Engineering Energy Expenditure Out
of the Workplace 113
Moving About: Transport and Urban Design..................... 115
Play and Leisure.. 118
The Burden Is Cumulative...................................... 120
Dr. Jekyll and Mr. Hyde, or Changing the Vicious to Virtuous 121

6   Individual Differences.. 125
Some Are "Squares," and Some Are Not........................ 125
Deciphering the Code, One Gene at a Time 126
Genes and Individual Susceptibility to Weight Gain:
The Experimental Findings 128
The Pimas.. 130
Genetic × Environmental Interactions: Conclusion................. 132

7 Is *Ad-Lib* Behavior Killing Us? 135
   A (Mis-)Match Made in America 135
   Like Our Genes, Our Mental Models Did Not Change............... 137
   Turning-Off *Automatic* Control and Asserting *Cognitive*
   Control 138
   It Can Be Done.. 140
   The Allure of the "Silver Bullet" 142
   Looking Ahead.. 144
   Notes.. 145

III We Can't Manage What We Don't Understand 167

8 The Energy Balance Equation: Reigning Intellectual Paradigm
   or Straitjacket?... 169
   The Magic Number 170
   From the Experts' Mouths to the Journalists' Ears to the
   Public's Mind 171
   We Like to Believe that We Are in Full Control.................. 173

9 What We Know that Ain't So 175
   Looking Back Versus Looking Forward 175
   The First Trap: Linear Thinking 177
      A Plumbing Analogy 180
   A Second Trap: Energy as a Single Currency 182
   We Need a Better "Map" 184

10 Closing the Loops on Energy Balance: Energy Output Side........... 185
   Tip of a Physiological Iceberg! 185
   "Under-the-Surface" Determinants of Energy Expenditure........... 186
   The System in Action: "Under the Surface" Responses to Energy
   Imbalance.. 191
   Implications for Treatment 193
      Failure to Account for Individual Differences 193
      How an Energy Deficit Is Induced Also Matters 195
   Seeing Through the Complexity 196
   Revisiting the Bathtub Analogy............................... 197
   Learning to "Squint" 199

11 Closing the Loops on Energy Balance: Energy Input Side 203
   Body Defenses on the Second Energy Front..................... 203
   Two-Tier System: Short-Term and Long-Term 204
      Short-Term Component.................................... 205
      Long-Term Component.................................... 206
   Two Asymmetries, Not One.................................. 208
   A Homeostatic System with a Difference 210

12 **Beyond Physiology: Closing the Behavior–Physiology Loop** 215
   Not Only Do We Eat Food, We Also Think About It 215
   Which Requires More Effort: To Do or Not to Do? 216
   Strength (and Weakness) Model of Human Self-Regulation 217
   A First Course in Managing Stocks and Flows 219
   The Evidence: To Use It Is to Lose It, at Least Temporarily 221
   A Challenge for the Self: How to Accomplish a Lot with a Little. 222
   Why Goals Matter, and How More May Be Less 224
   Weight Cycling: Not Once, Not Twice 230
   Understanding How Cycles Happen 231
   Longer-Term Risks 235
   Less Is More 236

13 **Looking Back and Looking Forward** 239
   Looking Back 239
   Understanding Is a First Step, But Far from Sufficient 240
   Looking Forward 243
   Notes 245

IV **We Can't Manage What We *Mis*-Predict** 263

14 **Learning by Doing** 265
   How Hard Can It Be? 266
   Trying Your Hand at Predicting Dynamics 267
      The Bathtub Exercise 267
      The Answer 269
      What Do These Results Tell Us? 271
   Beyond Bathtubs 274

15 **"Give Us the Tools, and We Will Finish the Job"** 277
   Sources of Complexity in Systems 277
   The KISS Acronym: "Keep It Simple, Stupid" 279
   Argument for a Calculus 281
   Leveraging Computer Technology 282

16 **A Microworld for Weight and Energy Regulation** 283
   Telescopes for the Mind. 283
   Simulation Models Are *Operational* Models. 284
   Overview of Model Structure. 287
   Energy Intake (EI) Subsystem 289
   Energy Expenditure (EE) Subsystem 290
   Energy Metabolism and Regulation Subsystem 291
      Glucose and Free Fatty Acid Metabolism 292
      Protein/Amino Acid Metabolism 296
      Exercise Metabolism 297
   Body Composition Subsystem. 298

Fat Mass (FM) 299

Fat-Free Mass (FFM) 301

Taking Off. 301

17 Experiment 1: Assessing Weight Loss—Reality Versus Fiction. 303

The Experiment 305

Experimental Results 306

Looking Inside a White Box 308

It Is Not Academic 310

18 Experiment 2: Going Ballistic—On a Diet 311

Chasing a Moving Target. 311

The Experiment 312

It Is No Passive Tool 314

19 Experiment 3: Understanding Why 250 Pounds Does Not Equal 250 Pounds 317

Individual Differences: More than Meets the Eye 317

The Experiment 318

Phase 1: Overfeeding 318

Phase 2: Dieting 320

114 kg $\neq$ 114 kg $\neq$ 114 kg!. 321

One Size Does Not Fit All 322

20 Experiment 4: Trading Treatment Options—Diet Versus Exercise. 325

Energy Is Not a Single Currency 325

Diet Versus Exercise: Do 500 kcal = 500 kcal? 326

Trading Exercise Intensity for Exercising Time. 330

Manipulating Diet Composition 332

Don't Trade . . . Integrate. 334

21 PhDs for the Masses? (That's *Personal Health Decision* support) 335

Notes. 337

V Prevention and Beyond 351

22 The Fat Lady . . . Models 353

23 The Third Path: Prevention 357

Can't Unscramble an Egg. 357

The Buck Starts Here 358

Make Healthy Choices the Easy Choices. 361

Public Works to Level the Playing Field. 362

Energy Input. 363

"Thought for Food" 364

Economic Incentives 365

Energy Output   367
Often Preventable But Rarely Prevented.   369

24   Location, Location, Location: Places to Intervene in Systems   371
Behavior Change Cannot Be Legislated   371
Lessons from Managing America's *Other* Energy Problem   372
Leverage Points   377
Leveraging Paradigms . . . and Succeeding   379
Back in the United States: A Challenge and an Opportunity.   383

25   It Will Take More Than Food Pyramids   387
"Educate Them and They Will Change"   387
Half a Century of Government Education   387
It Is Not Working.   389
It Is Deeper Than Just That   391
Information Is Not Enough to Change Mental Models   393
Learning from Experience: A Bad Second Option   397
Lessons from Business: Learning About Risky Stuff Without
Experiencing the Risk   400
Transforming Prevention from a Spectator Sport to a Contact Sport. . . .   403
"*Virtual* to Your Health"   407

26   Microworlds ʃl Us   409
Child's Play.   411
Learning About Healthy Behavior by Playing, Not by Lecturing   412
Double-Loop Playing   414
(Almost) Never Too Young to Think Systematically   414
At Home, the Real Risk Is in Expecting Too Little.   417
Shifting the Burden and Its Risks   418
Keeping the Burden   421
Teaching Children to Fish   422
Balance of Powers and Responsibilities   424

27   Beyond Prevention   425
Wellness Does Not Mean Only a Lack of Disease.   425
Beyond Prevention of Disease   427
Health Potential Programs for People?   429
The Second Flowering   431
    Advances in Molecular Biology: The Know-How.   433
    Computational Modeling of Physiological Processes: The Models   433
    Ubiquitous Computing and Intelligent Sensors: The Personal Specs . .   434
    The Internet: The Information Infrastructure   437
Not Automating,. . . Obliterating.   437
Notes.   441

Subject Index   463

Mismanaging the Obesity Threat
I

Like Boiled Frogs

1

Today's children may well be the first generation of Americans whose life expectancy will be shorter than that of their parents.[1,2] The culprit, public health experts agree, is obesity and its associated health problems.

For more than a century now, people's weights in the United States have been steadily rising. But the recent rise in obesity that started around 1980 is fundamentally different from past changes. In the early decades of the twentieth century, weights were below levels recommended for maximum longevity, and an increase in weight represented an increase in health, not a decrease.[3] The problem we now face arose because we did not know when to stop. Rather than leveling off, weight gain in the population has continued its rise unabated, leaping beyond healthy levels and leaving them in the dust. Today, Americans are much fatter than medical science recommends, and weights continue to increase. The worry is that if this trend is not reversed, it could start wiping out much of the progress that has been made in preventing some of the other major chronic health problems, such as heart disease, diabetes, and certain cancers.[4]

How the Problem Sneaked Up on Us

As the upward and outward trend in the population's weight and waistline was gradually accelerating in the late 1980s and early 1990s, most public health experts, as well as the public at large, failed to perceive the escalating threat. It is not difficult to see why: unlike old-fashioned communicable diseases such as AIDS, malaria, or tuberculosis, obesity exhibits no immediate symptoms. Initially, obesity affected a few people, and the numbers of the overweight and obese grew slowly enough that we have had time to get used to them.[5] Furthermore, in the 1980s and 1990s the science establishing links among diet, weight, and health was just developing.[6]

T.K.A. Hamid, *Thinking in Circles About Obesity*,
DOI 10.1007/978-0-387-09469-4_1, © Springer Science+Business Media, LLC 2009

On a personal level, weight gain also seems insidious to most people. And that too is understandable. Unlike the polar bear, people do not get fat by voracious fat eating in a short period.[7] Instead, weight gain typically occurs slowly, over decades. For example, the age-related upward drift in weight for adult men is, on average, only about half a pound per year.[8] Because of a lack of immediate adverse consequences, the early stages of weight gain often go unnoticed or may be viewed as innocuous and inevitable, or even as a sign of maturity.[9] And so a gradual increase in body weight might not be recognized until people are trapped in an unhealthy lifestyle, which can ultimately result in chronic obesity.[10]

It would take years for the nation to take notice. Not until the tail end of the 1990s did we begin to pay much attention to obesity and the effects of a poor diet and a sedentary lifestyle on health and well-being.[11]

Maladaptation to slowly building threats is by no means limited to obesity, and neither is it uncommon. Human beings are exquisitely adapted to recognize and respond to threats to survival that come in the form of sudden, salient events. "We are here today, as a species, because when something went bump in the night in the primeval forest, we noticed and reacted."[12] Our fixation on jolting events, it has been argued, is part of our evolutionary programming.[13] Change that is slow and gradual, however, is less perceptible to our cognitive apparatus. It is why, for example, we are much less likely to notice signs of aging in someone we live with (e.g., spouse or child) than we are in people we see intermittently (e.g., distant relatives). It is not that we are incapable of sensing continuous, gradual change; indeed, we often do. (For example, as a sailor I know I have no problem tracking every change in cloud formation of an approaching storm front while at sea.) But because our attention span is not unlimited, while the number of life's events competing for our attention is quite large, we tune in only to the changes we perceive as particularly important or threatening.[14] In the case of obesity, a lack of immediate adverse consequences often means that it is off our radar screen.

Societal maladaptation to creeping threats has been so pervasive and enduring in human affairs that it has been enshrined in social and public policy circles as the parable of the boiled frog:

> If you place a frog in a pot of boiling water, it will immediately try to scramble out. But if you place the frog in room-temperature water, and don't scare him, he'll stay put. Now, if the pot sits on a heat source, and if you gradually turn up the temperature, something very interesting happens. As the temperature rises from 70 to 80 degrees Fahrenheit, the frog will do nothing. In fact, he will show every sign of enjoying himself. As the temperature gradually increases, the frog will become groggier and groggier, until he is unable to climb out of the pot. Though there is nothing restraining him, the frog will sit there and boil. Why? Because the frog's internal apparatus for sensing threats to survival is geared to sudden changes in his environment, not to slow, gradual changes.[15]

The parable aims to highlight how subtle and insidious gradual change can be, and even if unhealthy and contrary to survival, it nevertheless can be tolerated over time and ultimately take life from the unsuspecting or complacent.

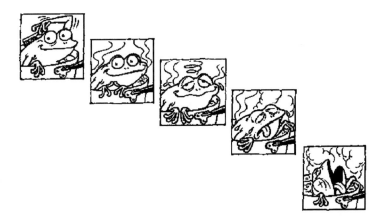

Figure 1.1 The boiled frog. (*Source:* www.crownresearch.com/RIJ.htm)

Early in our evolution as a species, our alertness to jolting threats had some powerful payoffs. The irony today is that the primary threats to our collective survival come not from sudden events but from slow, gradual processes.[16] The rise of religious militancy, environmental decay, global warming, and the depletion of the ozone layer are all slow, gradual threats, as is the growing obesity epidemic.

The Temperature Is Rising

Since 1960, five National Health and Nutrition Examination Surveys have been conducted to track health status and behavior in the United States.[17] Collectively, these surveys are considered the most definitive assessments of Americans' weight because of the duration and size of the studies and because they actually measure people's height and weight. The results of the latest survey (in 2004) reveal that two of every three American adults older than 20 (or 65 percent) are overweight, with a body mass index (BMI) of more than 25. The BMI is calculated as weight in kilograms divided by the square of the height in meters. This compares to fewer than one in four in the early 1960s.[18–19] This means that, currently, there are more than 130 million Americans who are overweight enough to begin experiencing health problems as a direct result of that weight. Even more concerning, close to half of them (approximately 60 million Americans) are heavy enough to count as clinically obese (with a BMI greater than 30); that is, they are so overweight that their lives will likely be cut seriously shorter by excess fat. A BMI of 30 (the threshold to obesity) roughly means being 30 pounds overweight for an average-height woman and 35 to 40 pounds overweight for an average-weight man.[20]

Not only has the speed at which obesity escalated in the population been alarmingly impressive, but so has its breadth. A recent study by researchers at the Centers for Disease Control and Prevention (CDC) found that "the rate of American obesity was increasing in every state and among both sexes, regardless of age, race, or educational level."[21] It seems hard to believe that a chronic condition like obesity could spread with the speed and breadth of a communicable disease epidemic, but it has.[22]

What is perhaps most ominous of all is that obesity is increasing even more rapidly among children and adolescents than it is among the adult population. Most of today's obese adults were not obese children, accumulating their extra pounds only after they were 25 or 30 years old. "But now we have more and more [young] people who are already obese at the age of 10, 15, or 20."[23] Today there are nearly twice as many overweight children and almost three times as many overweight adolescents as there were in the 1980s. The latest government data show that 30 percent of children and adolescents—about 25 million—are overweight or are at risk of becoming so.[24] That is the highest number ever recorded. All these overweight children and adolescents are on a course to fuel an even bigger national health problem as they mature into obese adults.

Even our pets are not immune. Almost 25 percent of America's dogs and cats are now obese. And the experts are saying our pets are gaining weight for many of the same reasons people do. "They're living longer . . . are often fed too much . . . and are increasingly confined to fenced-in suburbs with shrinking yards. Guilty owners, meanwhile, are showing their love not with walks, but [with] snacks."[25],[26]

If the rate of obesity in the general population continues to increase at the same pace it has for the past two decades, the *entire* U.S. adult population (and its pets) could be overweight within a few generations.[27] This is more than a red flag; this is fireworks going off.[28],[29]

Yet, despite all the grim statistics, obesity has not yet entered America's social consciousness. Rather than seeing a red flag (or fireworks), the general public continues to view obesity as a cosmetic rather than a health problem.[30] A recent study by Harvard University researchers found that most Americans are still not seriously concerned with obesity and do not view it as a major health concern either for the country as a whole or particularly for themselves. The general public's perceptions about health risks were instead found to be skewed by highly visible and more emotionally charged health issues, such as heart attacks and AIDS, which were ranked far ahead of obesity as the most serious health concerns. Interestingly, more than half the respondents in the Harvard study were overweight, yet few saw their own weight as a serious heath issue.[31]

The Heavy Burden of Obesity

All this would matter less if being overweight were beneficial or, at very least, safe. But in most cases it is neither. While the complications of obesity may not be as dramatic as those of HIV, for example, its burden can affect more people and is a source of far more deaths. According to the CDC, obesity now kills five times as many Americans as microbial agents—that is, infectious diseases.[32] In 2000, the most recent year for which CDC figures are available, obesity accounted for more than 112,000 deaths in the United States.[33] Experts predict that if current trends continue, with Americans smoking less but continuing to get fatter, obesity will soon overtake smoking as the primary preventable cause of death among Americans.[34]

In a new study, a group of Dutch researchers sought to quantify the mortality risk people face from being overweight. Specifically, they sought to assess the years of life lost (YLL) due to obesity, that is, the difference between the number of years one would be expected to live if obese versus not obese. The study was one of a few that actually tracked a group of individuals over an extended period and that helped identify the deleterious effects of obesity on health and longevity in ways that cannot be revealed by "snap-shot"-type studies that look at a cross-section of the population at one point in time. Their findings, based on a study of the health history of more than three thousand people over four decades (between 1948 and 1990), were portentously straightforward: getting fat, indeed, kills. And as the degree of overweight increases, the life spans contract. Somewhat of a surprise was the finding by the Dutch researchers that even moderate amounts of excess weight "conferred a noticeable diminution in life expectancy."[35]

Here are some sobering findings from this important study:[36]

- Nonsmokers who were overweight but not obese (which roughly means being 10 to 30 pounds above a healthy weight) lost an average of three years off their lives.
- Obese people (with BMI greater than 30) died even sooner:
  - Obese female nonsmokers lost an average of 7.1 years.
  - Obese male nonsmokers lost 5.8 years.

- For those who were obese *and* smokers, the double burden caused the loss to be significantly higher:
  - Obese female smokers died 7.2 years sooner than normal-weight smokers and 13.3 years sooner than normal-weight nonsmoking women.
  - Obese male smokers lived 6.7 years less than normal-weight smokers, and 13.7 years less than normal-weight nonsmokers.

To put these figures into perspective, just consider that completely eliminating all kinds of cancer in America would add only about 3½ years to life expectancy.[37]

Obesity, it is becoming increasingly clear, exacts such a heavy toll on longevity because it increases the risk of developing many chronic diseases at surprisingly low levels of excess fat—as little as 5 to 10 pounds above desirable body weight.[38] That's because surplus body fat, which was once thought of as little more than an inert storage depot, is, metabolically, a highly active organ, producing hormones and chemical substances that can flood the body, damaging blood vessels, causing insulin resistance, and promoting cancer-cell growth.[39]

A growing number of studies are now allowing us to quantify the links between obesity and coronary heart disease, diabetes, hypertension, and selected cancers, which are the major ailments most frequently associated with obesity.[40] In one recent study, for example, obese individuals were 1.7 times more likely to have heart disease, twice as likely to have hypertension, and three times as likely to have diabetes compared to normal-weight people.[41] Another study that investigated cancer risk found that excessively heavy men and women were three times as likely to develop kidney cancer compared with those of healthy weight, while obese postmenopausal women faced up to a 50 percent higher chance of developing breast cancer than nonobese women.[42]

These obesity-associated health risks increase in direct proportion to increases in a person's weight and the duration of a person's obesity. Research is also revealing that the *distribution* of the body's excess fat—the so-called body fat topology—has a bearing on health risks as well.[43] For example, people who carry excess weight in the abdomen (the so-called apple shape) are more likely to have diabetes and heart disease than are those built like pears, who deposit fat in their hips, thighs, and backsides.[44,45]

As science marches ahead and the methods for studying disease become more sophisticated, we can expect the news about weight and health to grow even worse.[46] New research, for example, already points to a link between excess body weight and the risk of death from most cancers. A recently published study by the American Cancer Society found that the higher a patient's BMI, the greater the risk of cancer death. The researchers attributed the higher death rates in obese cancer patients to several possible causes. For some patients, the cause was delay in diagnosis. That's because the cancers of obese patients may be under layers of the body fat and, thus, can be harder to detect (a person's fat can literally be too dense for x-rays or sound waves to penetrate). It was also recently found that in men, excessive body fat can suppress the prostate-specific antigen (PSA), the blood protein used to diagnose prostate cancer in its early stages. The resulting delay in diagnosis explains why in obese men, prostate cancer tends to be diagnosed in more advanced stages.[47] For others, the culprit can be biological mechanisms associated with obesity, such as increased levels of certain hormones (sex steroids, insulin, and growth factor I) that are believed to stimulate the growth of nascent cancer cells in various organs.[48]

For Older Americans, The Future Is Now

For obese people in their fifties and sixties, the physical burden of carrying excess weight can interfere with even the most routine activities. Physical tasks, such as climbing stairs, maneuvering into an automobile, sitting comfortably in a chair, and walking any distance, can become difficult and sources of pain and embarrassment.[49] A recent study to assess disability among older Americans (aged 50 to 69) found that difficulties in performing tasks such as bathing, eating, dressing, and getting in or out of bed rise by 50 percent in men who are moderately obese and threefold in those who are severely obese (BMI greater than 35). In women, the likelihood of such problems doubles with moderate obesity and quadruples with severe obesity.[50]

As baby boomers get older and fatter, they are also more likely to develop one of the double burdens of age and weight: arthritis. Survey data from the CDC suggest that the likelihood of experiencing arthritic pain increases fivefold in very obese people aged 60 and older, compared to those who are underweight.[51]

Putting on extra weight may also be far riskier for cognitive dysfunction than most people have imagined. Recent scientific studies have determined that weight gain may lead to degenerative changes in the aging brain and, quite possibly, Alzheimer's disease—a disease that many elderly and their families fear more than death itself.[52]

Such findings fly in the face of widely held assumptions that older Americans are getting healthier and that their disability rates are dropping. Instead, obesity-related ailments may very well be wiping out the recent health gains that the elderly have heretofore enjoyed from reduced exposure to infectious diseases and advances in medical care.

The Sociocultural Burden

Obesity not only affects long-term health and longevity, it is unique among chronic disease risk factors in that it also carries a sociocultural burden.[53] Indeed, to most of its victims it is through psychological pain that obesity has its most noxious effects.[54] The full public health burden of the obesity epidemic must thus be measured not only by the traditional measures of morbidity and mortality, but also by the psychological and social consequences experienced by those who suffer and by those around them.[55]

Using an imaginative new method they called "owning one's disability," two University of Florida (Gainesville) researchers, Rand and MacGregor,[56] sought to quantify the heavy psychological toll that obesity exerts on the psyche. They had patients answer a series of forced-choice questions as to whether they would prefer their current disability to a number of other handicaps.[57] In a sample of formerly severely obese patients who had undergone gastric surgery, Rand and MacGregor found that every single one of the patients they interviewed would prefer to be deaf, dyslexic, diabetic, or to suffer from very bad heart disease than to return to their morbidly overweight status. Ninety percent of the patients also preferred blindness to obesity, and 92 percent preferred having a leg amputated than to return to their overweight state. All patients preferred to be of normal weight than to have "a couple of million dollars" when given a hypothetical choice.

The extensive research done on obese people's quality of life suggests that the obese live in a world that often treats them with notable antipathy.[58] Some observers have gone so far as to characterize the disparagement of overweight and obese individuals as the last socially acceptable form of prejudice[59]—the last, perhaps, but certainly not the latest. "History shows that prejudice against obese individuals is not simply a product of society's current worship of a thin ideal. As early as the 12th century, Buddhists stigmatized obesity as the karmic consequence of moral failing."[60]

The frightening thing is that even small children are not immune from prejudice against the obese. Researchers have found that children "learn" at a very early age to associate obesity with undesirable personal characteristics. In one study, when children as young as 6 to 9 years of age were shown a fat person's silhouette and asked to describe the person's characteristics, they said: "lazy, lying, cheating."[61,62] And when shown black-and-white line drawings of an obese child and children with various handicaps, including missing hands and facial disfigurement, the participants singled out the obese child as the one with whom they least wished to play.[63] It is no wonder that "among the most prevalent consequences of obesity in children is the discrimination that overweight children suffer at the hands of their peers."[64]

Such discrimination is effectively robbing those overweight kids of their childhood, preventing them from doing the same kinds of activities that their leaner peers do.[65]

As children grow older, discrimination against the obese becomes more institutionalized.[66] Society's negative attitudes toward the obese take the form of discrimination in areas such as employment opportunities, college acceptance, and even marriage. In a study of college students, as an example, the eligible bachelors and bachelorettes rated embezzlers, cocaine users, and shoplifters as more suitable marriage partners than obese individuals.[67] Other studies found that obese young women were far less likely to marry than nonobese women, and those who did marry were more likely to marry "down"—that is, to marry someone of a lower social status—than were nonobese women.[68]

Feeling obesity's economic pinch can be even more direct, however. Insurance premiums, for example, rise in proportion to one's girth and could easily be double, triple, or up to five times the normal premium, even if one is otherwise in perfect health. And some severely overweight people may be declined insurance coverage altogether. To add insult to injury, this "fat tax" often falls on a slender wallet.[69] Studies consistently show that overweight job candidates are less likely to be hired than nonoverweight candidates (even when perceived to be equally competent on job-related tests).[70] And when hired, they often earn less.[71]

The physical and psychological consequences of obesity have profound economic ramifications for the nation as a whole. These economic ramifications take the form of direct costs, which include the costs incurred on preventive, diagnostic, and treatment services related to overweight and obesity, such as on physician visits, hospital care, and medications, as well as indirect costs that accrue to the wider economy because of time and productivity lost to sickness and premature mortality.[72] In 2000, the U.S. Surgeon General estimated these costs at $117 billion annually—an amount that's comparable to the entire gross national product of countries such as Portugal, Ireland, or Argentina.[73,74]

"Globesity"

The obesity problem is no longer just an American problem. The situation is nearly as dismal around the globe, with people in country after country following the American lead and growing heavier.[75] According to Dr. Stephan Roessner, a past president of the International Association for the Study of Obesity, "There is no country in the world where obesity is not increasing.

Even in developing countries we thought were immune ... the epidemic is coming on very fast. ... In some areas of Africa, overweight children outnumber malnourished children three to one."[76] Not even "paradise" has been spared. On some South Pacific islands, as many as three-quarters of adults are dangerously obese. These are levels so high that the magnitude of the disorder is changing and molding the very culture of these islands.[77]

"It has often been said that one of the great tragedies of human social evolution is that half the world's population worries about the consequences of overeating while the other half starves."[78] This is now literally true. Today, for the first time, the number of overweight people in the world has risen to match the number of undernourished: 1.2 billion.[79]

In her 2003 annual message, Dr. Gro Harlem Brundtland, the Director-General of the World Health Organization, was clearly alarmed:

> These are dangerous times for the well-being of the world. ... Too many of us are living dangerously—whether we are aware of that or not ... either because we have little choice, which is often the case among the poor, or because we are making the wrong choices in terms of our consumption and our activities.[80]

A Bucket Half-Empty?

The "temperature is rising," and like the frog, we are showing every sign of enjoying ourselves. "Our lives are characterized by too much of a good thing—too much to eat, to buy, to watch and to do, excess at every turn."[81] The risk we face, if we do not address the obesifying forces in our environment and patterns of behavior, is that these forces will get woven so tightly into our social fabric—our economic system, leisure and entertainment, health care, even education—that it will be difficult to reverse the damage,[82] not unlike the frog whose capacity to respond to the threat of boiling slowly atrophies with the slow rise in temperature, getting groggier and groggier until ultimately it becomes unable to climb out of the pot. We have got to be smarter than that boiled frog if we want to avoid that amphibian's fate.[83]

Reducing the national waistline will require a major shift in the way we think about managing our instincts and our environment. "Gone are the days when weight control was instinctual, when food was scarce and humans had to be active just to survive," says James Hill, director of the Center for Human Nutrition at the University of Colorado, and a leading researcher in the obesity field. As a result, says Hill, "we have to use our brains to restrict those instincts .... We have to teach people to override their biological instincts with their cognitive abilities."[84]

But how can this be done?

Scientists and health officials have long believed that the key to reversing obesity is information, offering the public more and better information about healthy food choices, for example. Most government programs aimed at weight control are based on this principle. This viewpoint relates to what the philosopher Karl Popper used to call "the bucket theory of the mind." When minds are seen as containers, and public understanding is viewed as a function of how much scientific facts are known, the focus naturally is on how many scientific facts public minds contain.[85]

An irony of America's obesity epidemic is that, at a time when Americans arguably know more about food and nutrition than at any time in their history, they are gaining more weight.[86] Despite all the diet books, the wide availability of reduced-calorie and reduced-fat foods, advice from weight-loss specialists, and the broad publicity about the obesity problem, the number of obese is not declining.[87] Something other than ignorance must be driving the trend.

What people need to realize is that effective self-regulation of health behavior, as in any other endeavor, requires certain cognitive skills. Knowledge (in the bucket) without the requisite decision-making skills will produce little change. Paradoxically, the recent advances in medicine have made these skills more critical, not less. Improved medical care and the elimination of infectious diseases have increased life expectancy, so that minor dysfunctions due to personal mismanagement have more time to develop into chronic diseases later in life. Gaining 30 or 40 pounds at the age of 20 or 30 may not have been too much of a concern a century ago, when the life expectancy was only 40. Today, the life expectancy of the U.S. population has nearly doubled, from 40 to almost 80 years (although the trend may be reversing), which means that there is ample time for those 30 or 40 pounds to translate into serious ailments.[88]

An old comedian once remarked: "Had I known I would live this long, I would have taken better care of myself." This is no longer a joke.

The Leverage (or the Impediment) Is with the People

In the United States today, most obese individuals attempting to lose weight do so themselves, without seeking professional help.[89,90] For example, dieting, the mainstay of obesity treatment, is most often undertaken as a self-directed process with instruction from a book or slimming club within the community, or often just by self-induced restraint. Experts expect this trend to continue, for several reasons. Given the sheer number of obese individuals who need help, it is clear that there are not enough health professionals available to provide intensive, long-term treatment.[91] A second important driver is the cost of weight-loss programs. At the moment, most insurance companies and health maintenance organizations do not consider obesity per se—that is, obesity uncomplicated by other conditions—a reimbursable expense. As a result, if dieters seek professional treatment, they usually must pay out of pocket for all or most of the cost of treatment (which can be as steep as $65 an hour for an average nutritionist).[92,93]

Third, weight has always been seen as a very individual, very personal thing. The wellness movement, which has taken hold of the health mentality of the U.S. population, is rooted in the concept of personal control over health. This focus on individual responsibility reaches extremes in the search for the perfect body. Because eating is under one's conscious control, most people consider weight "to be a matter of an individual's decisions, or perhaps of a failure to make decisions."[94] One (unfortunate) consequence is that individuals, like the culture in general, assume more control than actually exists. This perhaps explains why most people believe that every overweight person can and should achieve slenderness, and why obese people are stereotyped as lacking in self-control.[95]

Control over our bodies, however, must be considered within the context of biological realities, and the reality is that obesity is not simply a problem of willful misconduct—eating too much and exercising too little—as it continues to be (mis)viewed not only by the lay public but by health care providers and insurance companies as well. Obesity is a complex multifactorial disease involving genetics, physiology, and biochemistry, as well as environmental, psychosocial, and cultural factors.[96]

People must come to realize that in managing our health—and our bodies—we are decision makers who are managing a truly complex and dynamic system: the human body.

It Is Not Easy Becoming a *Top Gun*

To underscore the often hidden complexities of human weight regulation, I have often asked my students (many of them navy pilots) to think about the similarities and the differences between the task of managing their bodies (which they must do to stay "navy trim") and flying their state-of-the-art aircraft. There are several interesting parallels between the two tasks. Both our bodies and the navy's latest flying machines are marvelously complex systems. Yet, both are quite vulnerable in turbulent environments, and in both cases the "piloting" task is not a simple matter of making a single one-time decision. Rather, it is a dynamic decision-making process involving a series of decisions made over time. Furthermore, the decisions are not independent of one another since what we can or cannot do *now* is often constrained by decisions we have already made.

The analogy, while useful, is not perfect, however. Managing our bodies poses two subtle (and tricky) complications. For one, in managing our health we are not merely "flying" our bodies, we are also *redesigning* them in "flight." Our bodies are continuously changing over time, both autonomously (e.g., because of aging) and in reaction to our lifestyle choices. Managing our bodies is, therefore, akin to pursuing a target that not only moves but also reacts to the actions of the pursuer, which may explain why it can be an extremely challenging, and often frustrating, endeavor.

A second complication is time delay. Unlike with the controls on a supersonic aircraft, the time delay between taking an action (eating a piece of chocolate cream pie or smoking a cigarette) and its effect(s) on the state of our health can be quite long. Time delay complicates things because it means we can no longer rely on receiving timely feedback on the outcomes of our decisions and actions. And that makes it so much harder to learn and to adjust. (We shall see later that because many of obesity's health consequences are the result of the cumulative stress of excess weight over a long period of time, this issue has proven particularly troublesome for obesity prevention efforts.)

What would it take to become a "top gun" on this lifelong "flight"? Research in control theory and behavioral decision making suggests that effective control of a dynamic system, whether it is the energy regulation of our bodies, the energy regulation of an atomic reactor, or the flight attitude of a supersonic jet, requires two essential cognitive skills: the operator's ability to develop an adequate model of the system and the ability to "run" that model, that is, to infer how the system changes over time.[97–98] By the operator's model of the system is meant *structural knowledge*—knowledge of how the system's variables (such as the energy consumed and expended in the case of weight regulation) are related and how they influence one another and are influenced by the system's external environment. A perfect operator model without a capability to "run" it is of little practical utility however.[99] The ability to infer system behavior is essential if the decision maker (or pilot) is to know how actions taken will influence the situation or system and, thus, is essential in devising appropriate interventions for change. The two skills are needed *together*.

Unfortunately, living systems—the human body included—do not come with an operator's manual, nor are their structures always readily apparent, and so grasping a system's structure and its dynamic tendencies is never automatic. It requires skills to see *through* complexity to the underlying structures generating a complex situation or problematic behavior.

The good news, though, is that, while the skills are not necessarily innate, they can be successfully acquired.[100] It just may require reading an entire book to acquire them!

Let's see why.

States *In* Mind

People analyze many situations and make hundreds of decisions every day while at home, at school, at work, or on the road. Rarely, however, do we stop to think about *how* we think. No one's head contains a family, city, school, hospital, or business. All human decisions are based on models, usually mental models (of family roles and relationships, a city's layout of streets and neighborhoods, the power hierarchy in a business organization, etc.) created out of each person's prior experience, training, and instruction.[101] They are the deeply ingrained assumptions, generalizations, or even pictures or images we form of ourselves, others, the environment, and the things with which we interact. These cognitive constructs are not simply repositories for past learning; they also provide a basis for interpreting what is currently happening, and they strongly influence how we act in response.[102]

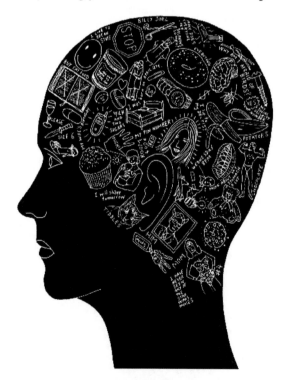

Figure 1.2 Mental models (*Source:* Courtesy of Peter Arkle.)

We like to think (and most us believe) that well-adjusted individuals possess relatively accurate mental models or perceptions of themselves, their capacity to control important events in their lives, and their future. Unfortunately, this is not the case, and what is more disturbing is that most people are unaware of this situation.[103]

A great deal of research in cognitive psychology has revealed that mental models are only simplified abstractions of the experienced world and are often incomplete, reflecting a world that is only partially understood.[104–105]

> Everyone, from the greatest genius to the most ordinary clerk, has to adopt mental frameworks that simplify and structure the information encountered in the world. ... [Mental models] keep complexity within the dimensions our minds can manage. ... But beware: Any [model] leaves us with only a partial view of the problem. Often people simplify in ways that actually force them to choose the wrong alternatives.[106]

This applies not only to "ordinary" people, but to scientists and professionals, as well. Sterman[107] provides some fascinating and, perhaps, troubling examples in the science and public policy domains. One example relating to global warming is particularly interesting because, like the obesity epidemic, it is a phenomenon with potentially grave consequences for humanity:

> The first scientific papers describing the ability of chlorofluorocarbons (CFCs) to destroy atmospheric ozone were published in 1974. Yet much of the scientific community remained skeptical, and despite a ban on CFCs as aerosol propellants, global production of CFCs remained near its all-time high. It was not until 1985 that evidence of a deep ozone hole in the Antarctic was published. ... The news reverberated around the scientific world. Scientists at NASA. ... scrambled to check readings on atmospheric ozone made by the Nimbus 7 satellite, measurements that had been taken routinely since 1978. Nimbus 7 had never indicated an ozone hole. Checking back, NASA scientists found that their computers had been programmed to reject very low ozone readings on the assumption that such low readings must indicate instrument error. The NASA scientists' belief that low ozone readings must be erroneous led them to design a measurement system that made it impossible to detect low readings that might have invalidated their models. Fortunately, NASA had saved the original, unfiltered data and later confirmed that total ozone had indeed been falling since the launch of the Nimbus 7.[108]

Sterman's summary of the lessons learned is both poignant and succinct: "[S]eeing is believing *and* believing is seeing."

People base their mental models on whatever knowledge they have, real or imaginary, naïve or sophisticated.[109] Once formed, these models shape not only how people make sense of the world (looking back), but also how they act and how they predict the outcomes of their actions (looking forward). Like the god Janus in Roman mythology (Figure 1.3), whose head has two faces, one facing forward and the other backward, human thinking goes in both directions whenever we put our minds to work on making a decision: looking backward to understand the past (e.g., explaining weight gain) and looking forward to predict the future (predicting a diet's outcome).[110] And we rely on our mental models to do both.

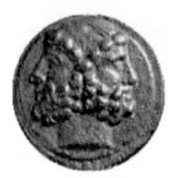

Figure 1.3 The god Janus in Roman mythology

Consider, as an example, the *energy-balance model* of body weight regulation, the implicit mental model by which many (if not most) dieters explain weight gain (looking backward) and predict diet outcomes (looking forward).[111,112] As is depicted in Figure 1.4, body weight is simply viewed as being dependent on the balance between energy intake (EI) and energy expenditure (EE), both of which are assumed to be under voluntary control. Unbalancing the energy-balance equation in the direction of weight loss, therefore, would appear to be straightforward: induce a caloric deficit (by reducing daily caloric intake below daily energy requirements, increasing energy expenditure through increased physical activity, or doing a little of both), and watch body weight drop in direct (linear) proportion to the energy deficit imposed.

Instructions in self-help books cannot be simpler: a weekly caloric deficit of 3,500 calories—induced through either dieting or exercise—induces a loss of 1 pound in a week, 10 pounds in 10 weeks (3,500 kilocalories [kcal] is the amount of energy in 1 pound of body fat).

The assumption here is that the there is a fixed energy cost of 3,500 calories per pound of lost tissue, and that the body's energy requirements remain steady as body size decreases.[113] The negative energy balance of 500 calories per day in the above example would, thus, shed about 50 pounds if extended for a year and almost 150 pounds over 3 years! The relationship is linear. It is also unbounded (taking weight loss projections to absurd values) and wrong.

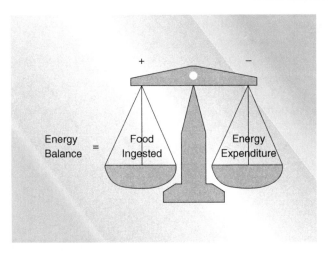

Figure 1.4 Energy (caloric) balance

In reality, losing weight has proven not to be that straightforward. Weight loss tends to decline with time, even if the prescribed diet *is* maintained, and people tend to lose less weight than they expect … much less. That's primarily because the two limbs of energy balance are *not* independent, but instead are physiologically linked, meaning that we cannot voluntarily change one, say, decrease energy input, and expect that the other (energy expenditure) will hold steady.

As we will see in later chapters, the complexities are neither capricious nor mysterious, and have a lot to do with the body's *homeostatic* processes—its adaptive (and defensive) mechanisms that continuously aim to maintain the body's internal stability in the face of internal or external threats to that stability. In dieting, when any significant weight is lost, the loss is interpreted by the body as a deprivation "crisis" that needs to be contained … and is. To restrain the rate of tissue depletion, the body compensates by slowing its metabolism (akin to the body changing its light bulbs to fluorescent lights to save energy). Additionally, as weight is lost, and both fat and fat-free tissue are shed, maintenance energy requirements, that is, the amount of energy the body requires to maintain the cells and sustain the body's essential physiological functions, drop, since there is simply less "stuff" to maintain.

The combined effect of these two energy conservation measures is to effectively shrink the diet's energy deficit, which in turn (and unfortunately for the dieter) dampens the rate of weight loss. For example, if a female dieter who expends a total of 2,000 calories per day cuts daily dietary intake to 1,500 calories, she would initially induce a daily caloric deficit of 500 calories. But (days or weeks later) as some weight is lost, the body's energy requirements also drop. The total energy expenditure level thus falls from 2,000 down to, say, 1,800 calories. As a result, the daily energy deficit effectively shrinks from 500 to 300 calories—a 40 percent decrease.

Weight loss during prolonged underfeeding is thus not linear but *curvilinear*. The changes in the body's composition and in its maintenance energy requirements constantly modify the subsequent pattern of weight loss until a new equilibrium body weight is reached, often at a level substantially higher than expected.

Ignoring the body's energy-sparing mechanisms that aim to limit tissue loss during caloric deprivation (as does the popularized energy balance model) may sell more diet books, but will inevitably lead to spurious predictions of treatment outcomes, which should be of concern because people's expectations about treatment outcomes and the degree to which they are met or not met are likely to affect self-efficacy—the belief in one's ability to accomplish one's goals—and in turn their long-term motivation and commitment.[114]

Emotions Play a Role

Our mental models are not only often incomplete, but they can also be biased by needs and emotions. Prior expectations and self-serving interpretations weigh heavily into how we view the world, and people's predictions of what will occur often corresponds closely to *what they would like to see happen* or to what is socially desirable, rather than to what is objectively likely.[115,116]

For example, consider people's *unrealistic optimism* about health. "It is consistently reported that people display an unrealistic optimism (also labeled *illusion of unique invulnerability*) in their assessment of perceived risk of occurrence of a variety of potential negative health and safety outcomes."[117] Such perceptions of relative invulnerability (the "it won't happen to me" notion) have been found across a wide range of diseases, hazards, and catastrophic events. Research in clinical and developmental psychology suggests that such positive illusions (several others will be discussed in later chapters) serve a wide variety of cognitive, affective, and social functions. For example, unrealistic optimism is often an attempt to avoid the anxiety one would feel from admitting a threat to well-being—a form of defensive denial. Illusions about unique invulnerability can also enhance a person's self-esteem. People may believe that vulnerability (say to tooth decay) is a matter of their constitution, so if the problem has not appeared, their bodies must be super-resistant. In problems like obesity or drug addiction, which many believe to be caused by behavior or personality, people may feel invulnerable because they would like to believe that they do not have the weakness of character that allows it to develop in them.[118] In short, even the well-adjusted individual appears to have the enviable capacity to distort reality in a way that enhances self-esteem and promotes an optimistic view of the future.

While the capacity to develop and maintain positive illusions may help make each individual's world a warmer place in which to live, it can be a risky business. Unrealistic optimism in matters of health and disease often leads people to ignore legitimate risks in their environment and avoid taking the necessary measures to offset those risks.[119] This, of course, can become a significant impediment to preventing conditions such as obesity. If people convince themselves that they are invulnerable to obesity, then they are unlikely to take measures to reduce their risk of gaining weight no matter how educated they are about the dire consequences of obesity. The "it won't happen to me" mindset gets in their way: why protect yourself from an event that will not occur?

The persistence and pervasiveness of deficient decision rules (such as about energy balance) and illusions (such as about invulnerability, among other things) suggest that raw, real-life experience is often not enough to correct people's mental models, and neither has been the mass-media–type educational campaigns (such as distributing copies of the *Dietary Guidelines for Americans* or the many similar educational materials on nutrition and exercise).[120,121] Indeed, the glut of information from many different sources may have backfired, as people have a tendency to retain information selectively in accord with their prejudices and to support their preconceived positions. For example, "All that many people did on low-fat and fat-free products was gain weight because they figured that fat-free gave them license to eat as much as they wanted, without regard to serving size and calories per serving."[122] Access to more information tends to increase *confidence* in judgment—people assume that the quality of decisions has improved because they can find information to support them—but it does not necessarily increase the *quality* of judgment.[123]

In a recently published study, psychologists Peter Ditto and David Lopez concocted a simple experiment that aptly demonstrates our bias to seek out information that supports our existing instinct or point of view, while avoiding information that contradicts it (the so-called confirming-evidence bias):

> [They] asked subjects to evaluate a student's intelligence by examining information about him one piece at a time. The information was quite damning, and subjects were told they could stop examining it as soon as they'd reached a firm conclusion. Results showed that when subjects liked the student they were evaluating, they turned over one card after another, searching for the one piece of information that might allow them to say something nice about him. But when they disliked the student, they turned over a few cards, shrugged, and called it a day.... By uncritically accepting evidence when it pleases us, and insisting on more when it doesn't, we subtly tip the scales in ... favor [of our preconceived notion or view].[124]

Consequently, many of us end up using information as a drunken man uses lampposts—for support rather than for illumination.[125]

Failure to Learn from Failure

Human beings learn many things by trial and error; we learn to walk, ride a bicycle, drive an automobile, and play the piano that way. We act, observe the consequences of our actions, and adjust. Which naturally brings up an interesting question: Why do we seem to have a "learning disability" when it comes to losing weight? Why, even after many trials (and many errors), do most people never seem to learn enough to become successful "losers" and often remain trapped in endless repeating rounds of (yo-yo) weight loss and regain?

Single-Loop vs. Double-Loop Learning

Like most behaviors, conscious human learning is *purposeful,* in that we regulate it according to our goals and objectives. So, assuming we have the will and the means, we'll continue trying, testing, probing, and accumulating experience on a task until we have satisfactorily resolved any perceived discrepancy between where we are (actual condition) and where we want to be (desired state).

All learning, thus, depends on *feedback:* we take an action that alters the real world in some way, we receive feedback about the consequences of that action, and then we take a new and different action to bring the state of the world closer to our goals.[126] We consider learning to have occurred when a mismatch between our intentions and outcomes is identified and is corrected.[127]

Often we find ways to move closer to our desired state without changing our mental model. In fact (as I relate from personal experience, below), it is possible for people to learn to adjust their actions and attain their goals in the context of existing, possibly incomplete (even faulty) mental models, such as when a dieter who fails to lose a desired amount of weight on some diet X (because of unrealistic assumptions about the weight/energy trade-off) switches to diet Y, then to diet Z, then perhaps experiment with appetite-suppressing drugs or combinations of dieting and exercising ... and ultimately achieves short-term success. All along, failure to achieve hoped-for weight loss or failure to maintain it rarely induces a reassessment of the dieter's underlying *operator's models* (such as the expectation that eliminating 500 calories from one's daily diet will result in a 50-pound weight loss in a year).

This apparent "learning deficiency" is by no means limited to weight loss and the obese. Learning to use life's raw experiences to adjust our entrenched worldviews is hard and, therefore, uncommon.[128] Experience, after all, provides only data, the raw ingredients for learning, not knowledge. People can turn data into knowledge only if they know how to evaluate the data.

This type of learning, where a mismatch between outcomes and intentions is detected and corrected without questioning or altering one's underlying worldview, is called surface or single-loop learning and is depicted by the top loop in Figure 1.5. In single-loop learning, we learn to tweak our decisions (e.g., switching from a diet X to a diet Y or to an exercise intervention) without altering our mental models or their associated decision rules. Single-loop learning can be compared with a thermostat that senses when it is too hot or too cold and then turns the heat off or on.

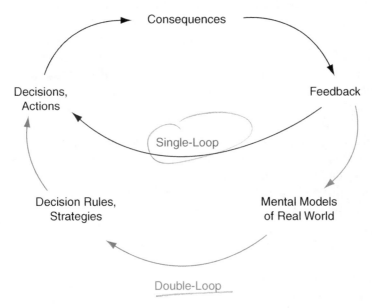

Figure 1.5 Single-loop and double-loop learning

By contrast, a more desired form of learning, called deep or double-loop learning, is achieved whenever we use the feedback information available to us to enhance our fundamental understanding of the decision task (as in the outer loop in the figure). Learning, in this deeper sense, is *discovery*—discovery of mental maps and decision rules that are better aligned with the decision task at hand. The same information filtered and processed through different decision rules now yields different, and, it is hoped, much better, decisions.[129,130]

An experience I had some years ago further illustrates the fundamental distinction between learning that challenges our worldviews and learning that does not (While the experience relates to sailing a boat [!!!] not managing my weight, it will help us here because, as we'll see later, there are intriguing parallels between steering a boat in stormy seas and managing one's weight in an obesifying environment.) While living on the East Coast during my college days, I used to sail a small sailboat I kept on Lake George in upstate New York. Even though the boat was a day-sailor, I had an autopilot installed in it so that I could sail it single-handedly. This worked in splendid fashion, reliably steering my boat to whichever destination I picked, and always doing it quite efficiently (i.e., steering the most direct course to a destination). When an error (mismatch) occurred, as would happen when the boat occasionally got bumped off-course by a strong gust of wind or by running into the wake of a fast ski boat, the autopilot would quickly detect the error and correct it.

After a few summers sailing on Lake George, I moved, with my beloved sailboat in tow, to the San Francisco Bay area when I accepted a faculty position at the Naval Postgraduate School. I, of course, knew that sailing in San Francisco Bay was going to be a more challenging (and wetter) sailing experience. (Not only were the winds much stronger, but more importantly—and unlike Lake George—the bay also had significant tidal currents.) But I looked forward to exhilarating weekly sails on the bay.

It did not take long, however, for exhilaration to turn to apprehension as my heretofore dependable autopilot started to mysteriously and repeatedly misbehave. On more than one scary occasion, while under autopilot control, the boat wandered significantly off-course and sometimes uncomfortably close to a navigational buoy or some other hazard.

What was happening was that my little boat was now being steered through a body of water that was not stationary, but rather was moving with respect to the bottom and the shore because of the current. The resultant motion of the boat was the net effect of these two motions combined, with regard to both speed and direction. When caught in a particularly strong current, the boat's actual motion over the bottom became markedly different from the course steered. For example, if the boat's heading was east, and there was a north to south current of comparable speed, the boat would sail in a southeasterly direction.

How did we (my autopilot and I) "learn" to react? The initial routine was something like this: I would start by setting the boat's course on a particular compass heading toward some desired destination, say, toward the famed island of Alcatraz, and the boat would initially start sailing in that direction. But, before long, we'd start drifting with the current and wander off course. It would take me a while, but eventually I would notice that we'd deviated from the desired course, and I would take action to correct it by resetting the boat's heading and the autopilot back toward the proper destination. And then the (single-loop learning) cycle would start again: drifting off course, detection by the skipper, and correction. The result was an inefficient zigzagging course such as that shown in Figure 1.6.

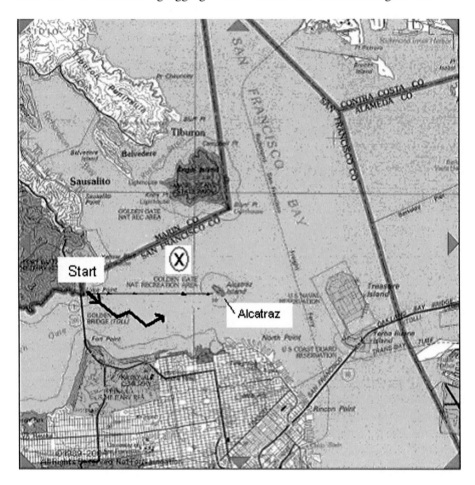

Figure 1.6 A day's sail to Alcatraz

The problem was that the autopilot's "mental model" was not updated to account for the new, *more complex* environment. Rather, it was constrained by its single-loop limitations to just act, sense, and react. Fortunately for my crew, the *skipper's* mental model ultimately was corrected. The trick for sailing a direct course to a desired destination in San Francisco Bay is to make due allowance for the estimated effect of the current. This means that the boat should be steered on a course somewhat *into the current* in the direction of point X in Figure 1.6, assuming the current is moving from top to bottom, and we are heading from the city front to Alcatraz. *That is a new decision rule,* as opposed to the "single-loop" approach of making a series of adjustments in response to veering off course. Provided the estimate of the current was correct, the boat would travel in a straight line because the current effects would be exactly countered by the course and speed offset from the intended track.

Controlling my sailboat in the turbulent waters of San Francisco Bay has some interesting parallels to how many dieters manage body weight in the current obesifying environment. Analogous to sea currents that lift all boats, our food-rich, activity-poor environment is "steering" us toward (the risky shoals of) positive energy balance. Our metabolic autopilots, which are fine-tuned over our evolutionary history to help us survive in an environment where a high level of physical activity was required for daily subsistence and the food supply was inconsistent, are failing us. And when we gain weight and then try to lose it, failure to achieve a desired body weight on the diet du jour often leads, as it did with the autopilot, to corrective actions (such as trying alternate diets) but not to a correction of people's underlying mental models (e.g., about their weight and energy regulatory system). And so, deficient mental models endure while people jump from one weight-loss "silver bullet" to another. The result is the weight cycling ("yo-yo dieting") phenomenon that many dieters experience (Figure 1.7).

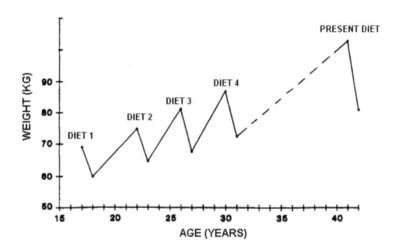

Weight and dieting histories of 31 women, all of whom had engaged in a minimum of four diets.

Figure 1.7 The results of a study that tracked the weight of 31 women over a 25-year period, in which the women (average age 40 years) dieted an average of five times. (Note that the figure looks like the mirror image of the zigzagging course to Alcatraz in Figure 1.6.) (*Source:* Wadden et al., 1992.)

Barriers to Learning

A significant barrier to deep learning about a complex system, such as human physiology, is that the deficiencies in our mental models are often not readily apparent. To see why, contrast learning to ride a bicycle, which most of us have learned by trial and error, with learning to regulate body weight. Consider first the bicycle case: the conditions for learning are excellent; the feedback we receive is immediate and unambiguous (albeit, sometimes painfully so). In one afternoon, we can try many different ways to ride and can easily determine which way works best. The bicycle's structure does not change in response to the rider's decisions, so what we learn does not become obsolete. Also, there are few, if any, confounding variables, and what others around us may or may not be doing is generally irrelevant.[131]

Now, let's consider a typical dieter scenario—a dieter who starts on diet X, expecting to lose 50 pounds in a year by eliminating 500 calories a day from her regular diet, but fails. In this case, the conditions for learning (for example, that her underlying energy rule is invalid) are more problematic. For one, the information feedback she receives is imperfect. She may not know with certainty, for instance, how many calories she *actually* consumed or expended during the diet. Such uncertainties alone are often enough for a frustrated dieter to explain away any mismatch between weight-loss expectations and actual outcome. In addition to imperfect information, there is also ambiguity. Ambiguity arises whenever changes (in this case, in body weight) resulting from our own decisions (in this case, going on a diet) are confounded by simultaneous changes in other variables that we do *not* control.[132] A host of other changes in our dieter's situation—in the amount and type of exercise she did, smoking initiation or cessation, travel, increased stress on the job, disease, medication, and even infection—may affect her outcome. Also, unlike in the bicycle case, the behavior of the dieter's family members does matter a great deal, changing the type, size, and frequency of meals served, television viewing habits, and so on. The bottom line is that there are too many ways to explain why a disappointing outcome occurred and to explain the mismatch between expectations and actual results. Thus, with all these reasonable explanations at her disposal, the dieter may not perceive a need to change her mental model.

Even when the evidence is clear enough that people should be able to learn from it, in situations such as dieting, where our self-esteem is on the line, we are naturally biased to interpret the evidence in a way that preserves our positive self-image, for example, to put the blame for our failure not on our unrealistic expectations, but on the shortcomings of the particular diet itself. Thus, in situations involving complexity, ambiguity, and imperfect information, misalignment between reality and people's perceptions of reality often endures. And endures.

What Is to Be Done?

"[T]he proper task of scientists is to diagnose and correct [such] misalignment," writes Edward Wilson.[133] This book, I hope, will be one small step to do just that.

At the public-policy level, it will require a shift in emphasis, from trying to stuff people's buckets with nutritional guidelines or to scare them into good health, to challenging people's deeply ingrained assumptions about health risk and well being and providing them with the conceptual skills (and the tools) they need to effectively exercise personal control over their health habits and their bodies.[134] That will entail a whole lot more than food-pyramid images or a new nutritional guideline. It will require us to *jump*.

Metanoia

Albert Einstein once observed that the significant problems we face cannot be solved at the same level of thinking we were at when we created them. We have to shift to a new level, a deeper level of thinking, to solve them.

Going back in history even further, the Greeks had coined a wonderful word for the mental "jumps" to new ways of thinking and acting that we often need to make: *metanoia*. It means a fundamental shift of mind or, more literally, transcendence (*meta* means above or beyond, as in "metaphysics") of mind (*noia,* from the root *nous,* meaning of mind).[135]

It may be time for a "metanoic" jump in addressing the obesity epidemic. In this book I argue for, and present, a different perspective for thinking about and addressing the obesity problem: a *systems thinking* perspective. It is a different way of thinking.

Synthesis, Not Analysis

A major shortcoming in much of the current debate on obesity has been the inability to integrate our knowledge of the multiple dimensions of the obesity problem, such as behavior, biology, and environment, into an integrated whole. Treatments of the problem, whether in academic or public discourse, invariably emphasize one aspect or problem area, such as nutrition, psychology, or metabolism. There is much attention on the separate mechanisms of human weight and energy regulation, but little on the whole bioenergetics system as an integrated operating system.

This fragmentation of knowledge is not a reflection of the way the world (and our body) works, but rather is the result of the analytic lens we impose—our natural predisposition when confronting a difficult problem to take things apart and treat the parts separately. In the case of obesity, this takes nutrition out of the context of lifestyle, biology out of the context of behavior, and behavior/lifestyle out of the context of the environment.

While breaking things apart is integral to the process of simplification—an effective strategy that scientists use to find points of entry into what may otherwise be impenetrably complex problems—we often forget that it is only a lens.[136]

> The difficulty arises when the method itself is reified into ... a "true" and "complete" representation of reality (i.e., "the world is like the method" rather than "the method helps us understand some aspects of the world").[137]

The performance of any system (whether it is an oil refinery, an economy, or the human body) obviously depends on the performance of its parts, but a system's performance is never equal to the sum of the actions of its parts taken separately. Rather, it is a function of their interactions.[138] These interactions (and their properties) are destroyed when the system is dissected, either physically or theoretically, into isolated elements. Breaking a system into its component pieces and studying the pieces separately is, thus, usually an inadequate way to understand the whole.

No matter how exhaustively one studies a particular component in isolation, there is usually no way to know what its true properties will be when it is put back in association with other parts of its ensemble.[139] An important, if not the most important, aspect of a part's performance is how it interacts with other parts to affect the performance of the whole. Forgetting that can only be at our peril or even death. In medicine, for example, the effect of one chemical frequently depends on the state of another, as when each of two medications may be helpful, but exposure to both in combination could be fatal.

It is important to emphasize that what I am saying here goes beyond the popular phrase, "The whole is greater than the sum of its parts." When dealing with systems, whether living or technological, the whole is *different from*, not *greater than*, the sum of the parts, because the essential properties of a system are properties of the *whole*, which none of the parts have.[140] For example, no part of an automobile can transport people, not even its motor. Therefore, when an automobile or any system is taken apart, it loses its defining function, its essential properties. "A disassembled automobile cannot transport people, and a disassembled person does not live, read, or write."[141]

The emergence of systems thinking in the middle of the last century was a profound revolution in the history of Western scientific thought. The great shock of twentieth-century science has been that systems cannot be under-stood by analysis.

> To understand things systematically literally means to put them into a context, to establish the nature of their relationships.... This is, in fact, the root meaning of the word "system," which derives from the Greek *synhistanai* ("to place together")....
> Thus the relationship between the parts and the whole has been reversed. In the systems approach the properties of the parts can be understood only from the organization of the whole.[142]

The challenge to us today in addressing the obesity epidemic—or, indeed, many of our persistent societal problems—is to "put things back together" again, after they have been examined in pieces. Such a holistic perspective does not imply denying the independent roles of the separate factors (nutrition, psychology, metabolism), but rather entails integrating them into a broader framework that incorporates the interactions between them—interactions that tend to get lost when the individual mechanisms are examined in isolation.

In this book, I will emphasize how the human body is a conglomerate of interrelated and interdependent control processes and subsystems. Taken together, they constitute a complex and dynamic marvel of system integra-tion, where changes in one subsystem can be traced throughout the entire body. A good example is appetite, a phenomenon arising out of and main-tained by a biopsychological system that includes the external environment (cultural and physical), the behavioral act of eating, the processes of inges-tion and assimilation of food, the storage and utilization of energy, body composition, and the neurohumoral system.[143] All these various factors are interconnected, pushing on each other and being pushed on in return. Appetite shapes body weight, and body weight influences appetite. Weight reflects activity levels (which are also shaped by the socioeconomic environ-ment), and activity levels reflect weight, and on and on.[144] Though all of these influences are always there, they are usually hidden from view, and because we are part of that lacework ourselves, it is doubly hard for us to see.[145]

Explaining things in terms of their context means explaining them in terms of their environment, and thus we can also say that all systems thinking is environmental thinking.[146] This contrasts with the atomistic and indivi-dualistic perspective in the analytical paradigm, in which objects are viewed as separate from their environments and people as separate from each other and from their surroundings.[147] Applying such a systems perspective in health is ushering in a sea change in the approach epidemiologists are taking to disease; they are looking less to the individual alone for answers, and more to the symphony of behavior–biology–environment interactions.

The strength of the systems approach lies in its capacity to integrate variables that otherwise would be isolated from each other. It allows us to integrate our knowledge of the multiple dimensions, and to examine the interactions between them, such as between the physiological and the behavioral, and between people and their external environment. Although the tools now associated with systems thinking (such as computer modeling tools used on large systems studies) are new and advanced, the underlying worldview is extremely intuitive. Even young children can learn systems thinking very quickly.[148]

We have been able to do this because of two innovations over the past half-century. The first innovation was the development of theory and concepts relating to the dynamic behavior of complex systems, that is, the understanding of how a complex system's behavior arises from the "organizing relations" of its parts.

As system science emerged as a serious field of study after World War II, early analyses revealed that different systems, whether biological, engineering, social, or economic, shared common principles in the ways in which their components work together to perform some well-defined function.[149] An important breakthrough came when theories about feedback control emerged from engineering (as in the study of servomechanisms during and after World War II) and served to explain self-organizing processes in human systems. Pioneering work in the mid–twentieth century[150] demonstrated that the same feedback mechanisms that govern how the components in an engineering system (such as in an autopilot) work together to perform a function also govern the goal-oriented behavior of human and other living systems.

> For example, the mechanism that the human body uses to maintain a constant body temperature of 98.6 degrees Fahrenheit resembles the control machinery designed to stabilize an airplane's altitude during flight. Both of these systems function to keep some quantity (blood temperature in one case, and altitude in the other) within narrowly defined limits under a wide range of possible disturbances (temperature variation in one instance, and atmospheric turbulence in the other).[151]

Like the autopilot or chemical refinery, the human body, we now understand, is a conglomerate of interrelated and interdependent information-feedback processes, which together constitute a dynamic and highly complex system.[152] Although not directly visible to us, these feedback processes are key governing mechanisms by which many of the body's systems are controlled and regulated. Human energy and weight regulation, as we shall see in this book, is no exception. It is a complex of nested feedback processes at multiple levels (the homeostatic processes at the physiological level, between the physiological and the behavioral, and between people and their external environment).

What Is Feedback?

Feedback is the process in which an action taken by a person or thing will eventually affect that person or thing: the situation of X affecting Y and Y in turn affecting X, perhaps through a chain of causes and effects. More generally, feedback is the transmission of information about the outcome of any process or activity back to its source.

Feedback is the processes encompass many of our conscious and subconscious decisions and underlie all goal-oriented behavior. In the human body, a multitude of involuntary hormonal-based feedback processes are crucial to maintaining the body's internal stability (its goal) in the face of changes in its external or internal environment. For example, in maintaining its core temperature, the body relies on the transmission of sensory information to detect any deviation from the desired core temperature level of 98.6 degrees Fahrenheit (its goal). If a deviation is detected, the body should rise, impulses from the brain are transmitted through the nerves to stimulate the sweat glands. This induces sweating, and the evaporation of the sweat cools the body down. Conversely, if a body temperature drops, the heartbeat increases and induces shivering. The heat-producing muscle contractions raise the body's temperature back to normal.

Essentially all organs and tissues of the body perform regulatory functions that help maintain the body's internal stability, even under extremes in our natural environment. More than a century ago, the French physician and physiologist Claude Bernard correctly attributed this internal stability to "the exquisite capacity of the body to monitor its internal state and to make adjustments to compensate for any perturbation of that stability."[153] In 1939, Walter Cannon, an American investigator, coined the term *homeostasis* to characterize this remarkable ability that is key to the survival of humans and most other living organisms. Indeed,

> [i]f one had to describe, with a single word, what physiology is all about, that word would be *homeostasis*. . . . [I]t refers to [feedback] mechanisms by which biologic systems tend to maintain the internal stability necessary for survival while adjusting to internal or external threats to that stability. If homeostasis is successful, life continues; if it is unsuccessful, disease and, perhaps, death ensue.[154]

Circles, Not Straight Lines

The feedback lens of systems thinking provides a powerful conceptual leverage in understanding and effectively managing complex systems (and that includes human energy and weight regulation, as we shall see). It is a decidedly a different way of thinking, however.

Most people, experiments have consistently shown, are predisposed to thinking in straight lines (linear thinking).[155] That is, we tend to view the world in terms of unilateral causation, independent and dependent variables, origins and terminations. Examples are everywhere: as when we think that appetite affects weight, parents socialize children, desires affect actions. Those assertions are incomplete (wrong) because each of them demonstrably also operates in the opposite direction: weight affects appetite, children socialize parents, and actions affect desires. In every one of these examples causation is circular, not linear.[156]

An open-loop, straight-line view of causality aptly characterizes how most people think about and seek to manage their energy balance "problem" as well. To lose weight, they set a weight-loss target, calculate a diet's caloric deficit, and launch. The results often disappoint.

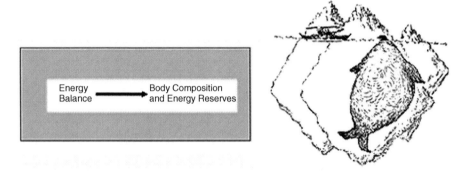

Figure 1.8 The energy balance equation shows only the tip of a physiological iceberg

Usually forgotten is the fact that our actions (dieting) alter the system (our body), which effectively alters the original situation (or problem) we are trying to resolve. Specifically, the caloric restriction we impose on our bodies when we go on a diet triggers involuntary energy conservation measures, as was explained, that act to restrain the rate of tissue depletion, and these homeostatic adaptations lower the body's energy requirements, effectively shrinking our diet-induced energy deficit. This link from effect back to cause closes the open loop (Figure 1.9).

Weight loss can therefore be viewed not only as the consequence of an initial negative energy balance, but also as the mechanism by which energy balance is eventually restored.[157] The causation is circular not linear: just as energy expenditure drains the body's energy stores, it is simultaneously regulated by them.

It is precisely these homeostatic (feedback) adaptations that can help us both understand as well as anticipate the curvilinear-type pattern of weight loss that has frustrated many a dieter: the (brief) initial phase of gratifying loss

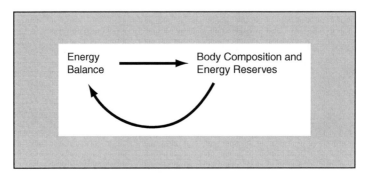

Figure 1.9 There is much more under the surface

in weight that invariably tapers off with time, ultimately leveling-off at a new steady-state weight that is substantially higher than expected or hoped for.

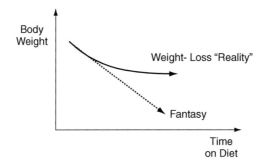

Figure 1.10 Linear versus curvilinear weight loss

In later chapters we shall see that there is much more "under the surface" than just one feedback link from body composition and energy reserves to energy balance. Because of the importance of ensuring sufficient energy for survival and reproduction, our body does not leave energy metabolism to chance; lack of energy would mean failure to thrive, and often, failure to survive.[158] A multitude of overlapping (sometimes redundant) physiological pathways are, thus, in place to regulate *both* sides of the human energy balance equation—the energy input side as well as energy expenditure.

There is also much more "over the surface." The adaptive feedback signals that regulate much of what we do are not limited to the physiological; they also characterize many of the interactions between the physiological and the behavioral, and between people and their external environment.

Indeed, in thinking about health and its determinants, the reciprocal influence of individual and environment cannot be overstated. People influence their settings, and their settings then act to influence their behaviors (including health behavior). As Winston Churchill once observed (while commenting on the design of the House of Commons), "We shape our environment, and then our environment shapes us."

Yet much discussion of the people–environment interactions, whether in academic or public discourse, continues to cast such interactions in terms of one-way causal connections. There is perhaps no more poignant example of the bankruptcy of linear thinking than the mutual finger pointing between the food industry and obesity researchers.

Food and beverage companies argue that they create new products in response to consumer demand and that (offering) choice is what a free society is all about.

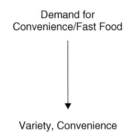

Demand for
Convenience/Fast Food

Variety, Convenience

But it would be just as true to describe the other half of the process. From the health industry's perspective, the food industry is a real culprit. It is more than a misnomer, many health experts argue, to suggest that it is simply a person's freely chosen lifestyle to eat nonnutritious, high-fat, energy-dense fast foods when healthier foods are much more expensive or altogether unavailable.

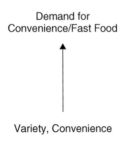

Demand for
Convenience/Fast Food

Variety, Convenience

But both statements are equally incomplete. The more complete statement of causality is that influence is mutual rather than one-way. The two linear relationships interact to create a closed loop in which the variables mutually influence one another. The consumer responds to lower prices, convenience, and variety by increasing consumption of those foods. This fuels growth and innovation in the industry, leading to more attractive products that are attractively priced (as market competition and economies of scale drive prices lower), and that are offered at more locations—all of which further increase demand (Figure 1.11).

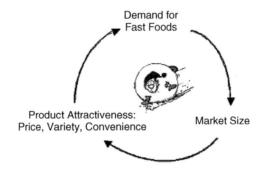

Figure 1.11 The two linear relationships interact to create a closed loop

Seeing this is terribly important, for it is the mutual influence—the closing of the loop—that creates a self-reinforcing (snowballing) dynamic that can escalate a problem or trend, such as fast food, to troublesome levels. With each trip around the loop, the phenomenon strengthens as the process feeds on itself, and given enough time an initial small "event" can morph into a major development. That is essentially how all epidemic scenarios arise.

The discipline of closing the loops helps us see such escalation structures—structures in which we may be "trapped." Many times such structures are of our own creation, but this has little meaning until those structures are seen. As long as we remain unaware of such structures, they continue to hold us prisoner.[159]

To think "straight" about systems, is to think in circles, and I mean this literally.

Dynamic, Not Static

People manage their bodies ballistically (like the firing of a cannonball: setting a weight-loss target, calculating a diet's caloric deficit, and launching). No wonder that they all too often miss their target. Managing our bodies is akin to pursuing a target that not only moves but also reacts to the actions of the pursuer.

While the operation of a static equation such as the energy balance equation may be reasonably obvious (a daily caloric deficit of 500 kcal

sheds off 1 pound in a week, 2 pounds in 2 weeks, and so on), predicting the
real behavior of the body's web of interconnected feedback processes can be
intellectually daunting (Figure 1.12).

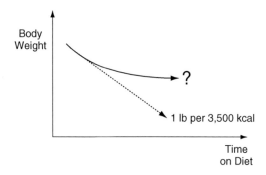

Figure 1.12 Predicting where a nonlinear system ends up is tricky

So, initially, the same features that made the feedback systems approach
attractive—putting things back together and recognizing the feedback interactions
between them—also made them somewhat slippery and elusive.[160] As inquiry
extended to more complex systems, it became more and more apparent that a
system of dynamic "bookkeeping" was necessary. The digital computer—the
second innovation referred to above—has provided that system.

Today, thanks to the availability of affordable, high-quality computing
capabilities, we can construct silicon surrogates of complex real-world processes such as human energy/weight regulation. Such computer models are
referred to as simulation models because the computer program simulates or
mimics the system under study.[161] No longer, in John Casti's words,[162] do we
have to live "in the shadow world of hypotheticality," or feel obligated to break
systems into manageable analytical "bites" and study these fragments in isolation with the hope that we can then reassemble these chunks of partial knowledge into an understanding of the overall system itself.

Engineers long ago learned to use computer models to learn about the
behavior of complex technological systems. So did pilots, who rely on flight
simulators to learn how to fly advanced new aircraft. Our bodies are as complex
as many technological systems. Why, then, do we not use the same approach
that engineers and pilots use, and create and use models of our human physiology to learn about and manage ("fly") our bodies?

The concern is often stated that the average person's knowledge and skill is
grossly insufficient for properly using models of a system as complex as the
human body. But what justification can there be for the apparent assumption
that ordinary people do not know enough to use models of their health, but
believe that they *do* know enough to directly intervene in managing their
weight and energy regulation?[163] I contend (and substantial supporting

evidence is beginning to accumulate) that people *do* know enough to use such tools. And with increasingly user-friendly software, ordinary people, for the first time in history, have access to and can learn to make effective use of models of systems as complex as their own bodies.

In this book, I argue for the development of computer-based models as laboratories for personal learning about obesity and weight management. Simulation models, also called "microworlds," are perhaps the only way we can discover how our complex bodies work since experimentation on our bodies in the real world is infeasible, expensive, and risky. A microworld allows us to see more clearly the long-term consequences of our lifestyle decisions, such as the slow, gradual physiological changes that accompany weight gain. They are the only practical, and safe, way to "experience" disease in advance of the real thing.

To rely instead on real-life experience for learning about how best to manage our health is a bad second option. Not only is it rarely effective, but when it comes to health, the cost of relying on trial and error to learn a good lesson may simply be too high. Often, we have just one shot at doing the right thing.

In addition to being laboratories for learning, computer-based tools also can serve as *personalized* health decision support systems, allowing people to assess treatment options and predict treatment outcome. As we will discuss in Part IV, the quantity and quality of weight loss, whether by dieting or exercising, depends on a host of personal factors that can vary significantly among individuals (e.g., initial body weight and composition, past history of weight gain, stamina and fitness). Because computer-based tools can be highly "personalized," they can provide specific, tailored solutions to dieters' individual needs.[164]

Obliterating, Not Automating

The expanding repertoire of information technologies coupled with the explosive growth of computer-based electronic communication is opening enormous possibilities for empowering people with the tools they need for personal health management, with potentially far-reaching transformative consequences. To date, however, we have done little more than use our fancy new technology to mechanize old ways of doing business. The shift to Information Age health management will involve much more than just putting our current health education pamphlets up on the Web, or using information technology to simply substitute one medium for another.

It is time to stop paving the cow paths! Instead of embedding outdated processes (legacy of earlier times when we were computationally poor) in silicon and software, we should obliterate them and start over. We should use information technology not to automate existing processes (like the ubiquitous BMI and caloric balance calculators) but to enable new ones.

In this book, I argue for and aim to demonstrate the feasibility and utility of a new generation of dynamic tools that support interaction and customization for personal health and wellness management. We are in a position to do this because of the great advances in systems sciences, medicine, and computer technology over the last few decades. It is a truly new development.

The book, thus, aims to bring the twin innovations of systems thinking and information technology together in a form that is accessible to the general reader, with the hope that it would have a profound influence on how ordinary people think about and manage their health and well being.

Notes

1. Brownell, K.D. and Horgen, K.B. (2004). *Food Fight.* Chicago: Contemporary Books.
2. Pollan, M. (2003, October 26). The (agri)cultural contradictions of obesity. *New York Times Magazine,* p. 41.
3. Cutler, D.M., Glaeser, E.L. and Shapiro, J.M. (2003). Why have Americans become more obese? *Journal of Economic Perspectives,* 17(3), 93–118.
4. Grady, D. (2003, November 11). What should we eat? *New York Times,* p. D6.
5. Pool, R. (2001). *Fat: Fighting the Obesity Epidemic.* Oxford: Oxford University Press.
6. Brownell, K.D. and Horgen, K.B. (2004). *Food Fight.* Chicago: Contemporary Books.
7. Bjorntorp, P. (2001). Thrifty genes and human obesity. Are we chasing ghosts? *Lancet,* 358, 1006–1008.
8. Weigle, D.S. (1994). Appetite and the regulation of body composition. *FASEB Journal,* 8, 302–310.
9. Grundy, S.M. (1998). Multifactorial causation of obesity: implications for prevention. *American Journal of Clinical Nutrition,* 67(suppl), 563S–572S.
10. Bjorntorp, P. (2001). Thrifty genes and human obesity. Are we chasing ghosts? *Lancet,* 358, 1006–1008.
11. Brownell, K.D. and Horgen, K.B. (2004). *Food Fight.* Chicago: Contemporary Books.
12. Richmond, B. (1991). *Systems Thinking: Four Key Questions.* Hanover, NH: High Performance Systems, Inc.
13. Senge, P.M. (1990). *The Fifth Discipline: The Art and Practice of the Learning Organization.* New York: Doubleday/Currency.
14. Hogarth, R. (1987). *Judgment and Choice.* Chichester, NY: John Wiley.
15. Senge, P.M. (1990). *The Fifth Discipline: The Art and Practice of the Learning Organization.* New York: Doubleday/Currency.
16. *Ibid.*

17. Five large-scale national surveys conducted in the United States between 1960 and 2004 provided estimates of the extent of overweight and obesity in the nation. These surveys were the National Health Examination Survey (NHES I, 1960–1962); and the four National Health and Nutrition Examination Surveys (NHANES I, 1971–1974; NHANES II, 1976–1980; NHANES III, 1988–1994; and the ongoing NHANES IV, which began in 1999). Beginning in 1999, NHANES became a continuous survey without a break between cycles. In each survey a nationally representative sample of the U.S. civilian noninstitutionalized population is selected using a complex, stratified, multistage probability cluster sampling design. In contrast to other surveillance studies, the NHES and NHANES involve measured heights and weights, from which BMI was/is calculated.

18. Daviglus, M.L., et al. (2003). Body mass index in middle age and health-related quality of life in older age. *Archives of Internal Medicine*, 163, 2448–2455.

19. Manson, J., et al. (2004). The escalating pandemics of obesity and sedentary lifestyle. *Archives of Internal Medicine*, 164(3), 249–258.

20. In some subpopulations the problem is worse than in others. For example, data from the National Health and Nutrition Examination Surveys clearly show that the rates of obesity in the United States follows a socioeconomic gradient, such that the burden of the disease falls disproportionately on people with limited resources, racial-ethnic minorities, and the poor. (The data show that the lowest educated groups having a prevalence of obesity that runs about 5 percent higher than more educated subpopulations). Reference: Speakman, J.R. (2003). Obesity: Part one: the greatest health threat facing mankind. *Biologist*, 50(1), 11–14.

21. Schlosser, E. (2002). *Fast Food Nation: The Dark Side of the All-American Meal*. New York: Perennial.

22. Analysis of recent data from the National Health and Nutrition Examination Surveys—conducted by CDC's National Center for Health Statistics—suggests obesity rates have been leveling off since 1999–2003. At this point, however, no one knows whether the pause will become permanent or whether it is simply a temporary reprieve, perhaps a statistical aberration, before the rates start upward again. Researchers need to see a few more years of data before declaring whether this is a true plateau in prevalence or just a temporary lull. In the meantime, most agree, it remains critical to help those who are already overweight and work to reduce the number of overweight Americans. Far too many children and adults are still overweight and at risk of illness and death unless we commit to reversing not just stabilizing the epidemic.

23. Reuters News Service, May 29, 2003.

24. Children are obese if their body mass index is equal to or greater than the 95th percentile of the age and gender-specific body mass charts compiled by the Centers for Disease Control and Prevention. A child who is in the 85th percentile is overweight and at risk for obesity.
25. *Wall Street Journal*. (2003, November 14), p. W1.
26. "Dogs and cats are classified as overweight when their body weight is 15 percent above what is deemed 'optimal' for their breed, and they are considered obese when their weight exceeds 30 percent above optimal" (Brody, J.E. [2006, July 18]. Wonder where that fat cat learned to eat? *New York Times*).
27. Hill, J.O. and Peters, J.C. (1998). Environmental contributions to the obesity epidemic. *Science*, 280, 1371–1374.
28. In the words of Keith Ayoob, a pediatric nutritionist at Albert Einstein College of Medicine in New York and spokesman for the American Dietetic Association. In: Hellmich, N. (2002, October 9). By the millions, kids keep gaining weight. *USA Today*, p. 9D.
29. Connelly, M. (2003, May 13). More children are obese, and more Americans know it. *New York Times*.
30. Manson, J.E. and Bassuk, S.S. (2003). Obesity in the United States: a fresh look at its high toll. *JAMA*, 289(2), 229–230.
31. Lee, T. and Oliver, E. (2002). *Public opinion and the politics of America's obesity epidemic*. John F. Kennedy School of Government, Harvard University, Faculty Research Working Papers Series (RWP02–017).
32. Easterbrook, G. (2004, March 14). The nation: wages of wealth; all this progress is killing us, bite by bite. *New York Times*, p. 5.
33. Hellmich, N. (2005, May 3). Obesity surges among affluent, Gap with poor all but disappears. *USA Today*.
34. Manson, J.E. and Bassuk, S.S. (2003). Obesity in the United States: a fresh look at its high toll. *JAMA*, 289(2), 229–230.
35. *Ibid.*
36. *New York Times* (2003, January 6). Being fatter at 40 can shorten life by 3 years. *New York Times*.
37. Cohen, P. (2004, May 15). Forget lonely. Life is healthy at the top. *New York Times*.
38. Hill, J.O. and Peters, J.C. (1998). Environmental contributions to the obesity epidemic. *Science*, 280, 1371–1374.
39. Wall Street Journal (2000, January 11). Being overweight in midlife boosts heart risks. *Wall Street Journal*.
40. Brownell, K.D. and Horgen, K.B. (2004). *Food Fight*. Chicago: Contemporary Books.
41. Carlos Poston, W.S. and Foreyt, J.P. (2000). Successful management of the obese patient. *American Family Physician*, 61(12), 3615–3622.

42. McKay, B. (2004, August 24). Obesity is linked to cancer risk. *Wall Street Journal.*

43. Stipanuk, M.H. (Ed.). (2000). *Biochemical and Physiological Aspects of Human Nutrition.* Philadelphia: W.B. Saunders.

44. Grady, Denise. (2004, July 6). Fat: the secret life of a potent cell. *New York Times,* p. D1.

45. Many researchers think the culprit is visceral fat, meaning deposits inside the abdomen, as opposed to subcutaneous (under the skin) fat. An apple-shaped person is sure to have visceral fat, as well as subcutaneous fat in the abdominal area. Anybody with a belly has visceral fat, and the more you have the worse off you are. It is not clear why visceral fat is riskier; it may be more active metabolically and spew out more toxic substances. In addition, its secretions go straight to the liver and may interfere with its functions, which include helping to regulate blood glucose and cholesterol. Reference: Grady, Denise. (2004, July 6). Fat: the secret life of a potent cell. *New York Times,* p. D1.

46. Brownell, K.D. and Horgen, K.B. (2004). *Food Fight.* Chicago: Contemporary Books.

47. O'Neil, J. (2005, January 25). Testing: obesity may skew prostate test. *New York Times.*

48. Brody, J.E. (2003, May 6). Another study finds a link between excess weight and cancer. *New York Times,* p. D7.

49. Brownell, K.D. and Horgen, K.B. (2004). *Food Fight.* Chicago: Contemporary Books.

50. Rundle, R.L. (2004, March 9). Obesity issues for elderly may rise. *Wall Street Journal,* p. D3.

51. Wall Street Journal (2004, April 22). Weight loss may ease arthritis. *Wall Street Journal,* p. D2.

52. Fackelmann, K. (2005, August 25). Does diabetes lurk behind Alzheimer's? *USA Today,* p. 1D.

53. Kumanyika, S.K. (2001). Minisymposium on obesity: overview and some strategic considerations. *Annual Review of Public Health,* 22, 293–308.

54. Kirschenbaum, D.S. and Fitzgibbon, M.L. (1995). Controversy about the treatment of obesity: criticisms or challenges? *Behavior Therapy,* 26, 43–68.

55. Battle, E.K. and Brownell, K.D. (1996). Confronting a rising tide of eating disorders and obesity: treatment vs. prevention and policy. *Addictive Behaviors,* 21(6), 755–765.

56. Rand, D.S.W. and MacGregor, A.M.C. (1991). Successful weight loss following obesity surgery and the perceived liability of morbid obesity. *International Journal of Obesity,* 15, 577–579.

57. Brownell, K.D. and Fairburn, C.G. (Eds.). (1995). *Eating Disorders and Obesity: A Comprehensive Handbook.* New York: Guilford Press.

58. Bray, G.A, Bouchard, C., and James, W.P.T. (Eds.). (1998). *Handbook of Obesity*. New York: Marcel Dekker.
59. Wadden, T.A. and Stunkard, A.J. (Eds.). (2002). *Handbook of Obesity Treatment*. New York: Guilford Press.
60. *Ibid.*
61. Cassell, J.A. (1995). Social anthropology and nutrition: a different look at obesity in America. *Journal of the American Dietetic Association*, 95(4), 424–427.
62. Dietz, W.H. (1998). Health consequences of obesity in youth: childhood predictors of adult disease. *Pediatrics*, 101, 518–525.
63. Wadden, T.A. and Stunkard, A.J. (Eds.). (2002). *Handbook of Obesity Treatment*. New York: Guilford Press.
64. Shils, M.E., Olson, J.A., Shike, M., and Ross, A.C. (Eds.). (1999). *Modern Nutrition in Health and Disease*. Baltimore: Williams & Wilkins.
65. Hellmich, N. (2002, October 9). By the millions, kids keep gaining weight. *USA Today*, p. 9D.
66. Shils, M.E., Olson, J.A., Shike, M., and Ross, A.C. (Eds.). (1999). *Modern Nutrition in Health and Disease*. Baltimore: Williams & Wilkins.
67. Wadden, T.A. and Stunkard, A.J. (Eds.). (2002). *Handbook of Obesity Treatment*. New York: Guilford Press.
68. Allison, D.B. and Saunders, S.E. (2000). Obesity in North America: an overview. *Medical Clinics of North America,* 84(2), 305–333.
69. Epperson, S. (2003, September 8). The obesity charge. *Time*, 162 (10), p. 100.
70. Wing, R.R. and Greeno, C.G. (1994). Behavioral and psychosocial aspects of obesity and its treatment. *Baillière's Clinical Endocrinology and Metabolism*, 8(3), 689–703.
71. Seidell, J.C. (1998). Societal and personal costs of obesity. *Experimental and Clinical Endocrinology and Diabetes*, 106(suppl 2), 7–9.
72. Speakman, J.R. (2003). Obesity: part one—the greatest health threat facing mankind. *Biologist*, 50(1), 11–14.
73. Shell, E.R. (2002). *The Hungry Gene: The Inside Story of the Obesity Industry*. New York: Grove Press.
74. Squires, S. (2001, Dec 14). National plan urged to combat obesity. *Washington Post,* p. A03.
75. Brownell, K.D. and Horgen, K.B. (2004). *Food Fight*. Chicago: Contemporary Books.
76. *Ibid.*
77. Shell, E.R. (2002). *The Hungry Gene: The Inside Story of the Obesity Industry*. New York: Grove Press.
78. Widmaier, E.P. (1998). *Why Geese Don't Get Obese: How Evolution's Strategies for Survival Affect Our Everyday Lives*. New York: W.H. Freeman.

79. Grady, D. (2003, November 11). What should we eat? *New York Times*, p. D6.
80. World Health Organization. (2002). *The World Health Report 2002: Reducing Risks, Promoting Healthy Life*. Geneva: World Health Organization.
81. Easterbrook, G. (2004, March 14). The nation: wages of wealth; all this progress is killing us, bite by bite. *New York Times, p. 5*.
82. Brownell, K.D. and Horgen, K.B. (2004). *Food Fight*. Chicago: Contemporary Books.
83. (http://www.paperboat.com/calliope/hiddenad.htm).
84. Spake, A. (2003). The science of slimming: getting rid of all those unwanted pounds is as simple as calories in, calories out. *U.S. News and World Report*, 134(21), 34–38.
85. Pickstone, J.V. (2000). *Ways of Knowing: A New History of Science, Technology and Medicine*. Chicago: University of Chicago Press,
86. Oliver, J.E. and Lee, T. (2005). Public opinion and the politics of obesity in America. *Journal of Health Politics, Policy and Law*, 30(5), 923–954.
87. Pool, R. (2001). *Fat: Fighting the Obesity Epidemic*. Oxford: Oxford University Press.
88. According to the United Nations' Second Assembly on Ageing, a million people now turn 60 every month, a demographic revolution that will mean older people will soon outnumber the young for the first time in history. Reference: Daly, E. (2002, April 9). U.N. says elderly will soon outnumber young for first time. *New York Times*.
89. Dyer, R.G. (1994). Traditional treatment of obesity: does it work. *Bailliere's Clinical Endocrinology and Metabolism*, 8, 661–688.
90. Tate, D.F., Wing, R.R., and Winett, R.A. (2001). Using Internet technology to deliver a behavioral weight loss program. *JAMA*, 285(9), 1172–1177.
91. Battle, E.K. and Brownell, K.D. (1996). Confronting a rising tide of eating disorders and obesity: treatment vs. prevention and policy. *Addictive Behaviors*, (21), 755–765.
92. Tahmincioglu, Eve. (2004, May 23). Paths to better health (on the boss's nickel). *New York Times*.
93. In July 2004, Medicare abandoned its long-held official view that obesity is not an illness, opening the way for the government to pay for at least some obesity treatments—such as surgery. To be eligible for coverage, the government also declared, "treatments must be proved effective." It remains unclear whether treatments such as weight-control drugs, diagnostic tests, and counseling by dieticians would be covered. Because many insurers take their cues from Medicare's policies, Medicare's ultimate practices are almost certainly going to affect future practices in the insurance industry. Reference: Akst, D. (2004, July 25). On the contrary; shedding pounds with Medicare. *New York Times*.

94. Pool, R. (2001). *Fat: Fighting the Obesity Epidemic.* Oxford: Oxford University Press.

95. Brownell, K.D. (1991). Personal responsibility and control over our bodies: when expectation exceeds reality. *Health Psychology,* 10, 303–310.

96. Committee to Develop Criteria for Evaluating the Outcomes of Approaches to Prevent and Treat Obesity. (1995). Summary: weighing the options-criteria for evaluating weight-management programs. *Journal of the American Dietetic Association,* 95(1), 96–105.

97. Conant, R. and Ashby, W. (1970). Every good regulator of a system must be a model of the system. *International Journal of System Science,* 1, 89–97.

98. *Ibid.*

99. Sterman, J.D. (1994). Learning in and about complex systems. *System Dynamics Review,* 10, 291–330.

100. Sterman, J.D. (2000). *Business Dynamics: Systems Thinking and Modeling for a Complex World.* Boston: Irwin McGraw-Hill.

101. Hunt, E. (1989). Cognitive science: definition, status, and questions. *Annual Review of Psychology,* 40, 603–629.

102. Ann Chapman, J. and Ferfolja, T. (2001). Fatal flaws: the acquisition of imperfect mental models and their use in hazardous situations. *Journal of Intellectual Capital,* (2), 398–409.

103. Sterman, J.D. (2002) All models are wrong: reflections on becoming a systems scientist. *System Dynamics Review,* 18, 501–531.

104. Ann Chapman, J. and Ferfolja, T. (2001). Fatal flaws: the acquisition of imperfect mental models and their use in hazardous situations. *Journal of Intellectual Capital,* (2), 398–409.

105. Peterson, C. and Stunkard, A.J. (1989). Personal control and health promotion. *Social Science and Medicine,* 28, 819–828.

106. Russo, J.E. and Shoemaker, P.J.H. (1994). *Decision Traps: The Ten Barriers to Decision-Making and How to Overcome Them.* New York: Fireside.

107. Sterman, J.D. (1994). Learning in and about complex systems. *System Dynamics Review,* 10, 291–330.

108. *Ibid.*

109. Norman, D.A. (1988). *The Design of Everyday Things.* New York: Doubleday Currency.

110. Einhorn, H.J. and Hogarth, R.M. (1987). Decision making: going forward in reverse. *Harvard Business Review,* 65(1): 66–70.

111. McArdle, W.D., Katch, F.I., and Katch, V.L. (1996). *Exercise Physiology: Energy, Nutrition, and Human Performance.* Baltimore: Williams & Wilkins.

112. Whitney, E.N. and Rolfes, S.R. (1999). *Understanding Nutrition.* Belmont, CA: West/Wadsworth.

113. Weinsier, R.L., Bracco, D., and Schultz, Y. (1993). Predicted Effects of small decreases in energy expenditure on weight gain in adult women. *International Journal of Obesity*, 17, 693–699.

114. Foster, G.D., Wadden, T.A., Vogt, R.A., and Brewer, G. (1997). What is a reasonable weight loss? Patients' expectations and evaluations of obesity treatment outcomes. *Journal of Consulting and Clinical Psychology*, 65, 79–85.

115. Taylor, S.E. and Brown, J.D. (1988). Illusion and well-being: a social psychological perspective on mental health. *Psychological Bulletin*, 103, 193–210.

116. Peterson, C. and Stunkard, A.J. (1989). Personal control and health promotion. *Social Science and Medicine*, 28, 819–828.

117. Clarke, V.A., Lovegrove, H., Williams, A., and Macpherson, M. (2000). Unrealistic optimism and the health belief model. *Journal of Behavioral Medicine*, 23, 367–376.

118. Whalen, C.K., Henker, B., O'Neil, R., Hollingshead, J., Holman, A., and Moore, B. (1994). Optimism in children's judgments of health and environmental risks. *Health Psychology*, 13, 319–325.

119. Taylor, S.E. and Brown, J.D. (1988). Illusion and well-being: a social psychological perspective on mental health. *Psychological Bulletin*, 103, 193–210.

120. Nestle, M. and Jacobson, M.F. (2000). Halting the obesity epidemic: a public health policy approach. *Public Health Reports*, 115, 12–24.

121. Jeffery, R.W. (2001). Public health strategies for obesity treatment and prevention. *American Journal of Health Behavior*, 25(3), 252–259.

122. Brody, J.E., (2004, March 23). Sane weight loss in a carb-obsessed world: high fiber and low fat. *New York Times*.

123. Hogarth, R.M. and Makridakis, S. (1981). Forecasting and planning: an evaluation. *Management Science*, 27(2), 115–138.

124. Gilbert, D. (2006, April 16). I'm O.K., you're biased. *New York Times*.

125. A quote by Andrew Wang in E.J. Huth and T.J. Murray (2000). *Medicine in Quotations: Views of Health and Disease through the Ages*. Philadelphia: American College of Physicians.

126. Senge, P.M. (1990). *The Fifth Discipline: The Art and Practice of the Learning Organization*. New York: Doubleday/Currency.

127. Argyris, C. (1992). *On Organizational Learning*. Cambridge, MA: Blackwell Publishers.

128. Sterman, J.D. (2000). *Business Dynamics: Systems Thinking and Modeling for a Complex World*. Boston: Irwin McGraw-Hill.

129. Sterman, J. D. (1994). Learning in and about complex systems. *System Dynamics Review*, 10, 291–330.

130. The terms *single-* versus *second-loop learning* were coined by Argyris, an organizational learning theorist at Harvard University.

131. Sterman, J. D. (1994). Learning in and about complex systems. *System Dynamics Review,* 10, 291–330.

132. Sterman, J.D. (2000). *Business Dynamics: Systems Thinking and Modeling for a Complex World.* Boston: Irwin McGraw-Hill.

133. Edward O. Wilson has been a professor at Harvard since 1955, is a pioneer of sociobiology and biodiversity, and considered by many to be one of the world's greatest living scientists. He wrote *Consilience: The Unity of Knowledge* (1998).

134. Bandura, A. (1997). *Self-Efficacy: The Exercise of Control.* New York: W.H. Freeman.

135. Senge, P.M. (1990). *The Fifth Discipline: The Art and Practice of the Learning Organization.* New York: Doubleday/Currency.

136. Wilson, E.O. (1998). *Consilience: The Unity of Knowledge.* New York: Alfred A. Knopf.

137. Diez-Roux, A.V. (1998). On genes, individuals, society, and epidemiology. *American Journal of Epidemiology*, 148(11), 1027–1032.

138. Ackoff, R.L. (1994). Systems thinking and thinking systems. *System Dynamics Review*, 19(2–3), 175–188.

139. Jervis, R. (1997). *System Effects: Complexity in Political and Social Life.* Princeton, NJ: Princeton University Press.

140. Capra, F. (1996). *The Web of Life: A Scientific Understanding of Living Systems.* New York: Anchor Books.

141. Ackoff, R.L. (1994). Systems thinking and thinking systems. *System Dynamics Review*, 19(2–3), 175–188.

142. Capra, F. (1996). *The Web of Life: A Scientific Understanding of Living Systems.* New York: Anchor Books.

143. Brownell, K.D. and Fairburn, C.G. (Eds.). (1995). *Eating Disorders and Obesity: A Comprehensive Handbook.* New York: Guilford Press

144. Pool, R. (2001). *Fat: Fighting the Obesity Epidemic.* Oxford: Oxford University Press.

145. Senge, P.M. (1990). *The Fifth Discipline: The Art and Practice of the Learning Organization.* New York: Doubleday/Currency.

146. Capra, F. (1996). *The Web of Life: A Scientific Understanding of Living Systems.* New York: Anchor Books.

147. Laszlo, E. (1996). *The Systems View of the World: A Holistic Vision for Our Time (Advances in Systems Theory, Complexity, and the Human Sciences).* Cresskill, NJ: Hampton Press.

148. Senge, P.M. (1990). *The Fifth Discipline: The Art and Practice of the Learning Organization.* New York: Doubleday/Currency.

149. Roberts, N., Andersen, D., Deal, R., Garet, M., and Shaffer, W. (1983). *Introduction to Computer Simulation: A System Dynamics Modeling Approach.* Reading, MA: Addison-Wesley.
150. By Wiener, Forrester, and others. See (1) Wiener, N. (1948). *Cybernetics: Or Control and Communication in the Animal and the Machine.* Cambridge, MA: MIT Press; and (2) Forrester, J.W. (1961). *Industrial Dynamics.* Cambridge, MA: MIT Press.
151. Roberts, N., Andersen, D., Deal, R., Garet, M., and Shaffer, W. (1983). *Introduction to Computer Simulation: A System Dynamics Modeling Approach.* Reading, MA: Addison-Wesley.
152. Guyton, A.C. and Hall, J.E. (1996). *Textbook of Medical Physiology.* Philadelphia: W.B. Saunders.
153. Brownell, K.D. and Fairburn, C.G. (Eds.). (1995). *Eating Disorders and Obesity: A Comprehensive Handbook.* New York: Guilford Press
154. Johnson, L.R. (1998). *Essential Medical Physiology.* Philadelphia: Lippincott-Raven.
155. Sterman, J.D. (2000). *Business Dynamics: Systems Thinking and Modeling for a Complex World.* Boston: Irwin McGraw-Hill.
156. Weick, K. (1979). *The Social Psychology of Organizing.* New York: Addison-Wesley.
157. Wadden, T.A. and Stunkard, A.J. (Eds.). (2002). *Handbook of Obesity Treatment.* New York: Guilford Press.
158. Hargrove, J.L. (1998). *Dynamic Modeling in the Health Sciences.* New York: Springer.
159. Senge, P.M. (1990). *The Fifth Discipline: The Art and Practice of the Learning Organization.* New York: Doubleday/Currency.
160. Roberts, N., Andersen, D., Deal, R., Garet, M., and Shaffer, W. (1983). *Introduction to Computer Simulation: A System Dynamics Modeling Approach.* Reading, MA: Addison-Wesley.
161. *Ibid.*
162. Casti, J.L. (1997). *Would-Be Worlds: How Simulation Is Changing the Frontiers of Science.* New York: John Wiley .
163. Forrester, J.W. (1971). Counterintuitive behavior of social systems. *Technology Review,* 73(3), 52–68.
164. Gustafson, D.H. et al. (1999). Impact of a patient-centered, computer-based health information/support system. *American Journal of Preventive Medicine,* 16(1), 1–9.

How We Changed Our Environment, and Now Our Environment Is Changing Us

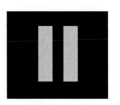

Unbalanced Act   2

Because eating is under conscious control—one can always decide not to put fork to mouth—weight has always been seen as a very individual, very personal thing. And being overweight, in turn, a matter of an individual's decisions—or, rather, of a failure to make decisions.[1] That is perhaps why most people believe that every overweight person can achieve slenderness and should pursue that goal, why obese people are stereotyped as lacking in self-control, and why being obese elicits scorn as often as sympathy.[2]

The inclination to explain health in terms of personal responsibility is deeply rooted in the Western culture, where both the power and responsibility of the individual are paramount.[3] And nowhere is this truer than in the United States. As Howard Leichter observes,[4]

> [T]he timelessness and persistence of holding the individual person responsible for his or her own health status has its genesis in one of the most distinguishing historical features of American culture and politics, namely the extraordinary emphasis on individuals' rights and responsibilities.

The *wellness movement*, which in the last few decades has taken hold of the health mentality of a large segment of the United States population, is rooted in this very concept of personal control over health. This is not surprising, as the notion of personal responsibility for our continual transformation, self-rejuvenation, and self-repair is certainly an appealing and almost irresistible one.[5] Perhaps the most striking expression of this focus on individual responsibility is Americans' quest for the perfect body. This obsession may explain why people with the "wrong" bodies are so poorly judged in American society, that is, considered self-indulgent, lazy, and lacking control, while those with the "right" bodies are seen as models of self-control.[6]

This individual-centered and (as we shall see) simplistic view of obesity's cause is not limited to laypeople. Health care professionals, it is disturbing to note, are among the chief offenders. Numerous studies of health care providers—dieticians, physicians, family doctors—reveal that many believe

T.K.A. Hamid, *Thinking in Circles About Obesity*,
DOI 10.1007/978-0-387-09469-4_2, © Springer Science+Business Media, LLC 2009

excess body weight simply reflects a lack of willpower, poor self-concept, and deep-seated psychological problems.[7] It is a disturbing finding because it has destructive results, including prejudice and discrimination toward the very patients for whom these professionals care.[8,9] In one study, for example, a survey of physicians found that they viewed their obese patients as weak-willed and even ugly and awkward. In another study, as many as 78 percent of the obese patients surveyed reported that they had "always, or usually, been treated disrespectfully by the medical profession because of [their] weight."[10]

"For every complex problem there is an [explanation] that is simple, direct, and . . . wrong."

—H.L. Mencken[11]

The individual-centered "theory" is an appealing proposition. For starters, it is a single-cause explanation and, hence, a simple one. And simple explanations can be very seductive to laypeople and experts alike. Cognitive theorists and philosophers argue that humans tend to seek simple causes for even the most complex problems.[12,13] Unfortunately, many of the simplifying short-cuts we habitually take have been shown to systematically lead to errors in judgment.

When explaining the causes of some behavior, for example, it is common for people to rely on factors that are most salient to them. The most salient thing in health behavior is the "actor" who is behaving. People are in the foreground; almost everything else—situational and environmental factors—is in the background. Hence the cognitive "trap."

> This over-readiness to explain behavior [not only in obesity, but for many dysfunctional behaviors] in terms of dispositional factors [such as abilities, traits, and motives] is so widespread and universal that it [has been] called "the fundamental attribution error."[14]

It is a tendency that often leads to attributions that are patently wrong. An example of biblical proportion is the one committed by the sailors in the Book of Jonah. "When a storm hit their ship, they didn't ascribe it to a seasonal weather pattern. They attributed the cause to Jonah's sinfulness, and responded by throwing him overboard."[15] In the case of health issues, the *fundamental attribution error* creates the bias of overattributing behavior to factors such as personal control, and grossly underweighing the influence of situational factors such as the socio-economic system in which we live.

As we have already seen in Chapter 1, experts are not impervious to such cognitive bias. In the past and still today, many in the health field have been engulfed by the overreadiness to explain health behavior in terms of individual-level drivers—the notion of *individualization*.[16] From the proponents of the long-standing behavioral model of disease, who view disease as stemming from the individual's choices and behaviors, to the more recent genetic model, in which disease is considered strongly influenced by an individual's unique genetic makeup,[17] this cognitive bias remains strong.

Biases—indeed most cognitive traps—thrive more easily and persist longer when there is subtlety and complexity, not when cause and effect are clear-cut, black-and-white affairs. In the domain of human health and disease, "grayness" and complexity remain, even today, the lay of the intellectual landscape.

There is no dispute, for example, that individual-level characteristics are important determinants of individual health and that our understanding of individual-level risk factors, from choices and behaviors to unique genetic makeup, has contributed greatly (and continues to contribute) to our understanding of health in populations. (A good example is the identification of lifestyle and biological factors associated with cardiovascular disease.) However, it has also become increasingly clear that a fixation on such determinants has limited our ability to examine and understand the full spectrum of disease causation.[18,19]

In the case of obesity, one consequence of the individual-centered fixation is the field's preoccupation with why individuals are obese and how to help them, rather than with why society is obese and how to help it.[20] Of the numerous diseases that have struck humanity throughout history, never has there been a disease as common as obesity. Many diseases were more deadly, for sure, but none as common. "[This] suggests that obesity develops through a mechanism which, unlike plague, tuberculosis, or AIDS, is induced by exposure to factors surrounding all of us in modern societies."[21] This may explain why, given the current environment, approaches to weight loss that focus on the individual have yielded less-than-impressive results.[22]

Another consequence of the individual-centered fixation is that individuals and the culture in general assume that they have more control than they actually do. Personal control is indeed important to human weight and energy regulation. However, we will see that control over our bodies must be considered within the context of environmental and cultural realities.

Part II provides a different conception of human health and disease, and, by extension, of the obesity problem. In contrast to the classical, individual-centered worldview, it is a systems-inspired worldview that adopts a much broader biopsychosocial perspective—one that looks beyond individuals' characteristics and behaviors for answers, to the symphony of behavior–biology–environment interactions.

The reason for this is scientific: our object of study demands it.[23]

Moving Beyond Individual-Centric Explanations

Obesity is not increasing because people are consciously trying to gain weight. Indeed, one of the major perplexities of this disease is that more and more people are getting fatter even in the face of broad publicity about the problem, tremendous pressure to be thin, and a titanic struggle by tens of millions of people to manage their weight. The fact that Americans spend some $50 billion annually on weight-loss products and services—services such as liposuction, which has become the most popular cosmetic surgery procedure in the country—shows that they can hardly be happy with the status quo.[24]

How, then, did we, as a society, get into this mess? To understand, we will need to go way back into our human history and evolution. An anthropological perspective, examining the problem and its root causes in the broader context of human history and cultural evolution, suggests that the obesity epidemic in Western cultures is caused by a mismatch between the modern living environment we share and a human physiology rooted in our evolutionary past.

"Civilization is but a filmy fringe on the history of man."

—William Osier

In the above quotation, Osier, the Canadian physician and historian, is saying that the past few millennia of human civilization represent a tiny fraction of the time since our human ancestors first appeared on earth.[25] Archaeological data suggest that it was not until approximately 12,000 years ago that some human groups started to shift from a food-foraging mode of existence to one of food production. This shift was driven primarily by ecological pressures from population growth and food scarcities, and it would prove to be of great consequence, as it was this relatively recent economic transformation that would ultimately allow for the evolution of complex societies and of civilization itself.[26]

But before that "filmy fringe" on our history and for hundreds of thousands of years, humans lived as hunter-gatherers dependent for their nourishment on the supply of game and on whatever fruits, nuts, berries, roots, leaves, and other vegetable matter was available.[27] While their diet was qualitatively adequate, food was scarce and the next meal unpredictable. In most prehistoric societies, starvation was a constant threat.[28]

Our understanding of life in the hunter-gatherer societies of antiquity is based not only on the abundant archaeological evidence that we have accumulated, but also on the anthropological study of *contemporary* hunter-gatherer populations. In what would surely qualify as a *Believe It or Not* story, there are today, at the dawn of the 21st century, some contemporary nonindustrial societies that are, in fact, "good approximations" of Stone Age humans of about 20,000 years ago—and not one or two, but a hundred or more.

Not surprisingly, they have all been the focus of intensive study by anthropologists. A cross-cultural ethnographic survey of a sample of more than a hundred such societies found seasonal food shortages for all of them, the same type of pattern that archaeological studies of excavated skeletal remains have revealed about the prehistoric hunter-gatherer societies. Shortages occur annually or even more frequently for roughly half of the societies, and the shortages are "severe" (approaching starvation-level) in nearly a third of them.[29]

That is the bad news. The good news, however, is that these best approximation surrogates for our human ancestors experience slow population growth, enjoy high-quality diets, maintain high levels of physical fitness, and are generally healthy. They are healthier, in fact, than many of the third-world populations currently undergoing the process of economic modernization or westernization.[30]

This is no accident. The interaction between any species and its food supply is one of the most important influences affecting biological adaptation and cultural evolution.[31] Because the struggle for survival of the human species has been driven by a lack, not an excess, of food, the human body has developed over the years to defend itself actively against this threat,[32] and it has succeeded.

In the hunter-gatherer mode of existence, where a high level of physical activity was required for daily subsistence and the food supply was inconsistent, the challenge to the body energy-control system was to provide a strong drive to eat to keep pace with energy expenditure and to rest when physical exertion was not required.[33] Because starvation was not only real but also a periodic threat, the greatest survival rates were among those who not only ate voraciously when food was plentiful, but who also stored the excess energy efficiently as a buffer against future food shortages.[34] Such individuals built up stores of fat that increased their survival prospects during famines, and they passed on these traits to their progeny, who, similarly, were more likely to survive.[35] For the females, whose reproductive fitness depended on their ability to withstand the nutritional demands of pregnancy and lactation, greater energy reserves provided a selective advantage over their lean counterparts in withstanding the stress of food shortage, not only for themselves but also for their fetuses and nursing children.[36,37]

It should not surprise, then, as Sharman Russell writes in his informative book, *Hunger: An Unnatural History*, that since human beings evolved to survive chronic threats of famine, we have grown afflicted by "chronic, troubling urges to gorge, grab, and hoard."

Our taste buds are also rooted in our evolutionary past. When, thousands of years ago, humans were hunting wild game and gathering wild plants for food, their primary food sources contained limited sugar, fat, and salt. But because these are essential to the proper functioning of the human body, it was always good for people to eat as much of them as they could find. In another adaptive response to human dietary needs, evolution equipped us with a nearly insatiable appetite for fat, salt, and sugar to encourage us to eat these foods. These strong taste preferences have been genetically passed on to us over the generations—and to good effect, until now.

> Fatty foods helped our ancestors weather food shortages. Salt helped them maintain an appropriate water balance in their cells, helping avoid dehydration. Sugar and the sweetness associated with it helped them distinguish edible berries from poisonous ones. By giving us the taste for fat, sugar, and salt, our genetics led us to prefer the foods that were most likely to keep us alive. It also led us to want to eat a wide variety of foods. The more types of foods we could eat, the more we were likely to consume the wide range of unknown nutrients we needed. Our natural inclination for variety made sure we got enough of these nutrients without us needing to know the difference between vitamin C, riboflavin, and a complex carbohydrate.[38]

In this evolutionary context, the usual range of human metabolic variation would have produced many individuals with a predisposition to become fat, but chronic food scarcity and vigorous physical exertion ensured that they never would.[39] Skeletal remains indicate that our human ancestors were typically more lean and muscular than we are today, and studies of contemporary hunter-gatherer populations are consistent with this finding. For example, studies of the !Kung San tribe in the Kalahari Desert show them to be lean, with skin fold thicknesses approximately half those of age-matched North Americans and suffering no obesity problem.[40,41]

This suggests that, despite seasonal fluctuations in food availability and a mode of existence characterized by vigorous physical exertion, the caloric intake and output of our hunter-gatherer ancestors were balanced over time.[42] Eating whatever animals they could kill or scavenge and whatever fruit and vegetable matter they could take from plants, early humans kept enough fat stores to make it through the occasional lean times, but not so much that it slowed them down significantly. Further, control of their body weight was largely accomplished through innate physiological processes and required little conscious effort. They did not have to think about how much to eat in order to maintain a desirable weight. Their bodies told them.[43]

Our current predicament, it turns out, is a direct byproduct of our early successes. Let's see how.

Evolved Asymmetry of Our Physiology

As mentioned, feeding behavior was a function that humans accomplished largely unconsciously and automatically. Given that obesity was not a common health problem throughout most of human history, it is not unreasonable that people instinctively believe that the body's regulatory system strives to maintain stability at some "natural" body weight, defending against both weight loss and weight gain.[44] Such a system would be symmetrical, defending against both positive and negative energy balances that threaten to cause weight change.

Unfortunately, this is a fundamental misconception that, because it remains quite common, seriously undermines (as we shall see in later sections) prevention efforts.

In reality, humans display a system of weight regulation that is *asymmetrical*. Because survival in a food-scarce environment is more acutely threatened by starvation than by obesity, evolution has selected our physiology and behavior to favor overconsumption rather than underconsumption. That is, our regulatory system has been organized by evolutionary selection to galvanize in a more robust way in response to deficient energy intake and stores than to excess energy.[45]

Before we see how this is accomplished, let's contemplate for just a moment the alternative: that of a *symmetrical* system that defends *equally* against weight loss or gain, while striving to maintain stability at some "normal" body weight. In a food-scarce environment, such a system would have probably led to extinction, because lower-than-average food levels would have led to a drop in weight to below "target." That's the downside. But an abundance of food would have exceeded the regularity system's "needs" (and capacity) to store it, leading to a maximum weight equal only to the target weight. This provides no upside to balance the downside.

Professor Sam Savage of Stanford University provides an interesting analogy that demonstrates how such a symmetric model would similarly lead to bankruptcy (cash starvation?) in business. Consider a hypothetical case of an entrepreneur considering building a manufacturing facility for a new product. She did extensive market analysis for her new product and expects average annual demand to be 100,000 units. A further analysis of construction and operating costs suggests that building and running a manufacturing facility with a 100,000 capacity would yield a healthy $10 million annual profit. What would happen if the demand of 100,000 units is indeed the correct average, but with year-to-year fluctuations between say 50,000 ("famine" market conditions) and 150,000 units ("feast" market conditions)? Intuitively, most people would expect that profit would still average out to $10 million: Some years it would be below, but those years would be compensated for by other years when it is above. Right? Wrong! Lower-than-average demand clearly leads to profits of less than $10 million. That's the downside. But greater demand exceeds the capacity of the new plant, leading to a ceiling on profit of $10 million. There is no upside to balance the downside. The result: an average profit much lower than the "target," perhaps leading to bankruptcy (extinction).

How Asymmetry Is Achieved by Our Physiology

The energy dynamic between organisms and their environments, that is, energy expended in the search for and consumption of food in relation to energy acquired and used for biological processes, is absolutely critical to survival and reproduction. This dynamic has important adaptive consequences for any organism's evolution.[46] Thus, it is not at all surprising that nature has worked so hard to make us succeed in a food-scarce environment. Indeed, we *have* succeeded, and this section explains how: how in humans, multiple redundant physiological systems evolved to ensure sufficient energy balance for survival and reproduction; and how humans display a system of weight and energy regulation that is *asymmetrical* not only in energy input (favoring overconsumption over underconsumption of food), but also in energy expenditure and storage.

Asymmetry in Energy Intake

In humans, feeding is controlled by two regulatory subsystems, one short-term and the other long-term. The short-term component controls the onset and cessation of feeding on a meal-to-meal basis. During the course of a meal, the body relies on an extensive array of receptors along the gastrointestinal tract to relay information to the brain about the amount and nutrient content of the food, such that the meal can be terminated when sufficient food has been consumed.[47,48]

Here's how this short-term subsystem works: as a meal is consumed, the presence of food in the gastrointestinal (GI) tract causes mechanoreceptors in the stomach to stretch, sending a message to the brain about the amount of food ingested. At the same time, the different nutrients of ingested food interact with chemoreceptors along the small intestine, triggering the release of GI hormones (such as cholecystokinin) to signal the nutrient content of the ingested meal. These neuronal and hormonal signals are decoded in the brain's feeding-control center (within the hypothalamus) to track the amount of food eaten and its nutrient content and to orchestrate the feelings of hunger/satiation that drive us to continue or to stop eating.[49]

A feeding episode—a meal—provides energy substrate to meet the immediate metabolic needs of the body. After a large meal, the unused portion of ingested food energy is stored, primarily in the body's depot of fat reserves. The function of the second long-term regulatory component is to monitor the depletion/repletion of these reserves—a function, it turns out, that's critical not only to our survival but also to our convenience.

To stay alive, humans, like all living organisms, need to continuously expend energy—literally every second of every day, whether we are awake or asleep. We must do that both to fuel physical activity and to sustain the body's basic metabolic and internal housekeeping functions. Our capacity to store energy long-term is what allows us to expend energy *continuously*, without having to constantly infuse energy into our bodies.

Consider for a moment how inconvenient it would be if that were not the case. It would be like running a retail business with some product on hand to sell but no additional inventory. Without the capacity to store energy long-term, energy output to sell but energy input would have to be tightly coupled; that is, for every calorie of energy *output* we expend, we would need a simultaneous infusion of a calorie of energy *input*. Since staying alive requires a continual exertion of energy, we would have to spend all our time finding and consuming food.

Thankfully, our energy stores—in a manner very much analogous to the role inventory plays in business—*decouple* energy-in and energy-out, so that energy expenditure can be continuous while energy input (feeding) does not have to be. That is what allows us to limit caloric consumption to just a few feeding episodes per day, with each one not only fulfilling our immediate energy needs, but also providing a little extra to supply our energy needs between meals and overnight, when there is no energy infusion.

Beyond the obvious convenience that this provides us on a day-to-day basis, our capacity to store energy is also key to our survival in a food-scarce environment. As with many other species that contend with a highly variable food supply, humans' energy regulation system is designed to maintain our energy reserves *at substantial enough levels* to provide a buffer against prolonged periods of food shortages.[50]

By contrast, species that live in an environment with a surplus of immediately available food—as many marine animals do, for example—do not need to maintain substantial energy stores.[51] The most striking example here might be the oyster. "[The oyster] only has to open its shell and filter the abundance of surrounding nutrients in sea water. [That's why the] oyster never gets fat; it is living in the midst of its food supply, and does not need to store energy."[52]

For species without constant access to food, conserving excess energy, primarily in the form of adipose tissue, is a necessary survival characteristic.

(*Adipose*, which is another word for fatty, comes from the Latin *adipatus*, meaning "greasy."[53]) These species include humans—and the polar bear.

> The main energy source of the polar bear is seal meat. The bear can only catch seals during the winter when the animals surface at the breathing openings in the ice. During the summer, with less ice, the polar bear cannot catch the seals, which are much more skilful swimmers than are bears. Throughout the winter the bears accumulate a massive amount of adipose tissue by preferentially selecting to eat the fat-rich parts of the seals such as the brains of the lean seal pups. The stored fat is then used for survival during the summer.[54]

Like the polar bear, human beings developed the ability to store energy in the form of fat during periods of surfeit to cope with the inevitability of periods of famine. In the words of Sharman Russell, this allowed our ancestors to survive not just a bad day of hunting, but a bad week of hunting, and not just a bad crop, but a bad year of crops.[55] Understanding how this is accomplished is important because it has direct bearing on obesity's etiology.

To regulate our energy stores at desired levels, the brain must perform two vital functions. First, it must sense the size of the fat stores and, second, it must be able to adjust hunger, satiety, and energy expenditure accordingly.[56] To do that, the brain relies on a lot of help from the body's fat mass.

In recent years it has become clear in recent years that the body's fat depot is not the passive receptacle of fat that it was once thought to be. Rather, the body's fat cells are highly active tissue that spins out a steady supply of nearly a dozen hormones—collectively known as adipokines—that carry messages to the brain and the rest of the body.[57] Because the concentrations of these hormonal secretions are proportional to the size of the body's fat mass, they serve as reliable signals to the brain about changes in (and the status of) the size of the body's aggregate fat stores.

Any time the brain detects a change in the status of the body's energy reserves—say a drop below desired levels—it triggers compensatory actions to adjust caloric intake and energy expenditure. An increase or decrease in caloric intake, for example, can be induced by adjusting the frequency or size of meals. This is achieved through the release of brain peptides (such as neuropeptide Y) from nerve terminals in the hypothalamus that serve to enhance or decrease the potency of the short-term satiety (or meal-ending) signals to the brain. In other words, the size of the fat reserves can turn up or turn down the *sensitivity* of the brain to the meal-generated satiety signals, which, as explained above, are part of the short-term regulatory subsystem. It is an elegant system, and it works.

> [A]n individual who has recently eaten insufficient food to maintain its weight will be less sensitive to meal-ending signals and, given the opportunity, will consume larger meals on the average. Analogously, an individual who has enjoyed excess

food and consequently gained some weight will, over time, become more sensitive to meal-terminating signals.[58]

This system of feeding regulation is asymmetric. This asymmetry results from the fact that the neuronal and endocrine factors generated when fat stores decrease (as a result of a prolonged negative energy balance) and that stimulate feeding are more potent than are the inhibitory signals generated when fat stores increase (as a result of overfeeding).

This was demonstrated more than twenty years ago in a clever series of experiments designed to reveal the differences in how humans compensate for increases/decreases in the energy content of their diet. In the experiments, Mattes et al.[59] surreptitiously diluted and then boosted the energy content of meals offered to free-living experimental subjects and observed how they compensated. What they found was rather surprising. When their subjects received lunches containing 66 percent fewer calories than their customary midday meal, the subjects compensated for the lunchtime deficit by ingesting additional nonlunch calories. As a result, their total energy intakes did not decrease. In contrast, when the subjects were covertly provided lunches containing 66 percent more calories than their customary midday meal, they did not adjust their nonlunch energy intake downward to compensate. As a result, total energy intake was significantly higher.

Humans, it thus appears, are "wired" to compensate for caloric dilution but not the reverse, exhibiting more tolerance for increases in caloric intake. Over the eons, this tendency served humans well since survival was more acutely threatened by starvation than by obesity.

The 1994 discovery of leptin by molecular biologists provided strong experimental support for this asymmetry in our regulatory system and significantly advanced our understanding of its biological underpinnings. Leptin is an amino acid protein synthesized in fat cells and secreted into the bloodstream in concentrations that are proportional to total fat stores. As such, it serves as a primary signaling mechanism to the brain about how much fat the body has stored. It has recently been shown experimentally that "when a person's fat stores shrink, so does [the body's] leptin production. In response, appetite increases while metabolism decreases."[60] The system, however, does not work quite the same in the other direction; that is, a rise in leptin does not necessarily lead to appetite reduction. The results "expose" the brain's true intentions in deploying leptin: it deploys it to track how much fat the body has stored *not to keep us from getting fat, but to keep us from getting too thin.*[61]

In summary, several principles may be deduced about human appetite regulation: (1) Feeding is controlled by two regulatory subsystems, one short-term and the other long-term. (2) The two systems are physiologically interdependent. (3) The two systems are not symmetric.

These principles provide prospective dieters with two crucial insights:

Firstly ... biological processes exert a strong defense against under-eating which serves to protect the body from an energy (nutritional) deficit. Therefore, under-eating must normally be an active and deliberate process. Secondly, in general biological defenses against over-consumption are weak or inadequate. This means that over-eating may occur despite efforts of people to prevent it.[62]

Asymmetry in Energy Expenditure

To adequately manage our energy reserves, it is not enough for the body's regulatory systems to manage the amount of energy input into the body. Just as in managing the financial budget of a business or a household, one needs to keep an eye on both sides of the ledger—what is coming in and what is going out—similarly with human energy regulation, the system needs to oversee how energy is stored and consumed. This subsection discusses energy consumption, and the next subsection explains how the body manages the status of its energy stores.

The body's total energy expenditure can be divided conceptually into three components. The smallest component (about 10 percent of daily energy expenditure) is the amount of energy expended in processing the food we eat—its digestion and absorption. A second component is the energy expended for muscular work. This typically accounts for 15 to 20 percent of daily energy expenditure, but can increase by a factor of two or more with heavy physical exertion.[63] The third and largest component is basal energy expenditure, also known as resting energy expenditure (REE), which is the maintenance energy required to keep us alive. This is the amount of energy required for the basic maintenance of the cells, maintaining body temperature, and sustaining the essential physiological functions (e.g., keeping the lungs inhaling and exhaling air, the bone marrow making new red blood cells, the heart beating 100,000 times a day, the kidneys filtering waste, etc.). In most of us the REE makes up about 60 to 70 percent of total energy expenditure.

As with the energy input side, the body's regulatory system for energy expenditure evolved to protect us against the frequent peril of food shortages and associated energy deficits, rather than energy surplus. The system evolved to complement the overconsumption bias (explained above) with the capacity to reduce the body's metabolic rate in response to negative energy balance and a bias toward conserving energy when physical activity is not required.[64] As Polivy and Herman[65] argue, it is an effective strategy that best ensures that the body's fuel reserves are conserved in lean times:

If there is a dearth of food available, the organism is better served by physiological adjustments that render what *is* available more useful—by means of what has come to be known as a *thrifty* metabolism—rather than by promptings to acquire more food when there simply is no more to be acquired, or when the energy expended in acquiring more might well exceed the energy content of the food itself. In short, in an ecology of scarcity, we are better served by metabolic adjustments than by behavioral adjustments.

As soon as the body senses an energy deficit, basal metabolism drops quite dramatically in order to conserve energy and restrain the rate of tissue loss. This is achieved chiefly through hormonal mechanisms that operate to decrease the metabolic activity at the cellular level, in essence enhancing the tissues' metabolic efficiency, as though the body were changing its light bulbs to fluorescent lights to save energy.[66] This homeostatic mechanism acts as a first line of defense against energy imbalance— a buffer, if you will, that helps spare the body's fat reserves in lean times. While, today, that may be bad news for dieters (because it limits weight loss), the survival value of an energy-sparing regulatory process that aims to limit tissue depletion during food scarcity is obvious.

The body's regulatory mechanisms work in reverse when confronted with a positive energy balance. Sort of. When a period of sustained positive energy balance induces weight gain, the body's basal or REE does rise. But experimental studies of human energy regulation have demonstrated that in this less-threatening case, the body's biological signals are relatively "muted."[67] That is, while the body does adjust its REE level upward when in positive energy balance, the adjustments do not increase energy expenditures enough to fully compensate for the imbalance.

The system clearly is not as robustly organized to galvanize in response to surplus energy balances (which are not particularly threatening to survival) as it is in responding to deficits (which are very threatening). This asymmetric bias in energy expenditure is in sync with the one we saw earlier on the energy intake side. Working in concert, these two limbs of our body's energy regulation system have effectively evolved us into what we are today: "exquisitely efficient calorie conservation machines."[68]

Asymmetry in Energy Storage

The third and final component in the energy equation is energy storage. Our primary source of energy is the food we eat. The human diet provides three energy-yielding macronutrients: protein, carbohydrate, and fat. The primary task of proteins is to provide the major building blocks for the synthesis of body tissue.[69] By contrast, fat and carbohydrate serve as the primary fuels to the body, fueling biological work and our physical activity, and replenishing our reserves. They are not equivalent, however—not by a long shot.

By a large margin, the primary form in which the body stores excess food energy is fat in the fat cells called adipocytes. This is no coincidence since fat is the more efficient way to store energy. When stored as fat, energy is stored at about 9 kilocalories (kcal) per gram of adipose tissue, which is almost 2½ times as many calories of energy as each gram of glycogen (the form in which carbohydrates are stored in the body). "In lean adults, fat reserves typically amount to some 10 kg, an energy reserve of 90,000 kcal, enough to survive about two months of near total food deprivation."[70] By contrast, the average person has only about 2,500 calories of carbohydrate reserves, stored mostly in liver and muscle.

Our fat stores allow us to store energy efficiently and in a compact form, making it possible for us to carry a substantial energy reserve without being slowed down. That is an enormous benefit when an individual (or an animal) must be highly motile to survive.

The two fuels are functionally different, as well. Carbohydrate-based fuel provides faster energy transfer and can be used anaerobically; that is, it can be metabolized to produce energy without the simultaneous use of oxygen. This makes it the ideal fuel to use for activities that need immediate bursts of energy (i.e., whenever we perform at a rate that exceeds the capacity of the heart and lungs to supply oxygen to the muscles), such as when we are trying to catch a bus or escape a charging rhino.

As already discussed, fat tissue is not just a static "spare tire" of energy around our waist. Rather, it is a highly dynamic tissue that is continuously secreting active substances (e.g., leptin) that play important roles in the body's weight-regulating system. As we have already seen, when it comes to its fat reserves, the human body is decidedly biased, with defenses against the depletion of its fat reserves that are more potent than the inhibitory signals it generates when fat reserves increase (as a result of overfeeding). There is a second asymmetry in the regulation of fat stores in humans: *when body fat is shed during weight loss, the size, but not the number, of fat cells dwindles.*[71]

The total amount of fat in a person's body is dependent on two factors: the number and the size of the fat cells in the body. When a person experiences a positive energy balance and starts to gain weight, initially the excess energy gets stored in the body's existing stock of fat cells, increasing their size. Fat cells can expand in size quite a bit, but they have a biological limit. When the cells approach maximal or "peak" size, a process of adipocyte proliferation is initiated, increasing the body's fat cell count. Thus, obesity develops when a person's fat cells increase in number, in size, or, quite often, both. *Once fat cells are formed, however, the number seems to remain fixed even if weight is lost.*[72,73]

This means that over time, and given the chance, an individual's total adipocytes are biased to creep upward in number. Worse yet, as the new cells fill up with fat, they work to achieve and then maintain nominal size. (The details of this mechanism are explained in Part III.) Long-term fat-cell proliferation results not only in an elevation of body weight, but also in the *defense* of that body weight,[74] and that is what makes *losing* excess weight so difficult.

Conclusion

Throughout much of human history, feeding behavior was set on "cruise-control," largely accomplished unconsciously and automatically, requiring little deliberate effort. Given that obesity was never a common health problem, it is quite understandable that people instinctively believe their body's feeding and energy regulation system is symmetrical, defending against both weight loss and weight gain. Unfortunately, this is but an illusion—and a risky one that may lull people into a false sense of invulnerability and seriously undermine obesity prevention.

In reality, as explained above, our weight regulation system is *asymmetric*. The fact that obesity was not a realistic possibility for our hunter-gatherer ancestors was a result of the "fit" between this asymmetrical design and their food-scarce environment—not the goal of the body's weight and energy regulation system.

Today, we are both lucky and unlucky. Most of us have ready access to food, but the very physiological adaptations that worked so effectively to keep us alive and in good form in a hunter-gatherer environment are resulting in a maladaptive response in our modern food-rich, activity-poor environment. With food becoming increasingly plentiful and the opportunities for physical exertion quickly diminishing, a persisting imbalance of energy intake and output is occurring in an ever-increasing proportion of the population.[75] It is an opportunity that was not anticipated by biology. Given the capacity of the human body to adjust to excess calorie intake by adding body fat, the potential for weight gain in today's population is enormous.[76]

But is it just a matter of time before the gears of evolutionary change recalibrate our weight and energy regulation processes to fit our new environment? Unfortunately, the answer is probably no. In the case of obesity,

> there do not appear to be strong biological mechanisms to oppose [it] once it is present. Even if the high levels of obesity seen today were sustained over generations within a population, there would be no selective pressure to remove [it]....
> [T]hat's because most chronic diseases associated with obesity generally occur well after reproductive age is reached.[77]

Human–Environment Interactions: Not One Way . . . and Not One-Way

3

Chapter 2 discussed how the energy dynamic between our human ancestors and their environmental circumstances has endowed us with multiple redundant physiological mechanisms to ensure us sufficient energy balance for survival and reproduction. We also saw how, as a result, the system of weight and energy regulation is three-way *asymmetrical*—in energy input, expenditure, and storage.

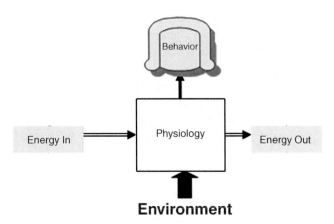

Figure 3.1 For much of human history, energy regulation was simple: the environment shaped our physiology, which, in turn, regulated our behavior

This environment → physiology interaction, however, is only a part of what is a far more complex and ongoing dynamic. As we shall shortly see, human–environment interactions are not one way—the pathways of inter-action are multiple—and they are not one-way—they are reciprocal. This is perhaps easiest to see on the energy input side, and so we pick up the story again and start with human feeding behavior.

One characteristic of humans is that we not only *eat* food, we also think about it. In humans, unlike, say, bears or oysters, eating behavior is

T.K.A. Hamid, *Thinking in Circles About Obesity*,
DOI 10.1007/978-0-387-09469-4_3, © Springer Science+Business Media, LLC 2009

controlled in accordance with biological states of need, and it is also a cognitively mediated activity. In other words, food is both a nutritional entity and a cognitive construct.

The human species is different from all others in that cultural and social conventions can be major determinants of food intake and can significantly affect the impact of metabolic and physiological signals.[78] For instance, cultural norms are the main reason we serve meals at particular times of day, and this occurrence, by itself, is what induces people to begin eating.[79] Besides time of day, our eating decisions take into account such things as appropriate meal size, whether other people are eating, our diet goals, our emotional state, and hunger and satiety.

The act of swallowing provides a natural demarcation that clearly delineates (and thus helps illustrate) the two worlds: the world of biology (post-swallowing) and the multidimensional biopsychological world (pre-swallowing). Post-swallowing is the world of ingestion and assimilation of food, the storage and utilization of energy, and body composition; it is a world of biology, physiology, and biochemistry. By contrast, the pre-swallowing choices about how much and what foodstuffs to ingest is a multidimensional biopsychological affair. Biological states of need do play their role by inducing, as explained, neurohumoral signals that regulate short- and long-term appetite levels. But it is far from a solo act. In our modern environment of abundance, purely physiological drives control feeding behavior only at the extremes of hunger or satiety. For most of us, that is a rarity. Rather, the choice of what and how much food to consume is increasingly about conscious human choice, environment, and culture (link "a" in Figure 3.2).[80]

A series of ingenious experiments on amnesic patients[81] dramatically demonstrates that external triggers such as social influences and visual cues

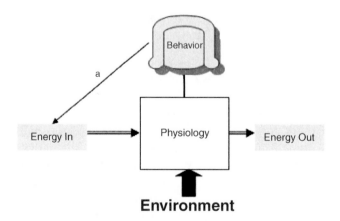

Figure 3.2 Personal choices/perferences play a role

have become more important than physiological state in determining eating behavior. The researchers wanted to find out how their amnesic patients would react when served a meal after just having consumed one.

> [The] amnesic patients who had no recall of what happened more than a few minutes before consumed a second full lunch and began a third, when each was served a few minutes after the prior meal was cleared away. The lack of memory for having just eaten a culturally appropriate, full meal, along with the presence of food, [was] sufficient to maintain eating.[82]

Once a person has started eating, the decision to stop depends on a different set of factors, and, again, energy balance is just a part of the story. Both the distension of the stomach and the food-triggered release of hormones from the gastrointestinal tract send satiety signals to the brain, but these are only suggestions, not orders. A man served his favorite dessert may eat on well past satiation. A woman on a diet may stop before her body says it is full in order to meet personal aesthetic objectives.[83] Besides personal preferences and goals, cultural and social conventions can be major determinants of meal termination, studies have shown. For example, experimental studies of human feeding behavior have revealed that a major reason humans end a meal is that they know they have already eaten an amount that constitutes an appropriate meal, as defined by the culture. For example, lunch can consist of soup, a sandwich, and a beverage.[84]

Clearly, then, human feeding regulation does not operate as an isolated physiological system. Rather, it is a complex biopsychological phenomenon with interactions between the physiological and the behavioral, and between people and their external environment.

Human Behavior Is Not Expressed in a Vacuum

As Chapter 1 pointed out, our choice of foods is not only a matter of personal preferences (captured by the link "a" in Figure 3.2), but also very much a function of what food is available in the variety of food outlets we have access to in our communities—the restaurants, supermarkets, and vending machines. Hence link "b" in Figure 3.3. The unavailability of certain healthful foods in the environment (home or school or neighborhood) obviously precludes their consumption. Thus, it is erroneous to imply that it is simply a person's freely chosen lifestyle to eat poorly when the food supply is characterized by an abundance of palatable, energy-dense fatty foods or when supermarkets have fled the neighborhood and been replaced by fast-food restaurants.[85,86]

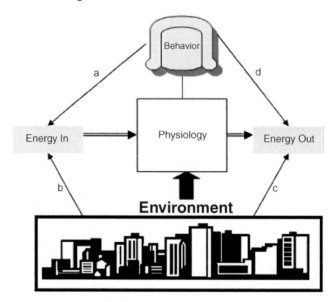

Figure 3.3 Personal choices as well as environmental factors affect energy in/out

Similarly, human behavior governing energy expenditure is simultaneously a function of lifestyle choices and preferences (link "d") and the opportunities we have to participate in leisure, occupational, or incidental activity (link "c"). For example, for most people, a sizable chunk of energy expenditure in conducting their daily business is the energy spent moving around. How our neighborhoods are built—with or without bike paths, foot paths, street lighting, and public transport—has a great influence on our choice to use, for example, active transport (walking, cycling) versus motorized transport (cars). Similarly, participation in active leisure activities is directly affected by the availability of community services such as recreational facilities, parks, sports grounds, and community clubs.[87]

Our physical and social environments provide the context within which people live their lives—what they eat, and how they work, play, and move around. All of these affect energy intake and expenditure.

All of these opportunities (or the lack of them), it is important to remember, are almost wholly of our own making.

It Is Not Just *Physical*

Unlike nonhuman systems, people are affected by more than matter and energy, that is, by the *physical* characteristics of their environment, such as the availability of foods, restaurants, and recreational facilities, as discussed above. Cultural and economic dimensions also play a role, shaping our attitudes, beliefs, and values relating to food and physical activity. That is why we must add the link "e" between the environment and our behavior, as shown in Figure 3.4.

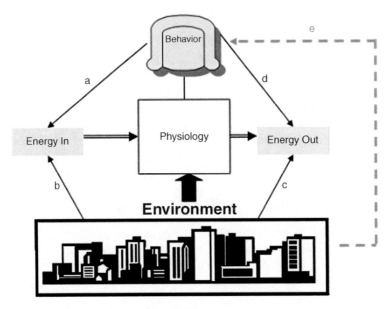

Figure 3.4 Cultural and economic dimensions also play a role

The social values that shape our ideals and aspirations about body weight and shape, for example, can greatly affect how much energy we try to ingest and expend. Sociocultural factors also play a large role in food *selection* (the quality as opposed to the quantity of the food we eat). In fact, to find out what foods another person likes and eats, the question to ask should be: What is your culture or ethnic group? "There is no other single question that would even approach the informativeness of the answer to this question."[88]

Socioeconomic factors also are important. The way food is marketed, distributed, and priced, and the value people place on convenience and price certainly affect what food and what amounts of it people choose to eat. Unlike the oyster and the bear, when making food choices, people consider the impact on the pocketbook, not just the impact on their stomach.

Socioeconomic factors similarly play a role in the energy expenditure side. For example, to many of us, socioeconomic parameters are the most powerful determinant in our choice of occupation. In our modern economies, these parameters drive many of us away from physical labor and toward knowledge occupations that require little energy expenditure.

We shape our environment, and then our environment shapes us.

—Winston Churchill

As we examine the role of the environmental systems in which we live in shaping our behavior and, ultimately, our health, we must not forget that many of the environmental characteristics we are discussing (urban design and infrastructure, architecture, technology) are almost wholly of our own making.

When it comes to human health and disease, as we will be discussing in great detail in the next two chapters, the relationship between the individual and the environment is *reciprocal:* people influence their settings, and their settings then act to influence their behaviors, including health behavior.[89]

> Man himself may be controlled by his environment, but it is an environment which is almost wholly of his own making.... When [we change our] physical or social environment "intentionally" ... [we play] two roles: one as a controller, as the designer of a controlling culture, and another as the controlled, as the product of a culture....

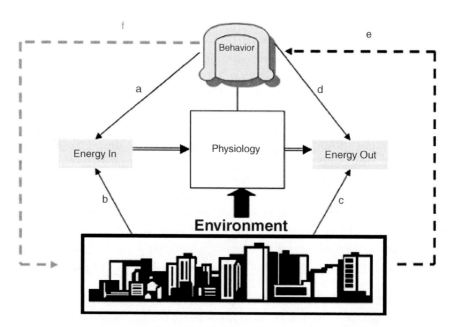

Figure 3.5 We shape our environment

There is much more to be said about man being guided by the systems of his own creation.[90]

This is the logic for adding the new link "f" in Figure 3.5, and to which we will turn our attention in Chapters 4 and 5.

A Symphony Out of Tune?

While the basis of obesity—positive energy balance—could not be more simple from a physiological point of view, the behavioral, cultural, and environmental factors affecting this energy imbalance are varied and complex.[91] These interactions include people's transactions with their physical environment (e.g., geography, architecture, and technology), as well as their sociocultural surroundings (e.g., cultural norms, economics, and politics).[92]

That is not to say that biology is not important.

> Moving beyond biologic and individual-based explanations does not imply denying biology, but rather involves viewing biologic phenomena within their social contexts and examining the tight interrelations between the social and the biologic at multiple levels. Neither does it imply denying individual-level explanations, but rather entails integrating them into broader models incorporating interactions between individuals, as well as group-level or society-level determinants.[93]

Figure 3.5 helps make the point that human energy regulation is a complex biopsychosocial phenomenon that is affected by a varied and complex array of cognitive, cultural and environmental factors. It is, however, a *still* picture and, as such, fails to capture one important dimension: time. While this is an unavoidable limitation given our medium, it is, unfortunately, a serious one, because the energy "imbalances" we are suffering as a society arise fundamentally out of interactions of biology and culture that have become out of sync because they are *occurring at different time scales*.

As we have argued, both biological adaptation and cultural evolution have important adaptive consequences for human behavior, but the two processes occur at vastly different tempos. In the case of biology, the evolutionary process is a relatively slow process, often with a long lag time between environmental change and evolutionary adaptation.[94] Indeed, our current physiology reflects evolutionary experience extending millions of years into the past. The tempo of cultural and socioeconomic change, however, is much faster—mere years or decades. It is this very substantial difference that has, in effect, knocked the symphony of "behavior–biology–environment" out of tune.

Tilting the Energy Balance: More Energy In

4

One of the few reasonably reliable facts about the obesity epidemic is that it started in the early 1980s. Any theory that tries to explain obesity in America has to account for this singular feature of the epidemic.

According to the National Center for Health Statistics, the percentage of obese Americans had been relatively stable at around 13 to 14 percent, but then unexpectedly and quite dramatically shot up in the 1980s (Figure 4.1).

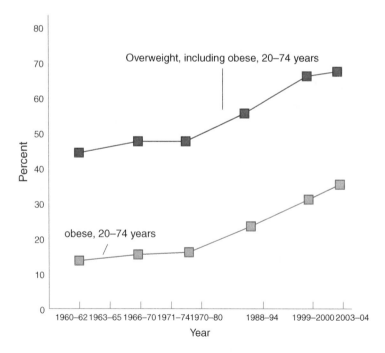

Figure 4.1 Overweight and obesity, United States, 1960–2004. (*Source*: Centers for Disease Control and Prevention/National Center for Health Statistics, *Health, United States*, 2006.)

T.K.A. Hamid, *Thinking in Circles About Obesity*,
DOI 10.1007/978-0-387-09469-4_4, © Springer Science+Business Media, LLC 2009

By the end of that decade, nearly one in four Americans was obese. The steep rise affected all segments of American society: all major racial and ethnic groups, all regions of the country, and all socioeconomic strata.[95,96]

The human body, like all systems, whether technological or biological, obeys the laws of thermodynamics, which define the immutable principle of energy conservation. Body weight can increase only if energy intake exceeds expenditure. Thus, the upward trend in the population's weight itself constitutes evidence that for an increasing proportion of the American population, the amount of calories consumed was exceeding the amount of calories burned.[97] However, this explains neither what started the trend nor why it has persisted. It also does not explain whether the imbalance is caused by eating too much food, not expending enough energy, or both.

These are the important questions that we aim to answer in this chapter and the next.

The Quantity of Food We Eat

There is growing evidence to confirm what many of us do not want to admit: "We're fat because we eat a lot—a whole lot more than we used to."[98] Empirical evidence from two different sources supports this contention.

One source of data on national food intake during the period when obesity started to escalate comes from the U.S. Department of Agriculture's twin surveys, the Continuing Surveys of Food Intake by Individuals (CSFII) that were conducted in 1977–78 and 1994–96. To track what and how much people ate, both CSFII surveys asked respondents to keep food diaries detailing their daily dietary intake (usually over a 3-day period). In addition, the researchers collected extensive demographic information about respondents, such as household size, income, race, age, and sex, to gain further insight into dietary differences among population subgroups, based on ethnicity and socioeconomic status, for example.[99]

The results of the twin surveys indicate that we are indeed fatter because we are eating more than we used to.[100] In the span of about two decades (from 1977–78 to 1994–96), the diaries indicate that per capita dietary intake increased by 10 percent.[101–103]

A 10-percent jump in a population-wide statistic is always a significant jump, especially over such a relatively short period of time. Even more worrisome is that this 10-percent jump, most experts believe, constitutes only a conservative estimate of the growth in America's appetite, because more recent studies have shown that self-reported food diaries tend to underestimate caloric intake. People often fail to record everything they eat, partly because most find it difficult to remember dietary details and partly because many are embarrassed about how much they eat.[104,105] Because of this difficulty, these reports of daily consumption are considered a conservative lower bound for Americans' daily consumption levels.

The data on the national food supply provide a second source of information on the nation's caloric consumption. These data, most experts agree, provide the most objective measure of the nation's caloric consumption. However, in contrast to the CSFII data on individual caloric intake, these data are highly aggregated, requiring careful analysis to tease out per-capita trends.

The national food supply data come from the Economic Research Service (ERS) of the U.S. Department of Agriculture (USDA), which annually calculates the amount of food available for human consumption in the United States as of July 1. Per capita consumption is then calculated by dividing the available food supply (measured as the sum of annual production, beginning inventories, imports minus exports, industrial nonfood uses, farm uses, and end-of-year inventories) by the total U.S. population as of July 1. In its annual calculations, the ERS also adjusts the aggregate supply data to account for the inevitable food loss due to spoilage and waste.[106]

As with the CSFII data, the national food supply data provide additional strong evidence of a demographic shift toward an increase in energy intake that has accelerated over the past three decades.[107] Unlike CSFII, which provides only a recent snapshot, the national food supply data have been collected for a much longer period, and thus give a more complete historical context for the trends.

Specifically, analysis of the national food supply data over the last 100 years indicates that per capita food consumption remained relatively steady between 1900 and 1965, albeit with occasional moderate declines, for example, during World War I and the Great Depression. Since 1965, however, the food supply has markedly increased, and particularly so in the last three decades. The USDA data indicate that between 1980 and 2000, the number of calories consumed per person per day in the United States (after adjusting for spoilage, waste, and cooking losses) increased by 23 percent, from 2,200 to slightly more than 2,700 calories.[108] That increase of about 500 calories is the equivalent of one Big Mac per person per day.[109] A 23-percent increase is more than double the increase seen in the CSFII survey's self-reported food diaries and is, most experts believe, the more accurate estimate.

Regardless of whether one leans toward the conservative 10 percent or the objective (and more reliable) 23 percent, either way, both sets of data point to two things: (1) after remaining roughly constant, the number of calories consumed has risen markedly and in lockstep with the recent escalation in obesity; and (2) the growth in energy intake is substantial enough to account for a significant chunk of the inflation we are witnessing in our aggregate "fat reserves."

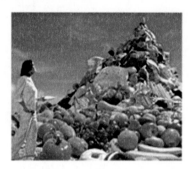

Figure 4.2 An overabundance of food choices confronts shoppers and diners every day. (Source: Adapted from Nestle, M. (2007). Eating made simple: How do you cope with a mountain of conflicting diet advice. Scientific American, 297(3), 60–69.)

The Causes Behind the Cause

Food abundance in the United States and in many other industrialized countries has afforded their populations an opportunity that humans had not previously had: "to eat food merely for pleasure and to consume more than the body needed to survive."[110]

Such an opportunity, however, while a *necessary* condition for overconsumption, is not a *sufficient* condition. Abundance, in other words, does not necessarily lead to increased consumption.[111] While more abundant food supplies may have facilitated increased caloric intake, it does not, by itself, provide a satisfying explanation for it.

Obesity and abundance are sort of analogous to lightning and thunder. Though related, lightning is not what *causes* thunder. Rather, both lightning and thunder are caused by an electric discharge (the fundamental cause) that we perceive first visually and then aurally. In a similar sense, to determine the fundamental cause behind the apparent causes of obesity, we need to go a little further.

Researchers in epidemiology and public health, as well as in economics and systems science, have mined almost a century's worth of nutritional data in search of answers. The emerging theory is that the trigger that induced obesity's escalation (and energy intake) was not a single factor, but, rather, the confluence of multiple socioeconomic and technological factors that came together and fed on each other in the second half of the 20th century. We now turn to those factors.

How America's Eating Habits Started to Change

As late as the 1960s, the primary cost of putting food on the table (as much as 60 percent of its total cost) was the time spent in the kitchen preparing it. Back then, most Americans cooked their own food at home using mainly raw agricultural products. That consumed a significant amount of time, with the typical American housewife spending more than 2 hours per day cooking and cleaning up.[112] America's eating habits started to change in the second half of the 20th century, when a growing number of women began to enter the labor force. According to David Cutler, Edward Glaeser, and Jesse Shapiro of the Institute of Economic Research at Harvard University, the resultant evolution of new roles for women turned out to be one of the most important developments affecting America's eating habits in the past 50 years.

What started drawing women into the labor force? In the decades after World War II, the U.S. economy experienced an important shift from an emphasis on the production of goods to the provision of services. Many of the new service-oriented jobs were white-collar jobs requiring little demanding physical effort; they were far removed from the dirty factory setting and, for these reasons, seemed more "appropriate" for women. Service industries such as banking, insurance, health, and education, which were growing rapidly, were more than happy to open their doors for more women to enter the labor force in order to sustain their rates of growth.

A number of other factors were also helping nudge more and more women through those doors. For example, the civil rights movement helped improve opportunities for and the treatment of women and minorities in the workplace, making paid work more attractive. Women's educational attainments were also, and at long last, catching up with those of men, allowing women more access to interesting and lucrative employment. And, last but not least, the women's movement helped accelerate the influx of married women into paid employment by making paid work appear more desirable to them.

As with many other social trends, the process can feed on itself. For example, in this case, women's increased employment opportunities led to a decline in the birthrate, which meant that women spent fewer of their adult years raising preschool-age children and, thus, had more years available to spend in paid employment.[113] By the end of the 20th century, women accounted for more than 60 percent of the labor force, up from 29 percent in 1950.

As more household time was diverted to outside employment, there was correspondingly less time and energy available for home activities such as food preparation and cleanup.[114] One important economic consequence of the growth of women's participation in the labor force was the increase in the economic value of their time; that is, their time spent in the household was more scarce and, thus, more valuable.

With less time to prepare meals, consumers would place a premium on fast and convenient food.

A confluence of technological innovations helped fuel these socioeconomic trends and reinforce the changes in women's lives and the structure of the American family. Comparable to the mass-production revolution

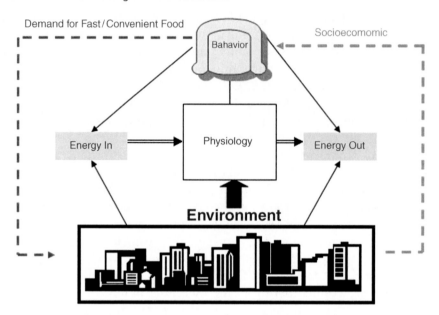

Figure 4.3 Socioeconomic forces induced growth of two-earner households, which spurred demand for fast/convenient foods

in manufactured goods that happened a century earlier, technological innovations in the preparation, packaging, and distribution of food were making it increasingly possible for firms to mass-prepare food, preserve it, and distribute it to consumers in convenient locations for ready consumption.[115,116]

As in many fields (in engineering, business, or medicine), revolutionary change rarely arises out of a single great innovation or invention. Rather, it often comes about when a diverse set of "ripe" technologies fit like pieces of a jigsaw puzzle to form new "ensembles" of technologies that allow us to do things we could not do before or to do them in a much better way.[117]

By the 1950s and 1960s, there had already been many important technological innovations in food processing, distribution, and home preparation. But most were developed separately and applied in isolation, offering marginal improvements. By the 1970s and 1980s, many of the pieces were in place, and when finally *integrated* they would make the modern convenience foods possible and revolutionize the food environment. For example, even after deep-freezing technology had been available for some time, frozen foods still were not widely used (except, perhaps, in the military, where they played an important role for the military during the war). But when integrated with technologies for vacuum packing, improved preservatives, and artificial flavors, they made modern convenience foods possible because they made them more available and tastier. In the home, microwave ovens (another "component" technology) allowed for rapid heating of those frozen and pre-prepared foods.[118]

Similarly, technological innovation was also revolutionizing the distribution of food.

> In order to produce food in one location that will be nearly ready for consumption in another location, [it was necessary to] surmount five main technological obstacles: controlling the atmosphere; preventing spoilage due to microorganisms; preserving flavor; preserving moisture; and controlling temperature. Innovations in food processing and packaging over the last three decades have improved food manufacturers' ability to address each of these issues.[119]

As technology made it increasingly possible for firms to mass-prepare, preserve, and distribute food to consumers for rapid consumption, market production of food increasingly became a substitute for household production of food.[120] By lowering the time price of food (i.e., the time needed for preparation and cleanup), the switch from individual to mass preparation was a godsend to the growing number of time-strapped, two-earner American households.[121]

Never had food been easier to prepare. Rising incomes allowed families to buy the latest appliances, from microwave ovens (in 83 percent of American homes by 1999) to nonstick pans and automatic dishwashers, which cut cleanup time.[122] By 1999, thanks to the abundance of processed foods and better kitchen appliances, the amount of time involved in meal preparation and cleanup was cut in half, from 2 hours per day in the 1950s to less than 1 hour.[123,124]

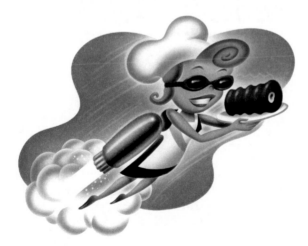

Figure 4.4 Illustration courtesy of Dan Picasso

Thus, postwar prosperity and technology were working together to create a climate that accelerated the reallocation of time from housework to outside work. With fewer hours needed to prepare food, women were freed up to do more wealth-generating activities outside the home. This, in turn, brought even more demand for convenience in food preparation and spurred the long-term trend toward eating out.[125] The two trends, in other words, fed on each other: The increased labor-force participation of women and the greater number of hours they worked stimulated the demand for inexpensive convenience and fast food, and vice versa.

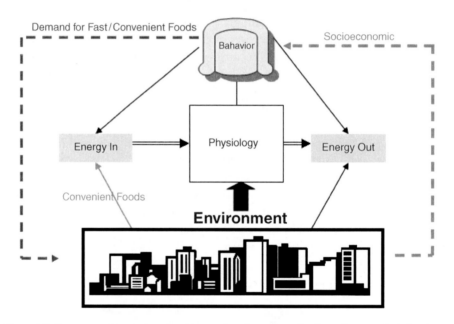

Figure 4.5 Consumer demand spurred innovation in and production of convenient foods

The socioeconomic-technological factors that changed family structures were also shaping *how* we eat. With both heads of the household working and the time available to prepare meals in short supply, fast and convenient foods were at a premium.

> Convenience [became] part of the unconscious cost-benefit analysis people make when choosing where and what to eat. Eating out increases, and with it comes deterioration in diet. What is eaten at home is also likely to be convenience foods.[126]

The public, thus, appears to have made an unconscious decision to accept the deterioration of their diet as a trade-off for convenience and time. Instead of the wife staying at home and having time to prepare healthy meals, the husband and wife opted to both work, gaining financial benefits, "even though they now may get their dinners at drive-through restaurants."[127] To students of behavioral decision making, this trade-off is neither surprising nor irrational.

Health is only one of many factors people consider as they make lifestyle choices such as what to eat, where to work, and how to play. The incentives of economics, convenience, and the value of time (to name a few) can be more important than health in influencing individual choices. Because health consequences are often long-term or may be perceived as low risk, they very often have less of an impact on our choices than factors with immediate influence, such as short-term financial reward and convenience.[128]

The issue here is not information or the lack of it (e.g., about the consequences of unhealthy eating), but incentives. Even when people know that eating home-prepared food is healthier, rational couples may elect to eat more convenient but less healthy food because they value their high-paying, two-career lifestyles and because they may not be willing to pay the price—in effort, expense, or time—for a traditionally cooked meal.[129]

What this effectively does is push the puzzle back a step. What we now need to explain is how the demand for and consumption of convenience and fast food induced an increase in calories consumed.

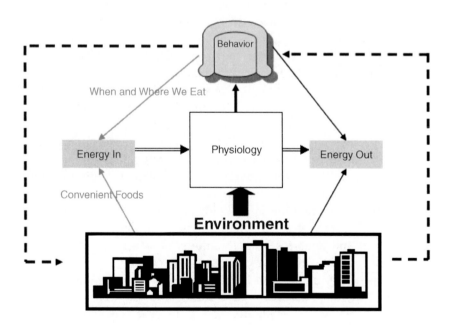

Figure 4.6 The availability of convenient foods affected when and where we eat

The increase in food/caloric consumption was induced through two mechanisms that relate to the *time* and *space* dimensions of how we eat:

1. The *time* mechanism relates to *when we eat,* and, because time is money, at what cost. It is about how convenience food provided affordability and convenience of eating anytime, all the time.
2. The *space* (or place) mechanism relates to *where we eat.* It is about how fast food provided the opportunity to eat anywhere, everywhere.

The First Mechanism: The *Time* We Eat

The switch from individual to mass preparation lowered both the time and monetary costs of food consumption. The decrease in the *time cost* of food, however, was the bigger deal.

As with any product or service, when thinking about the cost of food consumption, one tends to think in terms of monetary costs. But with food consumption, cost includes both time and money. Both of these cost components have declined over the last several decades, albeit at dramatically different rates. Consider first the monetary cost of food. According to the Bureau of Labor Statistics, with the exception of a spike during the oil shock in the 1970s, food prices have been dropping by an average of 0.2 percent a year since World War II.[130] Such a drop in food prices, while welcome, is too modest to have played a significant role in the upward jump in the population's caloric intake.[131] By contrast, the drop in the *time cost* of food has been quite dramatic, and thus of greater significance.

As already mentioned, back in the 1950s and 1960s, the primary cost of food for the average American household was the time spent in food preparation and cleanup. But that was before those technological innovations in convenience-food production and distribution had kicked in. As technology made it increasingly possible for firms to package and distribute mass-prepared foods, market production of food increasingly became a preferred substitute for household production of food.[132] Professional labor and capital in the supermarket and the factory replaced labor in the home, reducing food-preparation time. Time savings translate into cost savings, a translation that economists Cutler, Glaeser, and Shapiro estimate amounted to a 29-percent reduction between 1965 and 1995 in the per-calorie cost of food.[133]

Reductions in the time cost of food preparation led to an increase in the amount of food consumed through a standard price mechanism, just as reductions in any good's cost should lead to increased consumption of that good. When a meal takes 2 to 3 minutes to prepare, it is neither difficult nor expensive to eat anytime and all the time. A person on a diet is less likely to have a mid-afternoon snack if it requires a 10-minute walk to the corner store for ingredients and an hour of meal preparation and cleanup. That same person, though, is much more likely to have a snack if the vending machine is 10 yards away.[134]

Thus, while the dazzling array of new food technologies and the widespread availability of microwave ovens and vending machines have been a boon to the time-strapped American family, they have come at a cost. The increased convenience and reduced time between when we want a meal and when we can eat it would create a new and fattening pattern of eating.[135]

In a hunt for insights into exactly *how* Americans were consuming more convenience foods, Cutler, Glaeser, and Shapiro had to mine decades-worth of nutritional data, but, in the end, did find their answer: The escalation in caloric consumption has been most evident in America's growing *snacking* habit. The increased convenience (and variety) in our diet had provoked a shift in our eating patterns toward frequent "grazing"—small but cumulatively hefty snacks—as opposed to regular meals. In the last 30 years, the amount of energy we consume through snacks nearly doubled. Americans are eating more, in other words, because they are eating more frequently.[136]

Americans, across all age groups, are snacking more often and deriving more energy from snacks than ever before. Oliver[137] provides some revealing statistics on America's escalating snacking habit:

> In the mid-1970s ... Americans only got about 13 percent of their calories from snacking, a relatively small percentage. Today, men and women are getting almost 25 percent of their daily calories from snacking, the caloric equivalent of a full meal a generation ago. The average American male consumes more than 500 calories a day from snacks, the average female more than 346 calories a day.... Americans spend more than 38 billion dollars a year on snack foods, more than what they spend on higher education.

In the past 30 years, an enormous number of tasty snacks have been introduced into the U.S. food market, many falling into the nutrient-poor, high energy-dense categories.[138] These are distributed through vending machines that dot our workplaces, ensuring that cheap, high-fat, high-calorie snacks are no more than a few yards away.[139]

Snacking increases food consumption not only because people eat more times during the day, snacking on food that is often energy-dense, but also because snackers do not compensate for the snacks they eat by eating less at their regular mealtimes.[140,141] In one recent study that is typical of the many that have been conducted, researchers examined the impact of a snack consumed after a standard lunch on subsequent food consumption. "The researchers fed subjects a snack (400 kcal) at various times after a 1300-kcal lunch. [The result was that] the snack neither reduced the amount of food consumed at the dinner meal nor increased the time before the subjects requested their dinner meal."[142]

Studies that track longer-term energy intake are consistent with these findings. They show that total daily energy intake of adult snackers is, on average, 25 percent higher than that of non-snackers.[143] The average adult snacker, in other words, is eating the equivalent of four full meals a day, not three.[144]

Soft Drinks: The Liquid Snack

To quench our thirst, we don't just drink water anymore, which is a zero-calorie affair. We grab a soft drink instead. Each 12-ounce serving of a carbonated, sweetened soft drink provides about 150 kcal, all from sugars, and contains no other nutrients of significance.[145] A soft drink is the proto-typical junk snack.

The upward trend in per capita consumption of sweetened beverages correlates closely with the rising rates of obesity. Market research data show that since the 1970s, soft-drink consumption increased by more than 130 percent (or 200 calories), more quickly, in fact, than the consumption of any other food group.[146,147] Today, soft-drink consumption accounts for approximately 7 percent of the energy in our diet, with the average American drinking soda at an annual rate of about 56 gallons per person; that is nearly six hundred 12-ounce cans of soda per person per year.[148-150]

One reason the growth in soft-drink consumption is of concern to public health workers is that the intake rates are even higher among adolescents and children.

> [In the 1970s,] the typical teenage boy in the United States drank about seven ounces of soda every day; today he drinks nearly three times that amount, deriving 9 percent of his daily caloric intake from soft drinks. Soda consumption among teenage girls has doubled within the same period, reaching an average of twelve ounces a day.... Soft-drink consumption has also become commonplace among American toddlers. About one-fifth of the nation's one- and two-year-olds now drink soda.[151]

In 2001, a group of researchers from the Department of Medicine at Children's Hospital in Boston who were studying childhood obesity and its causes singled out childhood consumption of soda as their target.[152] The researchers tracked 548 ethnically diverse Massachusetts schoolchildren (average age, 11) for 19 months, looking at the association between their weight at the beginning of the study, intake of soda, and weight at the end of the study period. The results were quite revealing. For one thing, 57 percent of the children increased their intake over the study's 19-month period. The association between soda consumption and weight gain was so clear that the researchers could even link specific amounts of soda to specific amounts of weight gain. Each daily drink, the researchers calculated, added 0.18 points to children's body mass index (BMI), regardless of what else they ate or how much they exercised.

But perhaps the most interesting finding was that the children "were doing something with the soda that few people initially understood: . . . [T]hey were not compensating for those extra empty calories when they sat down for regular meals."[153] In other words, as with solid snacks, consumption of energy-containing beverages elicits little dietary compensation. The obvious implication: Because sugar-sweetened drinks represent energy added to, not displacing, other dietary intake, they must induce an increase in total energy consumption.[154]

Additional studies on adults confirmed that soft-drink consumers tend to have a higher daily energy intake than nonconsumers.[155] For example, one researcher "examined 7-day food diaries of 323 adults and found that energy from drinks added to total energy intake and did not displace energy ingested in [meals]."[156] In a Danish study, results showed not only a lack of compensation, but also how rapidly increased soft-drink consumption can affect weight.

> [The Danish] scientists studied overweight volunteers who were given soft drinks sweetened with either sugar or artificial sweeteners but were allowed to eat freely otherwise. During [the] ten-week study the people having sugared drinks consumed an extra 500–700 calories per day from the soft drinks. Those receiving the sugared drinks did not compensate for the extra calories and gained 3.5 pounds during the ten weeks.[157]

What particularly troubled the Danish researchers was that these results could occur in such a short time.

In a recent *Scientific American* article, Barry Popkin explained how evolutionary history may account for our imprecise and incomplete compensation for energy consumed in liquid form.

> For most of our evolutionary history, the only beverages humans consumed were breast milk after birth and water after weaning. Because water has no calories, the human body did not evolve to reduce food intake to compensate for beverage consumption. As a result, when people drink any beverage except water their total calorie consumption rises, because they usually continue to eat the same amount of food.[158]

Several other researchers postulated the specific physiological mechanisms that may account for this phenomenon.[159] It goes like this: Because liquid "meals" are of larger volume, lower energy density, and lower osmotic potential,[160] they are emptied from the stomach at a more rapid rate. The more rapid transit of fluids causes nutrient sensors in the gut to have a shorter exposure time to their nutrients and, as result, the signals influencing meal termination are weaker.

The Second Mechanism: *Where* We Eat

The forces that drove demand for convenience in food preparation—namely, the increasing scarcity and increasing value of household time—have also spurred the long-term trend toward eating out.

As moderately priced fast-food chains such as McDonald's and Howard Johnson's began spreading across the country in the postwar era, and with their new and increasingly popular credit cards in hand, many more Americans started dining out. Eating out, once done mainly by travelers and office workers, became another popular option for families to save time in the kitchen.[161]

- Today, Americans spend about half of their food budget and consume about one third of their daily calories on meals and drinks consumed outside the home, mainly at fast-food restaurants. That is nearly double the percentages in the 1970s[162] (Figure 4.7).
- "The average American eats out more than four times a week."[163]
- "On any given day in the United States about one quarter of the adult population visits a fast-food restaurant."[164]
- "The time spent by an average customer in a fast-food restaurant is a blistering eleven minutes."[165]

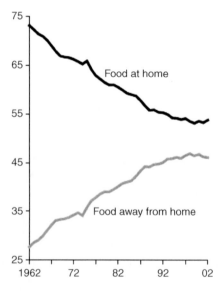

Figure 4.7 Share of total food expenditures (percent). (*Source*: Food Consumption (Per Capita) Data System, U.S. Department of Agriculture, Economic Research Service.)

Between 1970 and 2000, the number of fast-food restaurants grew from some 70,000 to close to 200,000, ensuring that Americans are not more than a few steps from immediate sources of a rich variety of fast foods.[166] Today, fast food pervades virtually all segments of society, including local communities, hospitals, and—in what to many is a troubling development—public schools. According to a survey by the Centers for Disease Control and Prevention (CDC), about 20 percent of the nation's schools offer brand-name fast food in their cafeterias.[167,168] Fast-food companies such as McDonald's and Pizza Hut have, for years, been offering schools financial incentives for allowing them to set up shop on school grounds. With many schools chronically short of funds for supporting academic programs and other activities, the financial incentive is understandably irresistible.[169]

The introduction of the drive-through window some 30 years ago made it possible to pick up fast food and eat on the run or take it home, which offered more time savings and quickly caught on.[170] Capitalizing on the trend, fast-food companies introduced menus and packaging to make it convenient for us to nosh on the road. Chips, candy, and soup are packaged in containers that snuggle neatly into car cup holders. In the newest wrinkle (and thanks to "cooperation" from the car manufacturers), those cup holders can heat and cool our meals or beverages to keep them at the right temperature.[171] Today, 60 percent of fast food sold in the United States is purchased at the drive-through.[172]

Fast Food: Eat Anywhere, Everywhere

The increasing frequency of fast-food use has undeniably increased Americans' total energy intake.

One of the most in-depth studies of the association between fast-food use and increased caloric intake was conducted by a group of epidemiologists at the University of Minnesota in 2001. The study involved almost five thousand adolescent students in thirty-one secondary schools and tracked their use of fast-food restaurants through daily dietary diaries. The results were striking:

> Fast-food restaurant use was positively associated with intake of total energy, percent energy from fat, [and] daily servings of soft drinks ... and was inversely associated with daily servings of fruit, vegetables, and milk. ... A boy who never ate at a fast-food restaurant during the school week averaged a daily calorie count of 1952; one who ate fast food one to two times a week (as did more than half of all the children in the study) consumed an average of 2192 calories a day (12% more); while those who ate fast food three times or more a week (one fifth of the studied) consumed an amazing 2752 calories a day (40% higher).[173]

For additional proof that these results were due to a causal relationship between fast food and energy intake and were not the consequence of some other unrecognized or incompletely controlled socioeconomic or demographic factors, additional studies were conducted in which subjects were used as their own controls, that is, comparing the energy inputs of the *same* subject on days with fast food versus days without fast food. The earlier results held. For example, in one of these studies, the child-subjects were found, on average, to eat 126 kcal/day more on days with fast food compared to days without fast food.[174]

Comparable findings of a strong association between frequency of fast-food restaurant use and total energy intake were observed for adults. In one representative study, total energy intake was 40 percent higher among men and 37 percent higher among women who reported three or more visits to a fast-food restaurant during the past week, compared to those who reported never eating at a fast-food restaurant during the past week.[175]

All of which raises this question: What is there about fast food that induces an increase in caloric consumption?

Several factors inherent to fast food seem to contribute to increased energy intake. Below, I categorize these factors along two broad dimensions: *qualitative* and *quantitative*.

The Qualitative Dimension

The first obvious mechanism is taste. Studies in humans demonstrate that taste is an important reason individuals choose the foods they do—often more important than healthfulness[176]—and that food consumption significantly increases with food palatability.[177]

Like any consumer product, fast food is "designed" for consumer appeal—specifically, to appeal to our primordial taste preferences for fats, sugar, and salt.[178] In his best-selling book, *The Omnivore's Dilemma*, Michael Pollan explains how adding fat, sugar, and salt to fast food is designed to push our evolutionary buttons:

> Add fat or sugar to anything and it's going to taste better on the tongue of an animal that natural selection has wired to seek out energy-dense foods. Animal studies prove the point: Rats presented with solutions of pure sucrose or tubs of pure lard—goodies they seldom encounter in nature—will gorge themselves sick. Whatever nutritional wisdom the rats (and men) are born with breaks down when faced with sugars and fats in unnatural concentrations—nutrients ripped from their natural context, which is to say, from those things we call foods.[179]

According to data gathered by the U.S. Department of Agriculture, fast foods contain on average 20 percent more fat than home-cooked meals,[180] which is a big jump for an average measure, and because it is an *average*, there are apt to be many fast-food items with an even higher fat content. For example, a Big Mac with a medium order of French fries has 1,020 kcal and 54 g of fat, which amounts to half the total recommended daily energy requirement and as much as 83% of recommended daily fat intake.[181] Besides the fat, fast foods, such as a Big Mac with French fries and a soda, are also higher in salt and sugar and much lower in fiber than home-cooked food.[182]

Food containing larger and more condensed amounts of fats and sugars is not only tastier, but is also more stable, meaning that it has longer shelf life and can better retain good "mouth feel" after an hour under the fast-food heat lamp.[183] All of this helps explain why the most popular fast-food items are generally high in fat, and why many of the lower-fat, so-called light fast-food options that some fast-food restaurants have recently introduced have not been popular with customers.[184]

Inducing *active* overconsumption of food through appetite stimulation may be the simplest explanation for why tasty fast food appears to promote excess energy intake and weight gain, but it is not the only mechanism.[185] Recent research on human appetite control and feeding regulation has revealed two additional mechanisms: the higher energy density of high-fat foods induces *passive* overconsumption, and the low thermic effect of fat allows us to retain more of it.

When people eat fat-enriched foods, they tend to consume more energy as a result of the higher energy density of fat. Because this does not appear to be consciously intended but rather occurs passively, without any apparent effort on the part of the eater, the phenomenon has been referred to as passive overconsumption.[186]

Perhaps the most illuminating work on this phenomenon has been the pioneering studies by Dr. Barbara Rolls and her team at Pennsylvania State University. Over the last two decades, Rolls's studies on human satiety have demonstrated that the number of calories in a given volume of food, that is, its caloric or energy density, makes a big difference in how many total calories people consume at a given meal, as well as throughout the day. That is primarily because people tend to consume a *constant volume* of food at a given meal, irrespective of its energy content.[187]

In a series of experimental studies, Rolls and her team have demonstrated that food volume has "the overriding influence" on satiety, that is, on what makes us feel full. Food bulk, not energy content, in other words, is the key to what makes our bodies say we have eaten enough. The corollary of that, of course, is that if people consume a constant volume of food at a given meal, then more total energy is consumed when the diets are high in energy density—as more calories are packed into a given weight or volume of food—than when they are low in energy density.[188,189]

Why would our system evolve to monitor weight and volume rather than energy or nutrient content? Blundell and King, two scientists at the BioPsychology Group at the University of Leeds in England, have a very plausible theory. They argue that because weight (before the advent of processed foods) was very often a good predictor of energy value and nutrient content, our system has "learned" to rely on weight as a reliable cue, that is, to associate the weight and volume of food consumed with its energy value and nutrient composition. Given the inability to sense visually the energy or nutrient content of food, it makes perfect sense that food weights and volumes become the important variables that we monitor subconsciously.[190,191]

> [This] ... does not mean that weight is fundamentally more important than energy content. ... [I]t does mean that humans [and animals] have learned during the course of their lives (and long-term exposure to food) that weight is very often a good predictor of energy value or nutrient content.[192]

Dietary fat is the most energy-dense macronutrient, containing more than twice as much energy per unit weight than either protein or carbohydrate (9 calories per gram for fat versus 4 calories per gram for both proteins and carbohydrates). Thus, a small quantity of food rich in fat has very high energy content.[193] In contrast, because water increases food volume without adding calories, foods such as vegetables and fruit, which have a high water content, cause us to feel full on fewer calories and lead to reduced energy intake.[194] After water, which has zero calories, fiber contributes the most to food volume for the fewest number of calories, supplying 1.5 to 2.5 calories per gram.[195]

A telling statistic that underscores the association between fast-food composition and caloric intake comes from the USDA, which calculates that if fast food had the same average nutritional composition (and so the same energy and fat density) as food prepared and cooked at home, Americans would consume approximately 200 fewer calories per day. That is an extra pound's worth of energy *every 20 days*.[196]

The fact that fast food is eaten ... well, fast, further contributes to *passive* overconsumption. Like any regulatory feedback process, the body's physiological system that regulates appetite takes time to kick in; it takes time for the body to sense that food has reached the stomach and to shut off the feeling of hunger.[197] After eating a full meal, the satiety signals that tell us we have had enough may not kick in for a full half-hour, that is, long after the blistering 11 minutes the average customer spends eating a fast-food meal.[198,199] By speed-eating fast food, we tend to stuff ourselves before our brains have the chance to slow us down, and the higher the energy density of the food we overeat, the higher the number of calories we ingest.

Active and passive overconsumption are the two primary mechanisms by which fatty fast food induces more energy consumption, in both cases, through inducing *intake*. Fast-food consumption contributes to the expansion of our fat stores in a third way: *When we eat fat-enriched foods, we tend to retain more of it*, because of the low thermic effect of fat.

When we overeat, the body needs to work, that is, expend some energy, to store those extra calories (whether ingested in the form of fat, carbohydrates or proteins) as body fat. Because, compared to the other two macronutrients, the pathway from dietary fat to body fat requires fewer metabolic steps, fat is the one that's stored most efficiently, that is, with the least amount of "losses." For example, storing excess energy from dietary carbohydrate or protein into body fat requires an expenditure of approximately 25 percent of ingested energy. By comparison, storing excess energy from dietary fat into body fat stores uses less than 5 percent of the ingested energy intake.[200] Thus, when the excess food we eat comes from fat-enriched fast food, we tend to retain more of it.

The *Quantity* Dimension

The fast-food quality issues are further compounded by a growing trend in the United States toward larger portion sizes. The explosive expansion we are witnessing in menu items with labels such as *big, mega,* and *super* is not some ploy by food companies to make us think we are getting more—we really *are* getting more (Figure 4.8).[201,202]

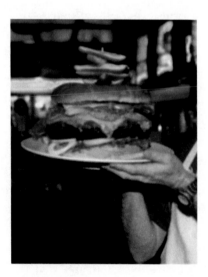

Figure 4.8 Fast food has become supersized

The portions of fast food we are now getting dwarf those of past generations; in some cases, the portions are two to five times larger than the portions our parents were served in the 1950s and 1960s.[203] Consider the following:

- A typical hamburger in the 1950s weighed 2.8 ounces and contained 200 calories. The typical hamburger today weighs 6 ounces and packs 600 calories.[204,205]
- A serving of McDonald's French fries ballooned from 200 calories in the 1960s to 450 calories in the mid-1990s to the present 610 calories.[206]
- Beverage sizes have also increased dramatically. "Soft drink containers morphed from eight ounces to twelve ounces to sixteen ounces and then to twenty ounces as the standard serving size."[207]
- Even our cookies are getting supersized, with some "monster" cookies today up to 700 percent larger.[208]

Interestingly, this massive supersizing trend appears to be mainly a U.S. phenomenon. When a group of University of Pennsylvania researchers compared restaurant and supermarket meals in the United States and in France, they found the French portion sizes to be significantly less hefty. A soft drink in France was a third smaller, a hotdog 40 percent smaller, and a carton of yogurt almost half as big. Even the croissant, perhaps the most iconic French food item, was smaller. A Parisian croissant is a 1-ounce affair, while in Pittsburgh it is 2 ounces.[209,210] (It is probably no coincidence that the French people are seriously leaner, and France's obesity rate is 7.4 percent, one fourth that of the United States.)

What underlies this American–Gallic disparity? Perhaps it is the cultural compulsion of Americans to get the most bang for the buck.[211] "More is better" seems to be a mantra for most Americans. We wanted bigger cars, bigger houses, and bigger portions, and more is what we got: "Portions big enough to feed a horse." [212] How did it all start?

The late David Wallerstein, a theater manager from Chicago and a long-time director of McDonald's, is sometimes credited with the supersizing trend.

> In the mid-1960s, Mr. Wallerstein realized that customers [at his theater] were reluctant to buy two bags of popcorn because they felt gluttonous, but would happily buy one jumbo bag. He later persuaded Ray Kroc, McDonald's legendary leader, to use the same strategy with French fries, and the race for ever-larger portions was on.[213]

It was a brilliant marketing strategy, one of those rare propositions that were win–win for both consumers and food sellers. From the consumer's point of view, large portions not only *seem* like bargains—they actually are.

For a relatively small increase in price, supersizing greatly increases the number of calories we get.[214] For example, a 16-oz soft drink at 7-Eleven costs just under 5 cents per ounce, while a 32-oz Big Gulp costs just 2.7 cents per ounce.[215] At McDonald's, it costs only 60 percent more to upgrade from a Quarter Pounder to a Medium Value Meal, which includes fries and a soda, for 125 percent more calories,[216] and an additional 87 cents buys almost three times as many French fries.[217]

From the restaurants' point of view, larger portions also proved a profitable option. Compared to the costs of marketing, packaging, and labor, the cost of the added ingredients to supersize a menu item is small.[218] On average, food accounts for about a third of the total cost of running a restaurant; labor, equipment, advertising, rent, and electricity make up the rest. So, while it may cost a restaurant a few pennies to offer 25 percent more French fries, it can raise its prices much more than a few cents and still offer the consumer a good deal. Smaller portions, by contrast, translate into lower profit margins; it is half the food, but it still requires all the labor. The result is that larger portions proved a reliable way to bolster the average check at restaurants.[219]

As the U.S. market size grew and as raw materials for food became even more abundant and cheap, food companies started competing for the consumer's dollar by increasing portion sizes rather than by lowering prices (which, of course, would have lowered revenues). Consumers responded predictably. They started favoring restaurants on the basis of portion size, which helped sustain and fuel the trend.[220]

With all this going for it, it is no wonder that the supersizing trend that began in the late 1970s has increased steadily ever since (Figure 4.9).[221] "As of 1996 some 25 percent of the $97 billion spent on fast food came from items promoted on the basis of either larger size or extra portions."[222]

Obviously, larger portions provide another opportunity for more caloric consumption, but can human appetite be expanded by merely offering more and bigger portions? The answer appears to be yes. Experimental studies on humans have established that there is, indeed, a significant positive association between portion size and energy intake, indicating that we eat more when served larger portions.[223] Supersized and "monster" meals, in other words, do encourage consumption of larger portions.[224]

In a 2001 study, nutritional researchers with Barbara Rolls's group at Pennsylvania State University demonstrated that the presence of larger portions *in themselves* "nudged" people toward eating more.

> Men and women volunteers, all reporting the same level of hunger, were served lunch on four separate occasions. In each session, the size of the main entree was increased, from 500 to 625 to 750 and finally to 1000 grams. After four weeks, the pattern became clear: As portions increased, all participants ate increasingly larger amounts, despite their stable hunger levels.[225]

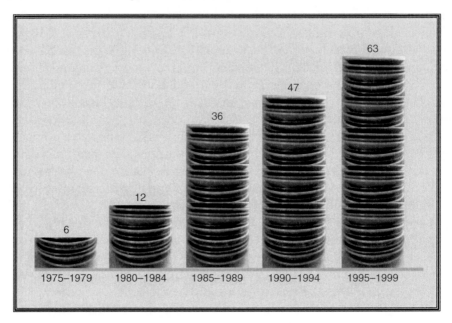

Figure 4.9 Supersize portions grow. The number of food items introduced in large sizes in the United States. (*Source*: Adapted from Nestle, M. (2007). Eating made simple: How do you cope with a mountain of conflicting diet advice. *Scientific American*, 297(3), 60–69.)

In the experiment, food intake was 30 percent higher when people were given the largest compared to the smallest serving, a significant increase, prompting the researchers to confidently conclude that, "human hunger could [indeed] be expanded by merely offering more and bigger options."[226]

But the researchers did not stop there. Additional studies that investigated the underlying mechanisms helped reveal something both interesting and hopeful for the future. They revealed strong cultural underpinnings to our apparent compulsion to eat more when served larger portions. The insights into the role of culture emerged from the work the Rolls group did with children. The experiments showed that before the age of 3, portion size does not influence a child's energy intake. However, that begins to change some time between the ages of 3 and 5 years as children develop and learn social and cultural conventions regarding food and eating.[227]

In a series of experiments, Rolls and her colleagues examined the eating habits of two groups of children, 3-year-olds and 5-year-olds:

Both groups reported equal levels of energy expenditure and hunger. The children were then presented with a series of plates of macaroni and cheese. The first plate was a normal serving built around age-appropriate baseline nutritional needs; the second plate was slightly larger; the third was what we might now call "supersized." The results were both revealing and worrisome. The younger children consistently ate the same baseline amount, leaving more and more food on the plate as the servings grew in size. The five-year-olds acted as if they were from another planet, devouring whatever was put on their plates. Something had happened. As was the case with their adult counterparts ... the mere presence of larger portions had induced increased eating.[228]

These results suggest that as children grow and develop socially, they shift from eating primarily in response to physiological signals of hunger and satiety—essentially, trusting their gut—to eating that depends more on environmental influences, such as the amount of food served, time of day, and social context. The older children had learned that cleaning the plate is what is expected and that they will be rewarded for doing so.[229]

As children grow into adulthood, they retain the expectations that the amount of food that others serve them is appropriate. As a result, many of us decide how much food to eat at a single sitting on the basis of how much food we are served. Indeed, in a survey conducted by the American Institute for Cancer Research, "67% of those polled said that, when dining out, they finish their entrees most or all of the time."[230] This is why experts tend to believe that it is no coincidence that Americans became fatter at the same time that they began eating out more and as restaurants began supersizing their portions.[231]

Thus, while we might like to believe that people will stop eating as soon as they feel full, it does not work that way. Human appetite, it turns out, is surprisingly elastic, a fact that, as with the asymmetric design of the system, also makes excellent evolutionary sense. Since our survival over the eons of human existence was more acutely threatened by starvation than by obesity, "it behooved our hunter-gatherer ancestors to feast whenever the opportunity presented itself, allowing them to build up reserves of fat against future famine."[232] Because starvation was not only a real but also a periodic threat, the greatest survival prospects belonged to individuals who ate voraciously when food was plentiful and efficiently stored the excess energy as a buffer against future food shortages.[233] Unfortunately, while the system represents a useful adaptation in an environment of food scarcity and unpredictability, it is problematic "in an environment of fast-food abundance, when the opportunity to feast presents itself 24/7. Our bodies are storing reserves of fat against a famine that never comes."[234]

A study of black bears in the Lake Tahoe basin on the California–Nevada border has found that those animals that live in and around cities and towns are heavier than those in wilderness... The culptit, say the wildlife experts who studied them,... is the garbage found at fast-food restaurants and in residential neighborhoods....

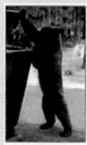

When the researchers tracked 59 bears, they found that the animals fell into two camps: country bears, which spent almost all of their time in wild lands, and city bears, which lived in residential areas, often right under people's noses.... The country bears, forced to roam over wild lands searching for pine cones, troves of berry bushes, or the occasional pery, spent more than 13 hours a day foraging. City bears, with all that rich garbage for the taking, spent much less time, an average of about 8.5 hours a day... And what does abundant food and relative lack of exercise do to the bears?

The bears that lived on garbage were heavier and taller than their country cousins... A normal adult male weighs 220 to 300 pounds, but garbage-fed males routinely reach 400 pounds or more,... and a few weighed 500 to 600—twice the size of some grizzlies.

Source: Henry Fountain, New York Times, November 25. 2003, and Cornelia Dean, New York Times, June 7, 2005.

Figure 4.10 The fast-food lifestyle is getting to the bears, too

Events Give Birth to Trends, But What Escalates Them Are Self-Reinforcing Processes

The forces discussed above were not just one-time socioeconomic shocks. Rather, what makes these forces particularly potent is that they are self-reinforcing dynamic processes that keep feeding on themselves, and on each other. Thus, instead of inducing a one-time spike in obesity in the population, they fuel a growing trend that continues to escalate.

This type of dynamic is typical of most tipping-point phenomena. Some major event or a confluence of events (e.g., postwar changes in employment patterns combined with advances in food production and distribution technology) provides the initial trigger, but then self-reinforcing processes take over and provide the energy that fuels the escalation, causing the initial event(s) to morph into an epidemic-type phenomenon. Because events are often salient, while the underlying reinforcing processes typically are not, this phenomenon is often difficult to appreciate.

The distinction is perhaps easiest to see in the archetypical tipping point: the spread of infectious disease such as the flu. In this case, the triggering event would be the introduction of the infectious agent, the virus, into the community. This initial infection, which may make the evening news, does not in itself ordain an epidemic. That will depend on the strength of the contagion *process*. Initially, most infectious diseases spread slowly, but as more and more people fall ill and become infectious, the number they infect can grow quickly (exponentially) as the process starts to feed on itself. As the number of infected people grows, there will be more opportunities for infected people to come in contact with and infect others, increasing the infectious population still further, and on and on.

Here is how we would depict such a *self-reinforcing* process (Figure 4.11, adapted from Senge[235]).

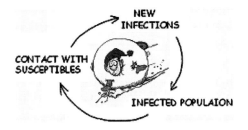

Figure 4.11 The self-reinforcing process that underlines the spread of epidemics

It is the strength of the self-reinforcing contagion process that will ultimately determine whether or not the initial infection leads to an epidemic. If the recovery period was short or the infectivity of the virus low, it is possible that people who get infected would recover quickly, before having the opportunity to infect others. In this case, the contagion process would be weak, and the population would resist the epidemic. However, the greater the infectivity of the disease or the higher the contact rate between individuals in the community, the faster and wider the epidemic will spread.[236]

Figure 4.11 shows how events in a reinforcing process can *snowball* as an initial change (e.g., infection in a population) builds on itself and is amplified, producing more and more of the same. This type of loop is known as a self-reinforcing (or positive) feedback loop because an initial change is amplified, producing further change in the *same* direction. You can follow this self-reinforcing process by walking yourself around the loop: More infected people mean more opportunities for contacts with susceptibles, which leads to still more infections, which means even more infected people, and so on.

Positive feedback processes can be mighty "engines" of change because with sufficient cycling, small deviations can be amplified into major escalations. In folk wisdom, we speak of them in terms such as "snowball effect," "bandwagon effect," or "vicious circle," and in phrases such as "the rich get richer and the poor get poorer."[237]

There is a second type of loop (one we already encountered in Chapter 1), known as a negative or deviation-counteracting loop. Negative feedback loops are different in that they counter and oppose change. The body's many homeostatic mechanisms that are tasked to maintain our internal stability (such as body temperature, blood pressure, and sugar and iron concentration) rely on this type of feedback process. Maintenance of body temperature (an example we discussed in Chapter 1) provides a good illustration for how negative feedback works to counteract deviation: if body temperature should rise → instructions from the brain are issued to induce sweating → the evaporation of the sweat cools the body, causing body temperature to drop back down.

Figure 4.12 best illustrates the difference between the two feedback effects. A system dominated by negative feedback is like a marble placed at the lowest point of smooth-sided bowl; pushing the marble off the equilibrium creates a force opposing the displacement.[238] A system dominated by positive feedback, on the other hand, is like falling off a cliff, in that the slightest disturbance causes the ball to fall off the peak and keep going.

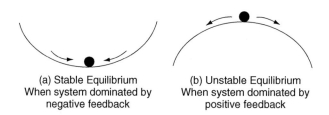

(a) Stable Equilibrium
When system dominated by
negative feedback

(b) Unstable Equilibrium
When system dominated by
positive feedback

Figure 4.12 (*Source*: Sterman, J.D. (2000), *Business Dynamics: Systems Thinking and Modeling for a Complex World*, Boston: Irwin McGraw-Hill, with permission of the McGraw-Hill Companies.)

One of the important insights to come from the young field of system dynamics is that both positive and negative feedback processes are the key governing mechanisms that control and regulate systems of all kinds (biological, engineering, social, and economic).[239] Thus, understanding (and learning to recognize) feedback can be very helpful in understanding how and why systems behave the way they do, for example, why systems "fight back" and resist intervention (when negative feedback dominates), or escalate to troublesome levels (when positive feedback dominates). Our system of human energy and weight regulation is no exception.

Later chapters discuss how human energy and weight regulation are indeed a complex of nested feedback processes at multiple levels (the physiological homeostatic processes, between the physiological and the behavioral, and between people and their external environment), and how the simple concept of feedback can help us clear up significantly muddled public thinking about how the system behaves (or misbehaves).

But for now, we return to our discussion of the socioeconomic landscape and its processes.

As suggested, rather than being one-time socioeconomic shocks, postwar changes in employment patterns, together with advances in food production and distribution technology, fed on themselves and each other. Below, we examine some of the reinforcing pathways, first on the consumption (demand) side and then on the production (supply) side.

Demand–Pull

The simple loop in Figure 4.13 depicts one important mechanism that reinforced postwar changes in the U.S. employment patterns. As discussed earlier in this chapter, when more women entered the workforce, demand for and consumption of convenience and fast foods increased as working couples sought to reduce food preparation time. With two incomes, an increasing number of households could buy the latest kitchen appliances, from microwave ovens that allowed for rapid heating of frozen and pre-prepared foods, to nonstick pans and automatic dishwashers that cut cleanup time, freeing still more time.[240] The decrease in the time cost of food preparation, in turn, helped make it possible for even more women to enter the labor force and devote more time to wealth-generating activities.

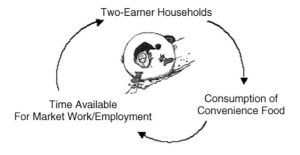

Two-Earner Households

Time Available
For Market Work/Employment

Consumption of
Convenience Food

Figure 4.13 Demand-pull loop

In other words, increases in labor force participation rates by women stimulated the demand for inexpensive convenience and fast food, and vice versa. The two trends fed on each other.

Thus, postwar prosperity and technology were working together, reinforcing each other in creating a climate that accelerated the reallocation of time from housework to outside work, and spurring the long-term trend toward convenience and fast foods.[241] As with most socioeconomic phenomena, such a reinforcing process is rarely an isolated phenomenon. Much like a swirling storm (which, by the way, is a feedback-driven weather system), as the consumption-technology reinforcing process fed on itself and grew over time, it left secondary reinforcing "eddies" in its wake. One example, depicted in Figure 4.14, is the longer-term effect that increasing reliance on convenience foods has had on children.

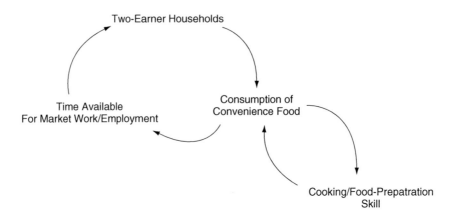

Figure 4.14 Food-preparation skills erode

The more parents rely on convenience food, the less opportunity their children have to acquire food-preparation skills and the more dependent on convenience foods they, in turn, become when they leave the home and start living on their own. Already, on many university campuses, we find students with rudimentary food-preparation skills drawn to convenience foods because it is their only feasible alternative. Perhaps none were as desperate as those at the University of Pennsylvania. Reporting on the grand opening of a new restaurant on campus called Cereality Cereal Bar and Café (with a menu of more than thirty cereals), *New York Times* reporter Lisa Foderaro was horrified to find the students consuming breakfast cereal "as if their grade-point averages depended on it—for breakfast, yes, but also for lunch, dinner and in between."[242]

Over time, more and more of the population becomes dependent on convenience food. This type of self-reinforcing feedback process is the classic pattern for how dependency, whether in individuals or in a society, grows into an "addiction."

Supply–Push

Similarly, reinforcing processes also operated on the supply side. As the market for convenience food picked up speed, market competition and economies of scale drove relative prices lower. Thus, fats and sweets provided in the form of snacks, beverages, or fast foods not only were convenient and palatable but also became huge bargains relative to other foods. Americans could eat pizza at about a thousand calories a dollar or consume a bag of potato chips or Oreo cookies from a vending machine at about 1,200 calories a dollar. By comparison, with fresh carrots at 250 calories a dollar, frozen orange juice at 170 calories per dollar, and spinach at about 30 calories a dollar, fresh foods were a relative rip-off![243,244]

Just as with taste and convenience, food prices do influence consumer food choices. In *Fat Land*, Greg Critzer tells about how Taco Bell, in the mid-1980s, cut prices and experienced a dramatic increase in business. The Taco Bell executives cut 25 percent off the average price of items, such as a taco, expecting that the average check size would drop, but that the drop would be compensated for by increases in the number of customers and visits per customer. They experienced something even better. Within 7 days of initiating the price reduction, the average check was right back to where it was before; instead of buying three items, customers bought four. "In other words, the mere presence of more for less induced people to eat more."[245]

In fact, as a recent University of Minnesota study demonstrated, it does not take that much of a drop in price to spur more sales. When the Minnesota researchers examined the effect of price reductions on sales of vending-machine snacks (at both work sites and at secondary schools), they found that, for some snacks, a drop of as little as a nickel spurred more sales. Not surprisingly, higher price reductions were associated with higher increases in sales—often significantly so. For example, reducing the price of snacks in vending machines by 50 percent increased sales by 93 percent.[246–248]

Thus, the lower relative prices of convenience foods further boosted consumption and market growth, completing the loop (Figure 4.15).

The supply-side reinforcing process, however, had even more going for it. Besides food availability and cost, food variety provided additional reinforcement.

Together with the gains in economies of scale, the growth of the convenience and fast-food industry allowed the industry to collectively devote more research and development resources to developing technologies that would make it possible to mass-prepare, preserve, and distribute an

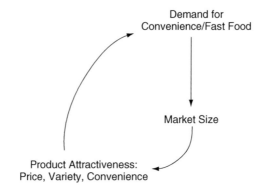

Figure 4.15 Supply-push loop

ever-increasing variety of foods. This fueled a steady increase in the variety of commercially prepared foods that continues today.[249] According to Productscan Online, the food industry is introducing new products at a whopping rate of 20,000 new products a year.[250]

More variety and convenience as well as bargain prices in the loop in Figure 4.15 stimulate more consumption. This was demonstrated in a clever study by researchers at the USDA Human Nutrition Research Center at Tufts University. Using advanced monitoring systems to track the eating patterns of free-living adult Americans, the Tufts researchers found that the higher the variety of snack foods present in their subjects' diets, the higher the number of calories from those foods the subjects would consume, and the higher would be the subjects' consequent body fatness.[251] Similar types of results were also obtained from controlled laboratory experiments. For example, in one such experiment, when human subjects were offered sandwiches with four different fillings, they were found to eat more than they did when they were given sandwiches with their single favorite filling. In a second experiment, when the subjects were served a four-course meal with meat, fruit, bread, and a pudding—foods with very different tastes, flavors, and textures—they ate 60 percent more food than those served an equivalent meal of only their favorite course.[252]

These results are stunning. Historically, the drive to eat a variety of foods had been a positive element in human evolution, helping early humans to increase and balance fuel intake, and, consequently, improve their metabolic, physical, and mental abilities.[253] Now, the same drive for novelty has turned unhealthful.

> In human prehistory, individuals who ... ate from a greater variety of foods may well have had a better micronutrient status than individuals who ate a lesser variety of foods because no single basic food supplies every essential nutrient ... [B]ecause the foods available to primitive hunters and foragers were both limited and intermittently available, those individuals who ate more total food when an increased

variety of foodstuffs could be found may have fared better than those who did not. Thus, under the conditions existing when early humans evolved, individuals with a strong drive to eat a variety of foods and to increase total food intake in the presence of dietary variety were likely to have benefited from the metabolic, physical, and cognitive advantages that a balanced diet provides. What can be termed the "variety principle" may thus have been strongly beneficial in human prehistory, becoming favored in genetic selection and predominating in the lineage from which modern humans descend.[254]

But, as the Tufts researchers noted in the summary of their findings, "[Today,] a drive to overeat when variety is plentiful is disadvantageous for weight regulation because dietary variety is greater than ever before and comes primarily from energy-dense commercial foods rather than from the energy-poor but micronutrient-rich vegetables and fruit for which the variety principle originally evolved. In short, variety had become the enemy."[255]

As with the demand-side loops, these supply-side reinforcing processes did not do their work in isolation. In most socioeconomic phenomena, various factors are often in play, all interconnected, all pushing on each other and being pushed on in return. The expanded diagram in Figure 4.16 incorporates an additional self-reinforcing process to the mix: the role of advertising.

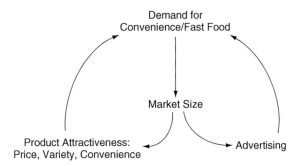

Figure 4.16 Adding the self-reinforcing loop of food advertising

Advertising and promotion have always been central to marketing in the U.S. food industry. As the market grew in size, the size and financial wherewithal of the major industry players grew with it, and so did the intensity of market competition. Increases in the advertising outlays naturally followed. Today, the U.S. food marketing system is the second-largest advertiser in the economy, after the automobile industry.[256] According to Professor Marion Nestle, chairwoman of the New York University nutrition and food policy department and the author of *Food Politics*, food companies spend $33 billion a year advertising and promoting their products—in effect, trying to persuade consumers to eat more.[257] These massive efforts by food manufacturers and restaurant chains to encourage us to eat more food appear to be working, and their success undoubtedly plays a role in increasing our caloric intake.[258] Social scientists are finding that our exposure to advertising messages that encourage food consumption does influence the amount the average person consumes.[259] Advertising also affects food choices, especially those of children.[260,261] A number of investigations have revealed, for example, that children's requests for foods were related to the frequency with which children saw the foods advertised on television. Repeated exposure to advertisements for particular types of foods fosters children's preferences for these foods.[262]

Putting It All Together

Figure 4.17 combines the demand-side and supply-side feedback loops, highlighting the interrelationships between them.

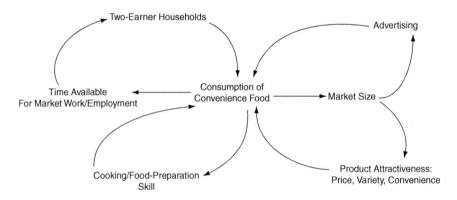

Figure 4.17 Integrating the multiple loops

These example feedback effects underscore how person–environment transactions occur in cycles in which people influence their settings (physically and socially), and how these changed aspects of settings then act to influence health behaviors.[263,264] Seeing this—I reemphasize—is terribly important. It is the mutual influence—the closing of the loop—that creates a self-reinforcing (snowballing) dynamic that can escalate a problem or trend, such as fast-food consumption, to troublesome levels. With each trip around any of these reinforcing loops, the phenomenon strengthens as the process feeds on itself, and, given enough time, an initial small "event" can morph into a major development. Because an event (or a confluence of events) that gives birth to a trend may no longer be what is sustaining it, often the leverage to affect change is in tackling the active reinforcing processes that are operating here and now.

Hurricane Obesa

Hurricane Obesa !!

A hurricane is weather system driven by the mighty force of positive feedback. Like the obesity epidemic, here too an event kicks start the process—in this case a tropical weather disturbance—but it is self-reinforcing feedback that escalates it.

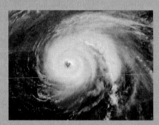

In the tropics, late in the summer months, warm ocean water evaporates and condenses into clouds. If there are no disturbances in the upper atmosphere, the atmospheric energy translates into your ordinary thunderstorm and quickly dissipates. However, if there is a trough of low pressure system or *front* then as the air rises and forms clouds it slowly begins to rotate/spin (counterclockwise in the Northern hemisphere), and move towards the center of the low pressure system. The incoming air must go somewhere so it rises. This rising air, which is saturated with water, cools and condenses to form more clouds. The condensation releases heat called latent heat of condensation. This latent heat warms the cool air aloft, thereby causing it to rise still higher. As the warmed air rises, more air flows into the area where the air is rising, creating strong winds.

This is the essence of a hurricane's feedback "engine" which continues to intensify the storm as long as there is warm water from which to draw energy. As more air moves in and more clouds form the cloud mass increases which increases the rotation. With increased rotation more air is pulled into the system, increasing the cloud mass further, which increases rotation, which increases the airflow... and on and on.

The "fuel" for a hurricane comes from the enormous amount of latent heat released from the warm ocean water. Once a hurricane moves over land, the large energy supply from the ocean is no longer available and the feedback no longer intensifies the storm. As it continues over land it begins to lose strength and eventually dissipates.

Sources:
http://science.howstuffworks.com/hurricane2.htm,
http://encarta.msn.com/encyclopedia_761565992/Hurricane.html,
http://www.odu.edu/webroot/instr/sci/tmmathew.nsf/pages/hurricanes

Figure 4.18 Like epidemics, a hurricane is sustained by positive feedback

Tilting the Energy Balance: Less Energy Out

5

The Water Is Boiling!

> When humans evolved, the challenge was survival in a world we could barely influence. Today, the hurricane and earthquake do not pose the greatest danger. It is the unanticipated effects of our own actions [that are killing us].[265]

The recent rise in the population's caloric intake could very well have been stifled had there been a balancing increase in energy expenditure. However, the population's increased energy intake has been accompanied by a decline in energy output. This energy "depression" is adding to our collective energy surplus, adding fuel to "Hurricane Obesa."

Like all technological and biological systems, the human body obeys the laws of thermodynamics, which define the immutable principle of the conservation of energy. Energy in the human body is not self-generated and does not dissipate into biological black holes; it merely changes from one form to another. When we eat, the chemical energy trapped within the bonds of the food nutrients is initially stored in its chemical form within the body's tissues. There, it is transformed into mechanical energy (and, ultimately, heat energy) by the action of the musculoskeletal system, or it is used to build body structures. If we eat too many calories or are too inactive relative to the calories we eat, the excess energy is stored, primarily in the form of body fat.

Maintaining a balance between energy intake and expenditure was not supposed to be a hard thing to do. Most species adapt and evolve to maintain a stable balance between energy expended and energy acquired, that is, between the energy expended in the search for food and its use for biological processes.[266] Because lack of energy means failure to thrive and, often, failure to survive, maintaining an energy balance between organism and environment is a critical aspect of survival and long-term ecological stability. It was no exception for early humans.

For our hunter-gatherer ancestors, there was a natural coupling between the input and output of energy. They could feast on more food, for example, only if they expended more muscular energy to hunt and gather additional foodstuffs. Conversely, a decrease in food availability meant death for some and, consequently, less energy consumption by the collective tribe. In the long-term, the caloric intake and output of those early humans tended to balance out, despite seasonal fluctuations in food availability and the ongoing need for high-energy output.[267] (Such a state of "stable equilibrium" is not unlike that marble placed at the bottom of the smooth-sided bowl in Figure 5.1. If nudged off its equilibrium, gravitational force would pull it back toward the bottom of the bowl.)

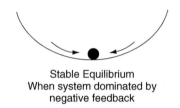

Stable Equilibrium
When system dominated by
negative feedback

Figure 5.1 (*Source:* Sterman, J.D. (2000), *Business Dynamics: Systems Thinking and Modeling for a Complex World*, p. 351. Boston: Irwin McGraw-Hill, with permission of the McGraw-Hill Companies.)

This balance has now been disturbed.

Today, in the United States, as well as in most other affluent nations, energy expenditure and energy intake have been largely decoupled. Unlike the hunter (whether man or beast), humans no longer need to exert themselves so much to obtain food energy. In terms of the calorie-to-effort return ratio (i.e., the human effort necessary to obtain a given amount of food energy), calories, from childhood on, are available at the lowest cost ever in human experience.[268]

This chapter explores how and why caloric expenditure has been dropping in the United States. We will see how the socioeconomic and technological changes that lowered the time and monetary costs of consuming calories (effectively reducing the real price of food and inducing an increase in food consumption) have contributed to the rise in obesity in a second way: by simultaneously raising the cost of expending calories and inducing a decrease in energy expenditure.[269] We also will look at how the time pressures that fueled the demand for convenient and fast food have increased our "need to get places faster, which causes us to drive rather than walk, to take the elevators instead of the stairs, and to look to technology for ways to engineer inefficient physical activity out of our lives."[270]

Figure 5.2 provides a roadmap for our discussion.

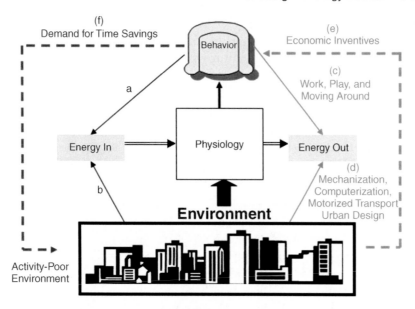

Figure 5.2 Stable equilibrium

Work: Engineering Energy Expenditure Out of the Workplace

As the U.S. economy continues to shift from an emphasis on the production of goods to the provision of services, fewer and fewer Americans are working at jobs that are "sweat-friendly."[271] Recent census data show that the proportion of the work force employed in occupations requiring heavy manual labor, such as farming, masonry, carpentry, and heavy manual factory work, continues to decline, while the proportion of the work force employed in more sedentary white-collar jobs is rising. Many of these new service-oriented jobs in industries such as banking, insurance, health, and education require little energy expenditure, often nothing more active than pressing keys on a computer.[272,273]

Meanwhile, even on the farm and on the factory floor, places that traditionally required a high expenditure of energy, we find that modern labor-saving technology is increasingly performing the tasks once performed by our bodies.[274] It is estimated that a hundred years ago, as much as 30 percent of the energy used in farm and factory work came from muscle power; today, only 1 percent does.[275]

In gradual, often subtle ways, physical exertion continues to be technologically engineered out of the American lifestyle. Even small savings add up over a year, a decade, and a lifetime. French et al.[276] worked out an interesting calculation to demonstrate how, in an office setting, the cumulative effects of small decreases in energy expenditure that occur by substituting e-mail for walking to a nearby office could be significant over long time periods:

> A 145-lb person expends 3.9 kcals/min walking and only 1.8 kcal/min sitting. Energy expenditure thus doubles by walking versus sitting. If one spends 5 min/day, 5 days/week, walking to coworkers' offices to interact, it would result in approximately 5000 kcals/year expended, compared with only 2500 kcals/year for the same amount of time spent sitting at the computer sending those coworkers e-mails. Walking versus sending e-mail could expend about a pound more energy per year.

Although the example is hypothetical, as the authors remind us, "the point is that small but consistent reductions in energy expenditure due to increased computer use could have a significant cumulative impact over time." In Figure 5.2, this trend to replace physical labor with modern technology is captured by the link "d."

The drivers underlying these trends are not just technological; they are economic as well. As is often said, "Economics craft institutions into energy-saving enterprises."[277] In many industries, minimizing physical labor and replacing it with technology has certainly been an effective strategy to save costs. While (on balance) this has been good for our pocketbooks, it has had profound (and unintended) consequences on the economic incentives that drive us to burn calories (link "e" in Figure 5.2).

Simply put, when work was strenuous, we were, in effect, being *paid* to exercise. Today, as more and more jobs become increasingly sedentary, we must *pay* for physical activity,[278] not only in the money we pay to get into the gym, but also in forgone leisure time.[279] To expend serious calories in our society today often involves a choice between going to the gym and spending time with our spouse or children.[280]

In the home, increasing reliance on prepared foods and the proliferation of labor-saving appliances, such as washing machines, dishwashers, microwave ovens, self-propelled lawn mowers, and automatic garage door openers, have caused household-related work also to decline markedly, further compounding the problem.[281] Here, too, the small savings from devices such as electric toothbrushes and TV remote controls become sizable when added up over a year, a decade, and a lifetime.[282] For example, Professor Andrew Prentice, head of the International Nutrition Group at the London School of Hygiene and Tropical Medicine, calculates that the seemingly insignificant switch to using a cordless phone robs us of the equivalent of a 10-kilometer walk each year (because it relieves us of going to a stationary phone). Using a television remote rather than getting up to change channels, he estimates, saves enough energy to add up to as much as an extra pound a year.[283]

Whether in the farm, factory, office, or home, technology is increasingly performing the tasks our bodies once performed. It is all adding up to an environment where fewer of us are expending the energy necessary to maintain a grip on our growing appetites.[284]

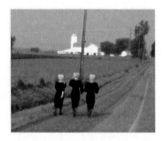

Figure 5.3 The Amish way of life. "Amish communities have very low rates of obesity despite having a diet that is extremely high in calories, sugar, and fat. What explains the Amish's secret? According to some researchers, it is an extraordinary amount of exercise. The Amish reject most modern technologies and live a physically demanding, agrarian lifestyle. In an Amish community, the typical man gets about ten hours of vigorous exercise and about forty-three hours of moderate exercise per week, the typical woman about three and a half hours of strenuous and thirty-nine hours of moderate exercise weekly. Even though the Amish diet consists of three full meals a day of rich and hearty foods such as ham, eggs, cake, and milk, their obesity rates were under 4 percent. [that's significantly] lower than the general American population." (*Source:* Oliver, J.E. (2006). *Fat Politics: The Real Story Behind America's Obesity Epidemic* (p. 143). Oxford, UK: Oxford University Press. Image courtesy of www.thespincycle.com)

Moving About: Transport and Urban Design

As we have already seen, culture and economics shape people's preferences relating to food and, in turn, energy intake. Similarly, human behavior relating to physical activity and energy expenditure is a function of both lifestyle preferences and the characteristics of our physical environment. How our neighborhoods are built—for example, with or without bike paths and footpaths, street lighting, and public transport—influences the use of active transport (walking, cycling) over motorized transport. Participation in active recreational activities is similarly affected by community services, such as the availability of recreational facilities, parks, sports grounds, and community clubs.[285]

As the "f" link in Figure 5.2 suggests, our modern urban environment is increasingly one of our own making.[286] We have created neighborhoods and communities that stifle rather than promote physical exertion. Nowhere is that more true than in how we get from place to place.

For decades, planners have designed our cities, towns, and suburbs on the assumption that every trip will be made by car. In many neighborhoods (including my own), sidewalks are a rare curiosity; what would be the point of having them, since most neighborhoods also lack stores and entertainment destinations within walking distance?[287]

> Even those willing to risk it are put off by the growing distance we have put between ourselves both from others, and from the places and things we need and desire. . . . Shopping centers are concrete islands surrounded by highways too treacherous to access by foot. Workplaces are inaccessible by public transportation. . . . Libraries, parks, and playgrounds are surrounded by acres of parking lot, making their access by anything but car if not out of the question, then at best unappealing.[288]

The pervasive availability of automobiles, combined with urban and suburban designs that make the automobile the most convenient transportation mode, has had a huge influence on how we choose to move around.[289] More than ever, the private vehicle is the dominant mode of transport for commuting, shopping, and other activities. In 2000, almost 90 percent of us drove to work.[290] Federal studies show that three out of four trips as short as a mile or less are made by car.[291] It seems as though we are conducting many aspects of everyday business without ever having to step out of our cars including eating our—you guessed it—fast food.[292] As stated earlier, it is estimated that up to 60 percent of fast food sold in the United States passes through the drive-through window.[293]

There are now more American households that own at least two vehicles (60 percent) than those that own one (30 percent).[294] As of 2002, only 10 percent did not own a private vehicle.[295] As cars proliferate their production costs and selling prices drop, which increases affordability and ultimately sales. In often subtle and indirect ways, this maintains the pressure to keep molding our communities for the convenience of automobile transport.

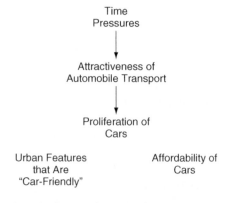

Figure 5.4 Can you complete the loops? The answer is in Figure 5.5

Moving around less is not just a problem for adults; children are not moving much either. A recent study, for example, found that fewer than 13 percent of students walk to school. That was partly because the schools were built on large sites at the edge of communities, beyond walking distance for most students.[296] But studies also show that even when schools are within walking distance, many school districts *prohibit* the children from walking to school because of safety and litigation concerns. With many communities lacking sidewalks for safe walking, who can blame them?[297]

Everywhere, it seems, there are obstacles to human exertion, and even those of us who try to sweat a little often find it difficult to expend the energy. The net result is a push toward collective positive energy balance and obesity.

That's precisely what researchers at San Diego State University's Active Living Program found when they conducted a large-scale field study to assess the impact of neighborhood characteristics on energy expenditure and the prevalence of obesity.

[The] researchers . . . surveyed residents in two neighborhoods in San Diego—one that was close to retail and public buildings and one that was far removed from those amenities. They found that people in the more "walkable" neighborhood took one to two more walking or biking trips a week on average than those in the less walkable neighborhood. . . . [And, surprise, surprise] about 60% of the respondents in the less walkable neighborhood reported being overweight, compared with 35% in the walkable area.[298]

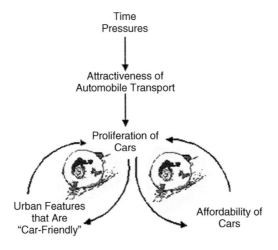

Figure 5.5 The completed loops

Play and Leisure

When it comes to our leisure-time activities, the United States can rightfully claim to be the "passive-entertainment" capital of the world,[299] an "honor" we would rather do without.

In the 21st century electronic frontier, Americans are spending most of their leisure time watching television, using computers, playing video games, e-mailing others, searching the Internet, and enjoying other electronic activities—all highly sedentary activities that require nothing more active than sitting for extended periods and pressing keys on a keyboard.[300]

Data from the *American's Use of Time Study* show that as the obesity epidemic was picking up speed in the 1980s, people were spending six times more time watching television than they did exercising or doing sports (close to 4 hours a day, every day).[301] Hardly anyone believes this to be just a coincidence. The typical American child now spends more time watching television than doing any other activity except sleeping.[302] The sad statistic for an educator like myself is that "[by] the time American children finish high school, they have spent nearly twice as many hours in front of the television set as in the classroom."[303]

Television has been present in virtually every household in the United States for some time, but what is new (and of concern to some) is the dramatic increase in recent years in the percentage of households with two or more television sets. In the 1960s, for example, "only 12% of U.S. households had more than one television set, [but] by 2000, 76% of U.S. households had more than one television set (and more than half of those, or 41% of all households, had three or more sets)."[304] Many of those extra sets are going into children's bedrooms, along with computers and video game consoles. In many homes, children's bedrooms are changing into little media arcades. A recent survey of children in grades 3 through 12 found that a record 68 percent have TVs in their rooms.[305] "Even the nation's youngest children are watching a great deal of television. About one quarter of American children between the ages of two and five have a TV in their room."[306]

A large number of studies (forty at last count) have demonstrated that TV time correlates with weight gain, and that the relationship is linear: the more hours of television viewed per day, the higher the prevalence of obesity.[307,308] Television watching contributes to weight gain, research findings suggest, through at least three mechanisms. First, television viewing is a completely sedentary activity that requires the viewer to expend very little energy—not much more, in fact, than the energy expended sleeping (the so-called resting metabolic energy rate).[309] Second, television watching is often associated with increased food consumption, because people like to snack while watching TV.[310] Worse still, what they eat is often the high-calorie, high-fat foods heavily peddled in TV commercials.[311] Third, television viewing replaces the time that could be spent on more vigorous physical activities. As Professor Norman Nie, director the Stanford Institute for the Quantitative Study of Society, likes to say, "time is hydraulic," meaning that time spent watching television is time taken away from other activities.[312] Quite simply, people who spend more time watching TV tend to exercise less.[313,314]

A recent report by the U.S. Surgeon General revealed that only 22 percent of adults in America engage in physical activity on a regular basis, while more than half of the adult population maintains an almost totally sedentary lifestyle. These are troubling findings, but not particularly surprising given the American public's persistent addiction to their "electronic tube."[315]

With the advent of the Internet and the availability of broadband connections, television viewing among children has started to decline (some estimate by as much as 18 percent from the 1980s levels). Unfortunately, the drop in television viewing is not translating into more calories burned. On the contrary, children are more than compensating for TV viewing time by using computers for surfing the Internet, instant messaging, or playing video games. It is estimated that the average child of ages 2 to 18 now spends close to 40 hours per week on these sedentary visual activities—the equivalent of an adult's full-time job.[316]

As after-school outdoor activities yield to computers, video games and television, parents are not fighting back; rather, many are embracing these modern-day baby sitters.[317] Beyond the usual concerns about time, money, and the need to rest, new parental concern about crime is a big reason why. Dangerous neighborhoods, or the perception of danger, discourage parents from permitting children to play outdoors.[318] Findings from a survey study suggest that close to 50 percent of all U.S. adults believe that their neighborhoods are unsafe. Such concerns only reinforce parents' inclinations to "bubble-wrap" their children, limiting childhood activity and spontaneous play. "What the surveyed parents were implying was utterly reasonable: TV-viewing may be bad, but at least my kid won't get shot, molested, kidnapped, or jumped into a gang while doing it."[319]

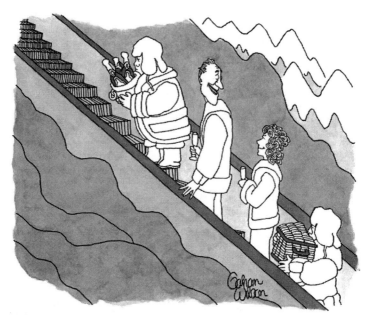

"I understand the Everest climb used to be quite a chore."

Figure 5.6 (© 2008, *The New Yorker Collection*, from cartoonbank.com. All Rights Reserved)

The Burden Is Cumulative

As a result of all of the factors discussed above, the energy expenditure for most adults in the United States now rarely climbs above the *resting level*. That's a level of energy expenditure that is equivalent to between 60 and 100 watts—the energy output of an ordinary light bulb! No wonder U.S. citizens have all too appropriately been termed *homo sedentarius*.[320]

It is a sad irony. The environment we toiled so hard to create for ourselves, while a very comfortable one, is one that our body's energy-regulating systems were never designed for. And an increasing number of people are paying the price[321]:

> It has often been said that humans are very adaptable creatures, and that is true. We can live in the Tibetan highlands, in the rain forests of Brazil, in Europe during the Ice Age, or in the Sahara Desert today. And because of this adaptability, we have always assumed that we could create almost any sort of environment for ourselves and thrive. We have also assumed that whatever environment we created for ourselves would likely be an improvement over what we had. Today, however, we have run smack into the limits of our adaptability. We have created for ourselves an environment—a food-rich, activity-poor environment—that makes a great number of us sick, and so far there has proved to be little we can do about it.

But let's not forget that, unlike a virus-induced disease, the structures underlying our obesifying environment are increasingly of our own making,[322] and so we can "unmake" them. However, before we can change those structures, we need to see them, for, as Peter Senge argues eloquently in *The Fifth Discipline*, "[societal] structures of which we are unaware hold us prisoner."

Exposing the societal structures underlying our obesifying environment is what we aimed to do in this chapter and the previous one.

Dr. Jekyll and Mr. Hyde, or Changing the Vicious to Virtuous

In the previous chapter, we saw how positive feedback loops self-reinforce, feeding on themselves and amplifying change—for example, causing a single infection to morph into an epidemic. It is important to emphasize that positive feedback loops are neither inherently bad nor inherently good. Deviation-amplifying processes, in other words, can be virtuous (i.e., in which they reinforce in a *desired* direction) as well as vicious. It is extremely important to understand this broader implication.

An even more subtle point is that the *same* feedback process can work both for and against us. Consider, as an example, the simplest of all investment systems, that of depositing money into a savings account at, say, a 10 percent interest rate compounded annually. The feedback structure of this system is shown in Figure 5.7.

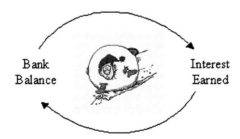

Figure 5.7 Compounding interest as a feedback structure

As interest is earned and reinvested, it is added to the original principal, increasing it. This boosts the interest earned the following year, adding further to the deposited amount, which increases our balance still further.

Now, consider what happens if the bank balance turns negative, such as when taking out a bank loan at a 10 percent annual interest rate. The same compounding (reinforcing) process now works in reverse, driving the negative account more and more into the red.

Our choices about exercise can work for us or against us in much the same way. Let's first see how it can work against us. As already mentioned, excessive television viewing by children replaces time spent in sports, increases food consumption, and promotes weight gain.[323] The gain in weight could then push the child further in the direction of decreased activity in a self-reinforcing vicious spiral. It is sad, but true that "among the most prevalent consequences of obesity in children is the discrimination that overweight children suffer at the hands of their peers."[324] Chubby children, for example, are less likely to be invited to participate in sports that leaner children play. Exclusion can also be self-inflicted, as when an obese child chooses to voluntarily withdraw because of embarrassment. Either way, lack of participation robs overweight children of the opportunity to practice and acquire skills; this→ accentuates their sporting ineptitude and → leads to further exclusion.

Biological mechanisms also add to this spiral of increased inactivity. As inactivity leads to weight gain, the added pounds often precipitate physiological complications that hamper the child's capacity to exercise (complications such as cardiovascular problems, respiratory difficulties, and osteoarthritis).[325]

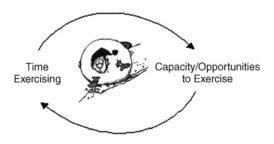

Time
Exercising   Capacity/Opportunities
                               to Exercise

Figure 5.8 Reinforcing process in exercising

But, as with the bank balance example, this very cycle can also virtuously work for us. Consider what happens if, in a different environment, we create the opportunity and incentives for the child to choose physical exercise, for example, opting to play soccer over watching TV. With play and practice, skill invariably improves. This, of course, can be tremendously self-rewarding, as it makes the child feel better about himself or herself and about exercising. In addition, becoming a more skilled player is apt to open up even more opportunities for future participation.

Exercising also causes physiological capacity to expand, such as increasing lung, heart, and muscle capacity.[326] As the physiological capacity of the body for physical exertion expands, children can play longer and harder, leading to further expansion of physiological capacity. This, in fact, is the reinforcing mechanism that underlies the notion of progressive training in many sports, an intuitive feedback practice that has had a long history, beginning with the Greek Olympian Milo.

> Milo of Crotona ... lived in Greece in the sixth century B.C. Milo is said to have hoisted a baby bull on his shoulders every day to improve his strength. As the bull grew heavier with age, Milo's strength also grew. Since that time, progressive resistance training has been an important part of the training programs of many athletes, from football players and track and field participants to swimmers and figure skaters.[327]

Learning to recognize and harness the power of positive feedback to one's advantage is a powerful conceptual leverage one gains from applying the systems approach.

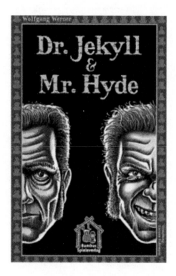

Figure 5.9 The story of Dr. Jekyll and Mr. Hyde, a novella written by the Scottish author Robert Louis Stevenson and first published in 1885 is an expression of the dualist tendency in culture. In mainstream discourse the very phrase "Jekyll and Hyde" has come to mean a person who may show a distinctly different character, or profoundly different behavior, in different situations. (*Source:* Illustration courtesy of Carsten Fuhrmann)

Individual Differences   6

Some Are "Squares," and Some Are Not

> [While] we are all becoming victims of the profound changes in the human environment, genetics modulates how quickly each of us falls off the cliff.
> —Andrew Prentice, head of the International Nutrition Group,
> The London School of Hygiene and Tropical Medicine

It is a common observation that there is much variability in how different people respond to life's health challenges. Obesity is no exception. For instance, some individuals more easily accumulate excess fat, always trying to lose those extra pounds, while others seem relatively well protected against the extra calories they ingest.[328]

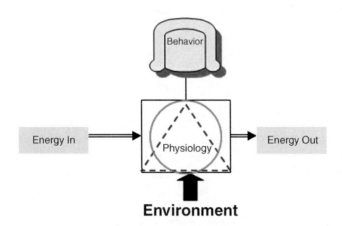

Figure 6.1 People come in different shapes and sizes

Personal differences arise from many sources. Individuals acquire different attributes, behaviors, and predispositions, and a lifetime of interactions with others and the environment magnify these differences.[329] Our genes also

T.K.A. Hamid, *Thinking in Circles About Obesity*,
DOI 10.1007/978-0-387-09469-4_6, © Springer Science+Business Media, LLC 2009

play a role. Because of differences in individual genetic makeups, we not only look different from one another, we also have different metabolisms and susceptibilities to disease, including the susceptibility to weight gain.

Genes, however, are not responsible for the obesity epidemic.[330] While genes will be involved in most diseases (if not hugely, at least to some extent), the population's obesity epidemic cannot be attributed to genetic factors.[331] This is simply because genetic changes in the population occur too slowly to account for the velocity with which obesity has accelerated over the last four decades. A period of time of a few decades is too short for the population's genetic makeup to have changed in any substantial way. Nor, in the case of the United States, is there evidence to suggest that the American gene pool has changed in a significant way as a result of immigration.[332,333]

Thus, while genetics may be helpful in explaining differences between *individuals*, it is not a satisfying explanation for changes in the *population*.

What has, of course, changed profoundly and in an incredibly short time is the environment that is acting on those genes.[334] It is, thus, safe to say, as the World Health Organization Consultation on Obesity has indeed declared:[335]

> [T]he prevalence of obesity in populations is largely determined by the environment (the social and cultural forces that promote an energy-rich diet and a sedentary lifestyle), whereas obesity in individuals in a given environment is largely determined by their genetic responses to that environment.

The distinct contribution of genes to individual variation in body weight and body mass index (BMI) and of environmental factors to the changes in populations was nicely framed in a recent review by John Murray. He wrote,

> In any individual's case, genetic factors play a role in determining body size but they tend to cancel out in large samples from a [stable] genetic pool, leaving levels and trends in body size that result from environmental factors.[336]

To the dismay of many, the promise of genetics as a convenient excuse for our growing waistlines simply has not panned out. Rather, the promise of genetics lies in two areas: in advancing our understanding of how (and the degree by which) genetic makeup contributes to individual susceptibility to obesity; and in its potential to help us personalize our approaches to both prevention and treatment, thus enhancing the effectiveness of both.

Deciphering the Code, One Gene at a Time

Much of the research, to date, on the genetic contribution to obesity has aimed to identify and characterize the genes that affect food intake and energy expenditure. The hope is that constructing the basic metabolic and nutritional pathways for energy and weight regulation will ultimately lead to new, high-leverage entry points to obesity treatment and prevention.[337]

The discovery of leptin in 1994 advanced our understanding of the biological underpinnings of the food intake part of the equation. Leptin, a product of the *ob* gene, is an amino acid protein synthesized in fat cells and secreted into circulation in proportion to fat-cell mass. Leptin's primary role appears to be signaling the brain when fat stores are depleted in times of deprivation (or dieting), thereby inducing an increase in appetite.[338,339]

Researchers are also studying how genes might influence weight regulation through their effects on energy expenditure. Progress has been made here, as well. For example, human studies are indicating that resting metabolic rate (RMR), which accounts for roughly 70 percent of daily energy expenditure for the average person, but can vary considerably from person to person, is also influenced by genetics.[340,341] The details of how exactly this is accomplished are not fully understood yet, but several candidate genes that code for protein products closely linked to energy-utilizing processes have been identified and may soon help explain the individual differences.[342,343]

All in all, since the discovery of the first obesity gene in 1994, scientists have pinpointed over 250 genes involved in human energy and weight regulation. "Some of them determine how individuals lay down fat and metabolize energy stores. Others regulate how much people want to eat in the first place, how they know when they've had enough and how likely they are to use up calories through activities ranging from fidgeting to running marathons."[344]

Fidgeting? Indeed.

What has become increasingly clear in recent years is that body weight and metabolism, unlike some physical traits such as eye color, which are the result of a single gene, appear to be regulated by a constellation of genes. It is an example of what scientists call a polygenic trait, a physical characteristic that comes from many different genetic sources.[345] Because energy regulation is so very critical for survival, Mother Nature, it appears, has worked hard to put in place not one, not even two, but multiple, redundant, and interlocking systems to ensure proper functioning.

Outside of a small percentage of people with specific genetic disorders, then, for most people there is no one "fat" gene that holds the key to shaping body weight.[346] Rather, there are literally thousands of possible genetic combinations that shape a person's weight,[347] and the particular scenario that results depends on the environment in which we live in.[348]

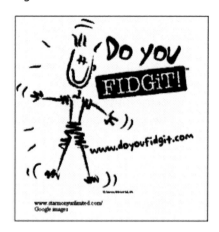

Figure 6.2 Scientists at the Mayo Clinic published research results in 2005 that suggest that fidgeting– the tendency to sit still or move around– is biological and infborn, governed by genetically determined levels of brain chemicals. Their study, published in *Science*, did not involve deliberate exercise, but it measured– with the help of the sensors–how much people moved about naturally and spontaneously. The difference in activity levels between lean people and overweight ones was striking. "The heavier ones tend to sit, while the lean ones were more restless and spent two more hours a day on their feet– standing, pacing around and fidgeting." The researchers could also show that the tendency to fidget influences weight, not the other way around. When the diets were altered to make the obseve people lose weight and the lean ones again it , the activity levels did not change. (*Source*: *New York Times*, May 24, 2005, *New weightLoss Focus: The Lean and the Restless*, By Denise Grady. Cartoon from www.starmonyunlimited.com)

Genes and Individual Susceptibility to Weight Gain: The Experimental Findings

Rather than focus on molecules, genes, and biochemistry, genetic *epidemiologists* aim to assess the degree to which obesity in individuals in a particular environmental setting is determined by their genetic responses to that environment,[349] that is, how much of an observed increase in obesity in a given population in a given environment is attributable to genetics? Researchers take a trait, such as BMI, and measure its so-called level of heritability, which, in essence, is a measure of how much of a trait's total variation among a group of people is caused by genes.[350]

Because of practical and ethical limitations on human experimentation, in researching heritability, genetic epidemiologists depend on *natural* experiments of familial aggregation, for example, measuring the level of heritability among adopted siblings growing up in the same home and twins reared apart. This, unfortunately, comes with a price. With such experimental designs, it is very difficult to fully tease out the genetic from the environmental determinants of obesity, because even when family members are reared apart, they are still raised in the same country, and often the same city, and are therefore exposed to very similar environmental influences growing up, such as similar foods, similar eating customs, and similar messages from the popular culture. Hence, an important proviso to keep in mind as we digest these results is that these heritability findings are calculated for groups of people growing up in roughly the same environment—the modern obesifying environment we all share.[351]

As early as 1923, Davenport published the results of a comprehensive (possibly the first) attempt to study the role of inheritance in human obesity. He concluded that BMI values were more similar among family members than among unrelated persons.[352] Eighty years later, we know quite a bit more. A large number of studies of familial aggregation have been conducted since Davenport's study to assess and better quantify the level of heritability of obesity.[353] Studies of individuals with a wide range of BMIs, together with information obtained on their parents, siblings, and spouses, suggest that obesity does indeed run in families. Broadly, these studies show the following:

- The BMIs of siblings are much more alike than the BMIs of people who are not related to each other.[354]
- Obesity in one parent more than doubles the risk that a child will be obese as an adult.[355]
- When both parents are obese, the chances that their children will be obese can be as high as 80 percent.[356]

Families, however, share many things besides genes; they share eating habits, leisure activities, financial resources, and so on. To make sure that observed similarities are not due simply to family members' having been raised in the same household and taught to eat the same way, researchers also compare adopted siblings who grow up in the same home but are not related and twins reared apart.[357]

In adoption studies, the results suggest that adults who had been adopted early in life have weights more closely resembling those of their biological rather than their adoptive parents.[358,359] Similarly, studies of twins reared apart show important gene effects. For example, BMI has consistently been shown to be similar between twins, with the similarity being greater in monozygotic (identical) than in dizygotic (fraternal) twins.

Similarities between twins were also found in the manner in which they respond to induced energy imbalances. For example, in one classic study, twelve pairs of identical twins were overfed by 1,000 calories a day for a 12-day period. At the end of the study, the mean weight gain for all the subjects was 18 pounds, but there was considerable variation among the individual subjects. The least that any of the subjects gained was 9 pounds, the most was 29, and the rest were scattered between those two extremes. "Within the pairs of twins, however, the weight gain was not nearly so random. Most subjects gained about the same amount of weight as their twin did, to within a few pounds."[360]

Clearly, these results demonstrate that human subjects have different genetic susceptibilities to environmental variables (such as overfeeding or inactivity) that lead to variability in the degree of positive/negative energy balance and, ultimately, weight gain/loss.[361] This explains why some individuals remain lean while consuming a high-fat diet and being inactive, while others gain weight, possibly a lot of it, in the same environment.[362]

What we should not conclude from these results, however, is that "it is the genes that make us do it."

> Our genes, except for very simple cases such as hair color or the shape of our noses, represent no more than possibilities or probabilities. The ultimate outcome [of how a developed person ultimately turns out]—which scientists call the phenotype, to distinguish it from the genotype, or the genetic instructions—depends on our interaction with the environment as we are developing.[363]

This interaction between our genotype and our phenotype can be seen in the following simple relationship:

$$Genotype + Environment \rightarrow Phenotype$$

Biology, in that sense, is not unlike language. Almost all humans inherit the capacity to speak and understand language, but which language they learn is entirely an environmental matter.

The epidemiological counterevidence to the notion of genetic determinism, as already argued, is the fact that while obesity prevalence has increased so dramatically in the last few decades, our biology as a species really has not—and could not have—changed (much).

And then, of course, there are the Pima Indians.

The Pimas

A striking example of genetic–environmental interaction is seen in the study of the two populations of Pima Indians—the Mexican Pimas living in a remote and mountainous part of northern Mexico (the Sierra Madre) and the American Pimas who live in Arizona. The two Pima Indian populations share the same ancestry, but are living in two very different environmental settings. As a result, they have very different lifestyles. While the Mexican Pimas are farmers, consuming food that they grow and engaging in high levels of physical activity, the Arizona Pimas, like many Americans, have a lifestyle characterized by an overabundance of food and limited physical activity.

Despite similar genetic backgrounds, the physiological differences between the two populations are rather striking. In the Arizona population, the prevalence of obesity is alarmingly high, as high as 80 percent, while, by contrast, their cousins over the border have no obesity problem at all.[364,365] Despite sharing the same genotype, the Arizona Pimas have a mean BMI that is seven to ten points higher than that of their counterparts in Mexico and are, on average, 55 pounds (25 kg) heavier.[366] The most serious distinction, however, may be this: the Arizona Pimas (but not their Mexican cousins) are afflicted with the highest rate of diabetes in the world.[367] What explains these differences? In a word: environment.

Two primary features that distinguish the lifestyles of the two communities are these: first, the amount of fat in the diet (23 percent in Mexico versus 36 percent in Arizona); and second, the tremendous amount of vigorous occupational physical exertion in Mexico compared with Arizona.[368,369]

Clearly, the low levels of physical activity and high intake of an energy-dense diet are the environmental factors precipitating obesity in the Arizona Pimas, "but it is the Pimas' genes that have made them particularly susceptible to these environmental factors."[370] The interaction between their particular genetic makeup and the characteristics of their modern U.S. environment has pushed their obesity and diabetes rates to extremely high levels, significantly higher than most other ethnic groups in the United States.[371]

The Pimas' unique genotype has come to be known as the "thrifty genotype." It is a constellation of genetic factors that encourages the conversion of calories into body fat.[372]

> For hundreds or thousands of years before the white man arrived, the Pimas had lived in the desert, dependent upon native plants and animals and whatever they were able to raise by farming along the Gila River. When the rains failed, as they did twice a decade on average, the crops dried up and even the desert was less bountiful. If a drought lasted more than a year or two, starvation loomed. So . . . the Pimas most likely to survive were those with efficient metabolisms and whose bodies stashed away a little something extra in times of plenty. . . . This caloric efficiency helped keep Pimas alive in times of famine, and it never really hurt them because their low-fat, low-calorie diets and their active lives kept them relatively lean even when food was plentiful. But in the second half of the twentieth century, when the Pimas' eating and exercise habits came to resemble those of the rest of the United States, the efficiency backfired.[373]

Obesity of the Arizona Pimas is, thus, the residue of genetic variants that were more adaptive in a previous environment. Their "thrifty gene" set enabled their ancestors, who farmed and hunted in a time of nutritional privation, to stockpile fat during times of plenty so they would not starve during periods of want.[374] These very genes that once protected their ancestors are today causing severe pathology and predisposing them to early death.

Genetic × Environmental Interactions: Conclusion

Genes load the gun, the environment pulls the trigger.[375]

The lesson to be learned from the experience of the Pimas is twofold: genetic-environmental interactions are both important and complex; and the genetic factor is not excess body weight per se, but rather a predisposition or vulnerability to obesity that is activated under suitable environmental conditions.[376] In our modern sedentary environment and with food beckoning on every corner, the genetically susceptible individual will gain weight, possibly lots of it.

What this means is that we cannot tell ourselves that our genes deserve 10 or 20 or 100 percent of the credit, or the blame, for our weight. Genes are very important, though not all-important, and so is the environment. The two interact in complex ways to create the people (and the nation) we have become.[377]

> [B]iology may explain which individuals in an obesity-prone environment will in fact become obese and may explain differences between people in the extent of obesity reached in response to a common environment. But biology does not

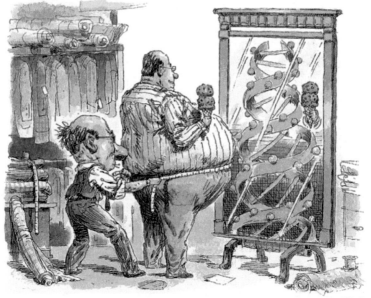

My Genes Made Me Do It   John Cuneo

Figure 6.3 (*Source*: New York Times, July 4, 2005, courtesy of John Cuneo.)

explain the world problem any more than understanding biological vulnerabilities in individuals explains why there is so much lung cancer. There is so much lung cancer primarily because of tobacco, and there is so much obesity because of a dangerous [obesifying] food and physical activity environment.[378]

Is *Ad-Lib* Behavior Killing Us?

7

In human feeding-behavior experiments, the free-living condition in which feeding is unrestricted and subjects (as in real life) are free to eat when they want and as much as they want, is called the ad-libitum (literally, the "at pleasure") condition.

A (Mis-)Match Made in America

xIn earlier chapters, we saw how as a species, we carry the physiological legacy of earlier times of privation, when the challenge to the body energy-control system was to provide a strong drive to eat in order to endure the periodic threat of famine and to maintain the high level of physical exertion needed for survival. We also saw how, in such an environment, an *asymmetric* system of energy regulation—one that favors overconsumption and strongly defends against negative energy balances and weight loss—drove early humans to eat voraciously when food was plentiful and stored the excess energy with great efficiency, aiding survival.

Yet, throughout most of human history, obesity was never a common health problem. The boom–bust cycles in food availability coupled with a mode of existence characterized by high-energy throughput, naturally balanced the caloric intake and output over time.[379]

Maintaining a healthy, normal body weight was not the goal of this asymmetric design; it was the result of the physiology–environment interaction. Today, we are not always so lucky. The same physiological adaptations that kept us alive and in good form in a hunter-gatherer environment are resulting in a maladaptive response in our modern food-rich, activity-poor environment. Our pro-consumption physiological system is still intact, and still encouraging us to overeat, and with constant access to an abundant supply of high-calorie, high-fat food and a sedentary

T.K.A. Hamid, *Thinking in Circles About Obesity*,
DOI 10.1007/978-0-387-09469-4_7, © Springer Science+Business Media, LLC 2009

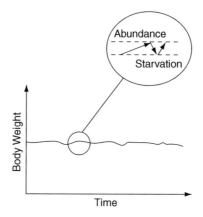

Figure 7.1 The way it was

lifestyle that has reduced our energy requirements, there is constant pressure on the system toward positive energy balance (and weight gain).

Figure 7.2, while admittedly highly simplified, does capture these key distinctions between the way it was and the way it is. Both then and now, the strong drive to overeat and efficiently store excess energy builds up fat stores and body weight in times of abundance, as in point A in both figures. Given the way it was, such fat stores would be called upon at least every 2 to 3 years during periods of famine. During these periods, body weight would drop, as in point S in the left figure, but not for long and typically without adverse consequences. As good times eventually returned, body weight and energy reserves were restored. And so it went.

In today's environment, our bodies are socking away a few extra calories day after day, year after year for a famine that never comes.[380] Furthermore, with a paucity of opportunities for physical exertion, our underactive lifestyle contributes to the positive energy imbalance, pushing weights even higher, to point A+.

This persistent imbalance of energy intake and output was not anticipated by biology, and given the capacity of the human body to adjust to excess

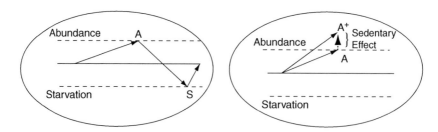

Figure 7.2 Left: The way it was. Right: The way it is

calorie intake by adding body fat, the upside potential for gaining weight in the population was enormous.[381]

The current epidemic of weight gain in many cultures, thus, is an understandable function of a changed relationship between biology and the environment.

> Living in a world of high-calorie, high-fat foods, always in plentiful supply, and with labor-saving devices that keep us from having to exert ourselves too much, sometimes our finely tuned internal machines fail us. They tell us to eat more than we need for a healthy, normal weight, and, if we listen to their advice, we get fat. This makes maintaining a healthy weight a very different matter than it was intended to be. Instead of it being a task that is accomplished unconsciously and automatically, it becomes something we have to think about.[382]

Like Our Genes, Our Mental Models Did Not Change

Today, people are prisoners not only to the physiology that was vital to our Pleistocene-era ancestors, but also to hunter-gatherer instincts that no longer apply.

Humans have learned to rely on (and trust) their bodies' self-regulatory mechanisms and signals to maintain many aspects of their bodies' internal environment (e.g., body core temperature, body fluid volume and tonicity, blood glucose, etc.). In feeding, humans have similarly learned to instinctively regulate behavior in accordance with the body's biological states of need: eat when hungry (when the body senses an energy deficit) and stop eating when feeling full (when energy depots are replenished). For most of our history, we did not have to think about how much to eat in order to maintain a desirable weight. Our bodies told us. As we know, obesity was not a common health problem throughout most of human history. So, it seems reasonable for people to instinctively believe that the body's automatic control system defends against both weight loss and weight gain while striving to maintain stability at some "natural" body weight.[383]

Today, most of us continue to instinctively cruise on "automatic feeding control." Our feeding behavior is largely unconscious and automatic, requiring little deliberate effort. This drives us to eat to our physiological limits when food is readily available and selectively focus on foods high in energy density.

Like our genes, our "ad-libitum" mental model has not changed, reflecting behavioral instincts that no longer apply. Indeed, the very instinctive processes that have served the human race well until now fail us in the current environment, And what's most disturbing is that too many people remain unaware of this situation and are paying the price.

Turning-Off *Automatic* Control and Asserting *Cognitive* Control

The torrent of obesogenic pressures that are affecting all of us in our modern environment has often been compared to fast and furious sea currents that lift all ships in a turbulent sea.[384] In many ways, it is a very apt analogy, and one that underscores several intriguing similarities. It aptly conveys, for example, how exposure to factors surrounding all of us in modern societies induces obesity in the population, just as a raging current can carry all ships out at sea. The analogy also nicely explains how and why our built-in asymmetric system for energy regulation worked for us so well and for so long but is failing us now.

Our hard-wired physiological system of energy regulation that is "steering" us toward overconsumption and that defends against negative energy balances can be likened to an automatic steering system (an autopilot) that helps steer a ship at sea. In the case of energy regulation, our asymmetric system keeps us in good form in an environment in which food is scarce and the next meal unpredictable, and that would be like relying on an asymmetric autopilot— one that's rigged to steer slightly to the left or to the west of north—to safely steer ships that sail in a west-to-east cross current (See Figure 7.3).

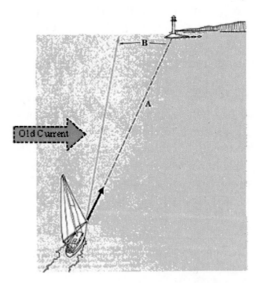

Figure 7.3 Old times. The system's bias to steer us left works for generations

Ultimate balance, in both cases, arises not out of a symmetric regulatory process or living in a stable environment, but from an *asymmetric* process that compensates for an unbalanced (biased) environment. It is not unlike in arithmetic when multiplication of two *negative* numbers produces a *positive* result.

This type of boat with this type of (biased) autopilot in this type of environment would safely make it, just as for thousands of generations our ancestors did with their energy "autopilots," until things started to change.

Now, let's take this analogy a step further. It is no longer a stretch, nor, sad to say, is it hypothetical to contemplate how human intervention may alter the weather environment in some significant or dysfunctional way. (Global warming, of course, comes readily to mind.) So, with tongue firmly in cheek, we keep our nautical analogy going and consider what happens if human intervention causes winds and the associated wind-driven sea currents to reverse direction, becoming east-to-west in the above scenario.

Figure 7.4 depicts what happens if we continue to steer by (biased) automatic control: we'll be blown out to sea.

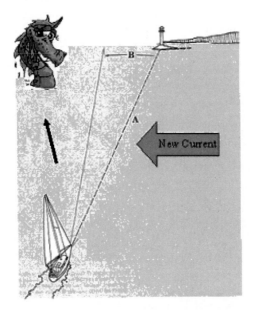

Figure 7.4 Current environment. The system's bias to steer us left is dysfunctional in the current environment

In an analogous manner, our innate asymmetric physiological drives are "steering" us to higher weights in our current food-rich activity-poor environment.[385] On the ocean, the solution requires a shift in strategy to override automatic control and take control of the helm. Similarly, reducing the national waistline requires a major shift in thinking about managing our instincts and our environment. At present and in the future, most of our population will maintain a healthy body weight only by replacing the passive model of involuntary (automatic) energy regulation and asserting cognitive control to proactively resist the "obesifying" aspects of the current environment.[386]

"Essentially," says James Hill, director of the Center for Human Nutrition at the University of Colorado, and a leading researcher in the obesity field, "we have to teach people to override their biological instincts with their cognitive abilities."[387] Here's the really hard part: it's not for a week, but for a lifetime.

It Can Be Done

> Perhaps our most important quality as humans is our capability to self-regulate. It has provided us with an adaptive edge that enabled our ancestors to survive and even flourish when changing conditions led other species to extinction. Our regulatory skill or lack thereof is the source of our perception of personal agency that lies at the core of our sense of self.[388]

Hill's statement at the end of the previous section comes not from a day-dreaming the theoretician, but from a pragmatic empiricist who knows first hand that it can indeed be done and how it can be done. Together with Dr. Rena Wing, a behavioral psychologist at Brown University, Hill founded the National Weight Control Registry (NWCR) to track and study—and learn from—people who were successful at long-term maintenance of weight loss. Today, the NWCR includes approximately five thousand individuals who have lost weight and kept if off for a long time. Essentially, these individuals have successfully reduced caloric intake and increased physical activity by relying primarily on intellect rather than instinct. They have, in other words, asserted *cognitive control* to restrict food intake, eat a low-fat diet, and engage in high levels of physical activity. The data from these "successful losers" demonstrate that obesity-susceptible individuals can sustain long-term weight loss through cognitive control strategies, even in the absence of macroenvironmental change.[389,390]

What makes this even more exciting is that the dividends of such a shift in thinking extend way beyond individual gain. As more and more of us start asserting cognitive control over our eating and physical activity, the impact of our collective healthy behavior will ultimately reshape our collective environment. For example, as Americans have begun demanding healthier, low-fat, higher-fiber food choices, more and more eating establishments have changed their food preparation procedures and menus accordingly. As competition intensifies among stores, restaurants, vending-machine companies, and fast-food chains, a wider variety of choices will become available at lower costs, further encouraging healthy eating.[391] A new *virtuous* cycle will be born. This reinforcing process is depicted as the right-hand-side positive feedback loop in Figure 7.5: higher demand for low-fat, high-fiber foods leads to the expansion of the market size for such foods, which leads to a decrease in prices and an increase in variety and availability, which spurs more demand, further increasing demand, and so on. What is of great import here is that this virtuous process will simultaneously weaken the existing vicious loop to the left, because, as the figure suggests, the two loops are *coupled* via market forces; a consumer shift to low-fat, high-fiber foods will (at least in part) mean a shift away from fast foods. The two loops are, in effect, "arm wrestling" for market share.

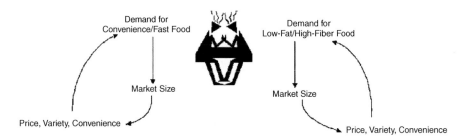

Figure 7.5 Left: The way it is. A vicious self-reinforcing process. Right: The way it could be. A virtuous self-reinforcing process

What will that do to the fast-food loop? The potential benefit from this can be enormous, since any significant shift away from fast food could potentially transform the fast-food loop trajectory from accelerated growth to accelerated decline. Why? Recall that in any positive feedback process, a change in one direction sets in motion reinforcing pressures that produce further change in the same direction, reinforcing and amplifying the original change. The direction of change, therefore, is significant, such as adding a deposit to an initially empty, but interest-earning, bank account, which will enable the account to grow exponentially over time. If, on the other hand, the original change is downward, such as taking a bank loan, the value of the account will keep decreasing, getting more and more negative over time as the interest we owe accumulates.

As Part V will explore in more detail (when we discuss prevention), public policy has an important role to play here, and that is to create supportive environments that make healthy choices the easy choices. In the above scenario, for example, government policy could help grease the shift to healthy eating by offering tax breaks that effectively subsidize healthy foods.[392] Similarly, public policy can do a lot of good on the energy-expenditure side by promoting active lifestyles. For example, public policy levers (such as building codes and regulations, zoning ordinances, and priorities for capital investment) may be deployed so that when communities are built or rebuilt, they would be designed "to the human scale, instead of to the automotive scale."[393] The trick, of course, is to do that without forcing society to go back in time. It is a challenge, as we will see in Part V, that many innovative communities have successfully tackled.

There is also a second challenge, one that may well prove to be the bigger challenge.

The Allure of the "Silver Bullet"

The greater challenge may well prove to be overcoming the human tendency to seek the quick fix rather than take on the difficult demands of exercising control. Americans, like those who live in the world's many other technological cultures, have grown accustomed to thinking in terms of medical miracles and quick fixes that require no effort on their part.[394]

With a disease like obesity, whose causality is complex and for which treatment options are confusing, often difficult, and always prolonged, it is doubly tempting to succumb to the allure of the "silver bullet."

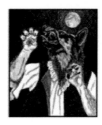

Figure 7.6 The allure of the silver bullet.
  "Of all the monsters that fill the nightmares of our folklore, none terrify more than werewolves, because they transform unexpectedly from the familiar into horrors. For these, one seeks bullets of silver that can magically lay them to rest. . . .
  And why a silver bullet? Magic, of course. Silver is identified with the moon and thus has magic properties. . . .
  And what could be more natural than using the moon–metal to destroy a creature transformed under the light of the full moon?"
  (*Source*: Brooks, F.P. (1987). No silver bullet: essence and accidents of software engineering. *Computer*, 20(4), 10–19.)

It is worth noting that in the movies, Hollywood often makes the werewolf a rather innocent character transformed against his (or rarely, her) will into a monster. In many ways, that is not unlike how many of us think about our fat.

It has been estimated that the tens of millions of American men and women who are currently attempting to lose weight spend approximately $50 billion annually on techniques for losing weight. Of concern is that a great chunk of the expense and the effort is wasted on ineffective, sometimes even harmful practices that extend beyond the merely unwise to the Faustian. The surging demand for a weight-loss "silver bullet" has fueled a rapid rise in fraudulent weight-loss schemes, including slimming soaps that slough off fat in the shower; miracle pills that get rid of excess pounds without dieting or exercise; plastic earplugs that curb the appetite; and even a glittering ring called Fat-Be-Gone that, when slipped on a finger, trims hips, buttocks, and thighs.[395]

But, as former Health and Human Services Secretary Tommy Thompson has bluntly declared, "There's not going to be a miracle weight-loss remedy or pill."[396]

Not only are there no silver bullets now in view, the multifactorial nature of obesity makes it unlikely that there ever will be any. As we look at the horizon, we see no single development—pharmacological or surgical—that, by itself, promises a solution. The redundancy and complex compensatory interactions that characterize human energy regulation are very difficult to interrupt. When a drug blocks one mechanism or peptide, another goes into overdrive to compensate. Moreover, in the human body, energy maintenance does not operate as an isolated island, but is intertwined with other functions. The gut hormone ghrelin is a good example of that. It not only makes us hungry, but it is also essential for tissue repair, bone strength, and muscle growth. Thus, intervening to suppress it may trigger a slew of unnerving (potentially life-threatening) consequences.[397]

Similarly, it is unlikely that surgical approaches will provide us with a "silver scalpel." Today, liposuction (a procedure in which surgeons break up fat deposits and vacuum them out) is the most common type of cosmetic surgery in the United States, with close to half a million procedures a year. According to recent research studies of the procedure (published in the *New England Journal of Medicine*), merely sucking fat out does not give the metabolic benefits (nor does it provide the protection from heart disease and diabetes) that result from losing the same amount of weight through diet and exercise.[398]

> One reason for the finding may be that liposuction removes fat only from under the skin, whereas dieting and exercise reduce deeper deposits in the organs and inside the abdomen; such deposits are believed to be more dangerous. In addition, while liposuction removes some fat cells, it does not shrink [the size of] the billions left behind. [That is very significant, because] studies have shown that larger fat cells are more active metabolically than small ones, and more likely to spew harmful substances into the bloodstream. Dieting does shrink fat cells, making them less prone to release harmful substances.[399]

Realism is not pessimism however.

While this dashes all hopes for a magical solution, our new view of obesity—its multifactorial nature and biopsychosocial determinants—is, in fact, the beginning of real hope. Let's not forget that only a century ago, we took the first step toward managing infectious diseases, replacing demon theories and humors theories with germ theory. That very step, the beginning of hope, in itself dashed all hopes of magical solutions. It told us that progress would be made stepwise, with great effort.[400]

So, I believe, it is with obesity today.

Looking Ahead

A shift in emphasis is desperately required, from seeking pie-in-the-sky solutions to providing people with the tools needed to exercise personal control over their health.[401] People must come to realize that in managing our health and our bodies, we are decision makers who are managing a truly complex and dynamic system: the human body. Effective self-regulation requires *skill*.

Effective regulation of any dynamic system, whether it is the energy regulation of our bodies or the energy regulation of an atomic reactor, requires that we do two things well: (1) understand how and why the system (our body) behaves the way it does; and (2) predict how it will behave in the future. The two skills—understanding and predicting—are interdependent, but conceptually different.

Understanding and prediction skills are the focus of the next two parts of the book. Part III examines understanding, helping ordinary people think systematically about the inner workings of human weight so they can better manage their own bodies and health. Part IV discusses prediction. While understanding helps us look backward to make sense of the past (e.g., explaining weight gain), we need prediction to look forward (e.g., to devise treatment strategies and assess treatment outcomes).

Notes

1. Pool, R. (2001). *Fat: Fighting the Obesity Epidemic.* Oxford: Oxford University Press.
2. Shell, E.R. (2002). *The Hungry Gene: The Inside Story of the Obesity Industry.* New York: Grove Press.
3. Brownell, K.D. (1991). Personal responsibility and control over our bodies: when expectation exceeds reality. *Health Psychology,* 10, 303–310.
4. Leichter, H.M. (2003). Evil habits and personal choices: assigning responsibility for health in the 20th century. *Milbank Quarterly,* 81(4), 603–626; cited in Schwartz, M.B. and Brownell, K.D. (2007). Actions necessary to prevent childhood obesity: creating the climate for change. *Journal of Law, Medicine and Ethics,* 35(1), 78–89.
5. Kolata, G. (2005, April 17). The body heretic: it scorns our efforts. *New York Times.*
6. Brownell, K.D. (1991). Personal responsibility and control over our bodies: when expectation exceeds reality. *Health Psychology,* 10, 303–310.
7. American College of Sports Medicine. (1995). *ACSM's Guidelines for Exercise Testing and Prescription.* Baltimore: Williams & Wilkins.
8. Wadden, T.A. and Stunkard, A.J. (Eds.). (2002). *Handbook of Obesity Treatment.* New York: Guilford Press.
9. Brownell, K.D. and Fairburn, C.G. (Eds.). (1995). *Eating Disorders and Obesity: A Comprehensive Handbook.* New York: Guilford Press.
10. *Ibid.*
11. Skrabanek, P. and McCormick, J. (1990). *Follies and Fallacies in Medicine.* Buffalo, NY: Prometheus Books.
12. *Ibid.*
13. Sterman, J.D. (2000). *Business Dynamics: Systems Thinking and Modeling for a Complex World.* Boston: Irwin McGraw-Hill.
14. Plous, S. (1993). *The Psychology of Judgment and Decision Making.* New York: McGraw-Hill.

15. Tierney, J. (2008, January 1). A 100 percent chance of alarm. *New York Times.*
16. Plous, S. (1993). *The Psychology of Judgment and Decision Making.* New York: McGraw-Hill.
17. Diez-Roux, A.V. (1998). On genes, individuals, society, and epidemiology. *American Journal of Epidemiology,* 148(11), 1027–1032.
18. *Ibid.*
19. Krieger, N. (1994). Epidemiology and the web of causation: has anyone seen the spider? *Social Science and Medicine,* 39(7), 887–903.
20. Wadden, T.A. and Stunkard, A.J. (Eds.). (2002). *Handbook of Obesity Treatment.* New York: Guilford Press.
21. Bjorntorp, P. (2001). Thrifty genes and human obesity. Are we chasing ghosts? *Lancet,* 358, 1006–1008.
22. Wadden, T.A. and Stunkard, A.J. (Eds.). (2002). *Handbook of Obesity Treatment.* New York: Guilford Press.
23. Diez-Roux, A.V. (1998). On genes, individuals, society, and epidemiology. *American Journal of Epidemiology,* 148(11), 1027–1032.
24. Cutler, D.M., Glaeser, E.L. and Shapiro, J.M. (2003). Why have Americans become more obese? *Journal of Economic Perspectives,* 17(3), 93–118.
25. Porter, R. (Ed). (1996). *The Cambridge Illustrated History of Medicine.* Cambridge, UK: Cambridge University Press.
26. Lawrence, P.R. and Nohria, N. (2002). *Driven: How Human Nature Shapes Our Choices.* San Francisco: Jossey-Bass.
27. Pool, R. (2001). *Fat: Fighting the Obesity Epidemic.* Oxford: Oxford University Press.
28. Lawrence, P.R. and Nohria, N. (2002). *Driven: How Human Nature Shapes Our Choices.* San Francisco: Jossey-Bass.
29. *Ibid.*
30. *Ibid.*
31. Eaton, S.B. (1992). Humans, lipids and evolution. *Lipids,* 27(10), 814–820.
32. Pi-Sunyer, X. (2003). A clinical view of the obesity problem. *Science,* 299, 859–860.
33. Peters, J.C., Wyatt, H.R., Donahoo, W.T., and Hill, J.O. (2002). From instinct to intellect: the challenge of maintaining healthy weight in the modern world. *Obesity Reviews,* 3, 69–74.
34. Brownell, K.D. and Horgen, K.B. (2004). *Food Fight.* Chicago: Contemporary Books.
35. Lawrence, P.R. and Nohria, N. (2002). *Driven: How Human Nature Shapes Our Choices.* San Francisco: Jossey-Bass.
36. *Ibid.*
37. Bray, G.A, Bouchard, C., and James, W.P.T. (Eds.). (1998). *Handbook of Obesity.* New York: Marcel Dekker.

38. Wansink, B. and Huckabee, M. (2005). De-marketing obesity. *California Management Review*, 47(4), 6–18.
39. Brown, P.J. (1998). Culture, evolution, and obesity. In: G.A. Bray, C. Bouchard, and W.P.T. James (Eds.). *Handbook of Obesity*. New York: Marcel Dekker.
40. Pool, R. (2001). *Fat: Fighting the Obesity Epidemic*. Oxford: Oxford University Press.
41. Bray, G.A, Bouchard, C., and James, W.P.T. (Eds.). (1998). *Handbook of Obesity*. New York: Marcel Dekker.
42. Eaton, S.B., Eaton, S.B., Konner, M.J., and Shostak, M. (1996). An evolutionary perspective enhances understanding of human nutritional requirements. *Journal of Nutrition*, 126, 1732–1740.
43. Pool, R. (2001). *Fat: Fighting the Obesity Epidemic*. Oxford: Oxford University Press.
44. *Ibid.*
45. Flier, J.S. (2004). Obesity wars: molecular progress confronts an expanding epidemic. *Cell*, 116, 337–350.
46. Leonard, W.R. (2002). Food for thought: dietary change was a driving force in human evolution. *Scientific American,* 287(6):106–115.
47. Walsh, B.T. and Devlin, M.J. (1998). Eating disorders: progress and problems. *Science*, 280, 1387–1390.
48. Shell, E.R. (2002). *The Hungry Gene: The Inside Story of the Obesity Industry*. New York: Grove Press.
49. Whitney, E.N. and Rolfes, S.R. (1999). *Understanding Nutrition*. Belmont, CA: West/Wadsworth.
50. Peters, J.C., Wyatt, H.R., Donahoo, W.T., and Hill, J.O. (2002). From instinct to intellect: the challenge of maintaining healthy weight in the modern world. *Obesity Reviews*, 3, 69–74.
51. Bjorntorp, P. (2001). Thrifty genes and human obesity. Are we chasing ghosts? *Lancet*, 358, 1006–1008.
52. *Ibid.*
53. Jungermann. K. and Barth, C.A. (1996). Energy metabolism and nutrition. In: Greger, R. and Windhorst, U. (Eds.). *Comprehensive Human Physiology*, Vol. 2 (pp. 1425–1457). Berlin, Heidelberg: Springer-Verlag.
54. *Ibid.*
55. Russell, S.A. (2005). *Hunger: An Unnatural History*. New York: Basic Books.
56. Thorburn, A.W. and Proietto, J. (1998). Neuropeptides, the hypothalamus and obesity: insights into the central control of body weight. *Pathology*, 30, 229–236.
57. Powell, K. (2007). The two faces of fat. *Nature,* 447, 525–527.

58. Woods, S.C., Schwartz, M.W., Baskin, D.G., and Seeley, R.J. (2000). Food intake and the regulation of body weight. *Annual Review of Psychology,* 51, 255–277.

59. Mattes, R.D., Pierce, C.B., and Friedman, M.I. (1988). Daily caloric intake of normal-weight adults: response to changes in dietary energy density of a luncheon meal. *American Journal of Clinical Nutrition,* 48, 214–9.

60. Marx, J. (2003). Cellular warriors at the battle of the bulge. *Science,* 299, 846–849.

61. Shell, E.R. (2002). *The Hungry Gene: The Inside Story of the Obesity Industry.* New York: Grove Press.

62. Blundell, J.E. and King, N.A. (1996). Overconsumption as a cause of weight gain: behavioral-physiological interactions in the control of food intake (appetite). In: Ciba Foundation Symposium (Ed.). *The Origins and Consequences of Obesity* (pp. 138–154). Hoboken, NJ: John Wiley.

63. Whitney, E.N. and Rolfes, S.R. (1999). *Understanding Nutrition.* Belmont, CA: West/Wadsworth.

64. Peters, J.C., Wyatt, H.R., Donahoo, W.T., and Hill, J.O. (2002). From instinct to intellect: the challenge of maintaining healthy weight in the modern world. *Obesity Reviews,* 3, 69–74.

65. Polivy, J. and Herman, P. (1985). Dieting and binging: a causal analysis. *American Psychologist,* 40(2), 193–201.

66. Shetty, P.S. (1990). Physiological mechanisms in the adaptive response of metabolic rates to energy restriction. *Nutrition Research Reviews* 3, 49–74.

67. Pi-Sunyer, X. (2003). A clinical view of the obesity problem. *Science,* 299, 859–860.

68. *Ibid.*

69. McArdle, W.D., Katch, F.I., and Katch, V.L. (1996). *Exercise Physiology: Energy, Nutrition, and Human Performance.* Baltimore: Williams & Wilkins.

70. Dalton, S. (Ed.). (1997). *Overweight and Weight Management: The Health Professional's Guide to Understanding and Practice.* Gaithersburg, MD: Aspen.

71. Pi-Sunyer, F.X. (1999). Obesity. In: Shils, M.E., Olson, J.A., Shike, M., and Ross, A.C. (Eds.). *Modern Nutrition in Health and Disease.* Baltimore: Williams & Wilkins.

72. *Ibid.*

73. Whitney, E.N. and Rolfes, S.R. (1999). *Understanding Nutrition.* Belmont, CA: West/Wadsworth.

74. *Ibid.*

75. Koplan, J.P. and Dietz, W.H. (1999). Caloric Imbalance and public health policy. *JAMA,* 282(16), 1579–1581.

76. Brownell, K.D. and Horgen, K.B. (2004). *Food Fight*. Chicago: Contemporary Books.

77. Peters, J.C., Wyatt, H.R., Donahoo, W.T., and Hill, J.O. (2002). From instinct to intellect: the challenge of maintaining healthy weight in the modern world. *Obesity Reviews*, 3, 69–74.

78. Anderson, G.H. (1993). Regulation of food intake. In: Shils, M.E., Olson, J.A., and Shike, M. (Eds.). *Modern Nutrition in Health and Disease*, 8th ed. Philadelphia: Lea and Febiger.

79. Baumeister, R.F., Heatherton, T.F., and Tice, D.M. (1994). *Losing Control: How and Why People Fail at Self-Regulation*. San Diego: Academic Press.

80. Germov, J. and Williams, L. (1996). The epidemic of dieting women: the need for a sociological approach to food and nutrition. *Appetite*, 27, 97–108.

81. Baumeister, R.F., Heatherton, T.F., and Tice, D.M. (1994). *Losing Control: How and Why People Fail at Self-Regulation*. San Diego: Academic Press.

82. Capaldi, E.D. (Ed.). (1996). *Why We Eat What We Eat: The Psychology of Eating*. Washington, DC: American Psychological Association.

83. Blundell, J.E. (1995). The psychobiological approach to appetite and weight control. In: Brownell, K.D. and Fairburn, C.G. (Eds.). *Eating Disorders and Obesity: A Comprehensive Handbook* (pp. 13–20). New York: Guilford Press.

84. Capaldi, E.D. (Ed.). (1996). *Why We Eat What We Eat: The Psychology of Eating*. Washington, DC: American Psychological Association.

85. Krieger, N. (1994). Epidemiology and the web of causation: has anyone seen the spider? *Social Science and Medicine*, 39(7), 887–903.

86. Blundell, J.E. and King, N.A. (1996). Overconsumption as a cause of weight gain: behavioral-physiological interactions in the control of food intake (appetite). In: Ciba Foundation Symposium (Ed.). *The Origins and Consequences of Obesity* (pp. 138–154). Hoboken, NJ: John Wiley and Sons.

87. Bray, G.A, Bouchard, C., and James, W.P.T. (Eds.). (1998). *Handbook of Obesity*. New York: Marcel Dekker.

88. Capaldi, E.D. (Ed.). (1996). *Why We Eat What We Eat: The Psychology of Eating*. Washington, DC: American Psychological Association.

89. Glanz, K., Rimer, B.K., Lewis, F.M. (Eds.). (2002). *Health Behavior and Health Education: Theory, Research, and Practice*. San Francisco: Jossey-Bass.

90. Forrester, J.W. (1979). System Dynamics: Future Opportunities. Paper D-3108-1, The System Dynamics Group, Sloan School of Management, Massachusetts Institute of Technology.

91. Foster, G.D. (2003). Principles and practices in the management of obesity. *American Journal of Respiration and Critical Care Medicine*, 168, 274–280.

92. Stokols, D. (1992). Establishing and maintaining healthy environments. *American Psychologist*, 47(1), 6–22.

93. Diez-Roux, A.V. (1998). On genes, individuals, society, and epidemiology. *American Journal of Epidemiology*, 148(11), 1027–1032.

94. Jervis, R. (1997). *System Effects: Complexity in Political and Social Life.* Princeton, NJ: Princeton University Press.

95. Olshansky, S.J., et al. (2005). A potential decline in life expectancy in the United States in the 21st century. *New England Journal of Medicine,* 352(11), 1138–1145.

96. Taubes, G. (2002, July 7). What if it's all been a big fat lie? *New York Times Magazine*, p. 22.

97. Nestle, M. (2002). *Food Politics: How the Food Industry Influences Nutrition and Health.* Berkeley, CA: University of California Press.

98. Nielsen, S.J. and Popkin, B.M. (2004). Changes in beverage intake between 1977 and 2001. *American Journal of Preventive Medicine*, 27(3), 205–210.

99. Puttnam, J., Kantor, L.S., and Allshouse, J. (2000). Per capita food supply trends: progress toward dietary guidelines. *Food Review*, 23(3), 2–14.

100. Nielsen, S.J. and Popkin, B.M. (2004). Changes in beverage intake between 1977 and 2001. *American Journal of Preventive Medicine*, 27(3), 205–210.

101. Young, L.R. and Nestle, M. (2002). The contribution of expanding portion sizes to the US obesity epidemic. *American Journal of Public Health*, 92(2), 246–249.

102. Nestle, M. and Jacobson, M.F. (2000). Halting the obesity epidemic: a public health policy approach. *Public Health Reports*, 115, 12–24.

103. McCrory, M.A., Suen, V.M.M., and Roberts, S.B. (2002). Biobehavioral influences on energy intake and adult weight gain. *Journal of Nutrition*, 132, S3830–S3836.

104. Cutler, D.M., Glaeser, E.L. and Shapiro, J.M. (2003). Why have Americans become more obese? *Journal of Economic Perspectives*, 17(3), 93–118.

105. Nestle, M. (2002). *Food Politics: How the Food Industry Influences Nutrition and Health.* Berkeley, CA: University of California Press.

106. Puttnam, J., Kantor, L.S., and Allshouse, J. (2000). Per capita food supply trends: progress toward dietary guidelines. *Food Review*, 23(3), 2–14.

107. McCrory, M.A., Suen, V.M.M., and Roberts, S.B. (2002). Biobehavioral influences on energy intake and adult weight gain. *Journal of Nutrition*, 132, S3830–S3836.

108. Oliver, J.E. (2006). *Fat Politics: The Real Story Behind America's Obesity Epidemic.* Oxford, UK: Oxford University Press.

109. Cutler, D.M., Glaeser, E.L. and Shapiro, J.M. (2003). Why have Americans become more obese? *Journal of Economic Perspectives,* 17(3), 93–118.
110. Brownell, K.D. and Horgen, K.B. (2004). *Food Fight.* Chicago: Contemporary Books.
111. *Ibid.*
112. Cutler, D.M., Glaeser, E.L. and Shapiro, J.M. (2003). Why have Americans become more obese? *Journal of Economic Perspectives,* 17(3), 93–118.
113. Dunn, D. (1997). Introduction to the study of women and work. In: Dunn, D. (Ed.). *Workplace/Women's Place: An Anthology.* Los Angeles: Roxbury.
114. Nestle, M. (2002). *Food Politics: How the Food Industry Influences Nutrition and Health.* Berkeley, CA: University of California Press.
115. Cutler, D.M., Glaeser, E.L. and Shapiro, J.M. (2003). Why have Americans become more obese? *Journal of Economic Perspectives,* 17(3), 93–118.
116. Chou, S., Grossman, M., and Saffer, H. (2001). An economic analysis of adult obesity: results from the behavioral risk factor surveillance system. Third International Health Economics Association Conference, York, England, July 23–25, 2001.
117. Burke, J. (1995). *Connections.* Boston: Little, Brown.
118. Cutler, D.M., Glaeser, E.L. and Shapiro, J.M. (2003). Why have Americans become more obese? *Journal of Economic Perspectives,* 17(3), 93–118.
119. *Ibid.*
120. Philipson, T. (2001). The world-wide growth in obesity: an economic research agenda. *Health Economics,* 10, 1–7.
121. Cutler, D.M., Glaeser, E.L. and Shapiro, J.M. (2003). Why have Americans become more obese? *Journal of Economic Perspectives,* 17(3), 93–118.
122. Bowers, D.E. (2000). Cooking trends echo changing roles of women. *Food Review,* 23(1), 23–29.
123. French, S.A., Story, M., and Jeffery, R.W. (2001). Environmental influences on eating and physical activity. *Annual Review of Public Health,* 22, 309–35.
124. Cutler, D.M., Glaeser, E.L. and Shapiro, J.M. (2003). Why have Americans become more obese? *Journal of Economic Perspectives,* 17(3), 93–118.
125. Bowers, D.E. (2000). Cooking trends echo changing roles of women. *Food Review,* 23(1), 23–29.
126. Brownell, K.D. and Horgen, K.B. (2004). *Food Fight.* Chicago: Contemporary Books.

127. Mitka, M. (2003). Economist takes aim at "big fat" US lifestyle. *JAMA*, 289(1), 33–34.
128. Hill, J.O., et al. (2003). Obesity and the environment: where do we go from here? *Science*, 299, 853–855.
129. Philipson, T.J. and Posner, R.A. (2003). The long-run growth in obesity as a function of technological change. *Perspectives in Biology and Medicine,* 46(3), S87–S107.
130. Raeburn, P. et al. (2002, October 21). Why we're so fat. *Business Week*, pp. 112–114.
131. French, S.A., Story, M., and Jeffery, R.W. (2001). Environmental influences on eating and physical activity. *Annual Review of Public Health*, 22, 309–35.
132. Philipson, T. (2001). The world-wide growth in obesity: an economic research agenda. *Health Economics*, 10, 1–7.
133. Cutler, D.M., Glaeser, E.L. and Shapiro, J.M. (2003). Why have Americans become more obese? *Journal of Economic Perspectives,* 17(3), 93–118.
134. Laigh, A. (2003, May 15). Increasing obesity: slim hopes for a culture that lacks self-control. *Sydney Morning Herald.*
135. Critser, G. (2003). *Fat Land: How Americans Became the Fattest People in the World.* Boston: Mariner Books.
136. Cutler, D.M., Glaeser, E.L. and Shapiro, J.M. (2003). Why have Americans become more obese? *Journal of Economic Perspectives,* 17(3), 93–118.
137. Oliver, J.E. (2006). *Fat Politics: The Real Story Behind America's Obesity Epidemic.* Oxford, UK: Oxford University Press.
138. McCrory, M.A., Suen, V.M.M., and Roberts, S.B. (2002). Biobehavioral influences on energy intake and adult weight gain. *Journal of Nutrition*, 132, S3830–S3836.
139. Franklin, B.A. (2001). The downside of our technological revolution? An obesity-conducive environment. *American Journal of Cardiology*, 87, 1093–1095.
140. Zizza, C., et al. (2001). Significant increase in young adults' snacking between 1977–1978 and 1994–1996 represents a cause for concern! *Preventive Medicine*, 32, 303–310.
141. Kenney, J.J. (2004). To snack or not to snack, that is the question. www.foodandhealth.com.
142. *Ibid.*
143. McCrory, M.A., Suen, V.M.M., and Roberts, S.B. (2002). Biobehavioral influences on energy intake and adult weight gain. *Journal of Nutrition*, 132, S3830–S3836.
144. Oliver, J.E. (2006). *Fat Politics: The Real Story Behind America's Obesity Epidemic.* Oxford, UK: Oxford University Press.

145. McCrory, M.A., Suen, V.M.M., and Roberts, S.B. (2002). Biobehavioral influences on energy intake and adult weight gain. *Journal of Nutrition*, 132, S3830–S3836.

146. French, S.A., Story, M., and Jeffery, R.W. (2001). Environmental influences on eating and physical activity. *Annual Review of Public Health*, 22, 309–35.

147. Oliver, J.E. (2006). *Fat Politics: The Real Story Behind America's Obesity Epidemic*. Oxford, UK: Oxford University Press.

148. Schlosser, E. (2002). *Fast Food Nation: The Dark Side of the All-American Meal*. New York: Perennial.

149. DiMeglio, D.P. and Mattes, R.D. (2000). Liquid versus solid carbohydrate: effects on food intake and body weight. *International Journal of Obesity*, 24, 794–800.

150. McCrory, M.A., Suen, V.M.M., and Roberts, S.B. (2002). Biobehavioral influences on energy intake and adult weight gain. *Journal of Nutrition*, 132, S3830–S3836.

151. Schlosser, E. (2002). *Fast Food Nation: The Dark Side of the All-American Meal*. New York: Perennial.

152. Critser, G. (2003). *Fat Land: How Americans Became the Fattest People in the World*. Boston: Mariner Books.

153. *Ibid.*

154. Taras, H., et al. (2004). Soft drinks in school. *Pediatrics*, 113(1), 152–154.

155. Critser, G. (2003). *Fat Land: How Americans Became the Fattest People in the World*. Boston: Mariner Books.

156. Ludwig, D.S., Peterson, K.E., and Gortmaker, S.L. (2001). Relation between consumption of sugar-sweetened drinks and childhood obesity: a prospective, observational analysis. *Lancet*, 357, 505–508.

157. Brownell, K.D. and Horgen, K.B. (2004). *Food Fight*. Chicago: Contemporary Books.

158. Popkin, B.M. (2007). The world is fat. *Scientific American*, 297(3), 88–95.

159. DiMeglio, D.P. and Mattes, R.D. (2000). Liquid versus solid carbohydrate: effects on food intake and body weight. *International Journal of Obesity*, 24, 794–800.

160. A measure of the potential of water molecules to move between regions of differing concentrations across a water-permeable membrane.

161. Bowers, D.E. (2000). Cooking trends echo changing roles of women. *Food Review*, 23(1), 23–29.

162. McCrory, M.A., Suen, V.M.M., and Roberts, S.B. (2002). Biobehavioral influences on energy intake and adult weight gain. *Journal of Nutrition*, 132, S3830–S3836.

163. Brody, J. (2002, July 16). How to eat without tipping the scale. *New York Times*, p. D7.

164. Schlosser, E. (2002). *Fast Food Nation: The Dark Side of the All-American Meal*. New York: Perennial.

165. Shell, E.R. (2002). *The Hungry Gene: The Inside Story of the Obesity Industry*. New York: Grove Press.

166. French, S.A., Story, M., and Jeffery, R.W. (2001). Environmental influences on eating and physical activity. *Annual Review of Public Health*, 22, 309–35.

167. Barboza, D. (2003, August 3). If you pitch it, they will eat. *New York Times*.

168. Story, M., Neumark-Sztainer, D., and French, S. (2002). Individual and environmental influences on adolescent eating behaviors. *Supplement to the Journal of the American Dietetic Association*, 102(3), S40–S51.

169. Buckley, N. (2003, February 18). Unhealthy food is everywhere, 24 hours a day, and inexpensive. *Financial Times*, p. 13.

170. Bowers, D.E. (2000). Cooking trends echo changing roles of women. *Food Review*, 23(1), 23–29.

171. Rothman Morris, B. (2005, October 26). Eating, drinking, cooking and, oh yes, driving, too. *New York Times*.

172. Shell, E.R. (2002). *The Hungry Gene: The Inside Story of the Obesity Industry*. New York: Grove Press.

173. Critser, G. (2003). *Fat Land: How Americans Became the Fattest People in the World*. Boston: Mariner Books.

174. Bowman, S.A., et al. (2004). Effects of fast-food consumption on energy intake and diet quality among children in a national household survey. *Pediatrics*, 113(1), 112–118.

175. French, S.A., et al. (2001). Fast food restaurant use among adolescents: associations with nutrient intake, food choices and behavioral and psychosocial variables. *International Journal of Obesity*, 25, 1823–1833.

176. McCrory, M.A., Suen, V.M.M., and Roberts, S.B. (2002). Biobehavioral influences on energy intake and adult weight gain. *Journal of Nutrition*, 132, S3830–S3836.

177. McCrory, M.A., et al. (1999). Overeating in America: association between restaurant food consumption and body fatness in healthy adult men and women ages 19 to 80. *Obesity Research*, 7(6), 564–571.

178. Bowman, S.A., et al. (2004). Effects of fast-food consumption on energy intake and diet quality among children in a national household survey. *Pediatrics*, 113(1), 112–118.

179. Pollan, M. (2006). *The Omnivore's Dilemma: A Natural History of Four Meals*. New York: Penguin Press.

180. French, S.A., et al. (2001). Fast food restaurant use among adolescents: associations with nutrient intake, food choices and behavioral and psychosocial variables. *International Journal of Obesity*, 25, 1823–1833.

181. French, S.A., Story, M., and Jeffery, R.W. (2001). Environmental influences on eating and physical activity. *Annual Review of Public Health*, 22, 309–35.

182. Drewnowski, A. (2003). Fat and sugar: An economic analysis. *Journal of Nutrition*, 133, 838S–840S.

183. Critser, G. (2003). *Fat Land: How Americans Became the Fattest People in the World*. Boston: Mariner Books.

184. French, S.A., Story, M., and Jeffery, R.W. (2001). Environmental influences on eating and physical activity. *Annual Review of Public Health*, 22, 309–35.

185. Poppitt, S.D. and Prentice, A.M. (1996). Energy density and its role in the control of food intake: evidence from metabolic and community studies. *Appetite*, 26, 153–174.

186. Blundell, J.E. (1995). The psychobiological approach to appetite and weight control. In: Brownell, K.D. and Fairburn, C.G. (Eds.). *Eating Disorders and Obesity: A Comprehensive Handbook* (pp. 13–20). New York: Guilford Press.

187. Drenowski, A. and Specter, S.E. (2004). Poverty and obesity: the role of energy density and energy costs. *American Journal of Clinical Nutrition*, 79, 6–16.

188. *Ibid.*

189. Hill, J.O., Wyatt, H.R., and Melanson, E.L. (2000). Genetic and environmental contributions to obesity. *Medical Clinics of North America*, 84(2), 333–346.

190. Stubbs, R.J., Prentice, A.M., and James, W.P.T. (1997). Carbohydrates and energy balance. *Annals of the New York Academy of Sciences*, 819(1), 44–69.

191. Blundell, J.E. and King, N.A. (1996). Overconsumption as a cause of weight gain: behavioral-physiological interactions in the control of food intake (appetite). In: Ciba Foundation Symposium (Ed.). *The Origins and Consequences of Obesity* (pp. 138–154). Hoboken, NJ: John Wiley and Sons.

192. *Ibid.*

193. Poppitt, S.D. and Prentice, A.M. (1996). Energy density and its role in the control of food intake: evidence from metabolic and community studies. *Appetite*, 26, 153–174.

194. Drenowski, A. and Specter, S.E. (2004). Poverty and obesity: the role of energy density and energy costs. *American Journal of Clinical Nutrition*, 79, 6–16.

195. Brody, I. (2004, October 5). With fruits and vegetables, more can be less. *New York Times*, p. D8.

196. Critser, G. (2003). *Fat Land: How Americans Became the Fattest People in the World*. Boston: Mariner Books.

197. Hazab, G. (2004, July 6). You are how you eat. *New York Times.*
198. Winter, G. (2002, July 7). America rubs its stomach, and says bring it in. *New York Times*, p. 5.
199. Shell, E.R. (2002). *The Hungry Gene: The Inside Story of the Obesity Industry.* New York: Grove Press.
200. Whitney, E.N. and Rolfes, S.R. (1999). *Understanding Nutrition.* Belmont, CA: West/Wadsworth.
201. Brownell, K.D. and Horgen, K.B. (2004). *Food Fight.* Chicago: Contemporary Books.
202. Franklin, B.A. (2001). The downside of our technological revolution? An obesity-conducive environment. *American Journal of Cardiology*, 87, 1093–1095.
203. *Ibid.*
204. Brownell, K.D. and Horgen, K.B. (2004). *Food Fight.* Chicago: Contemporary Books.
205. Nielsen, S.J. and Popkin, B.M. (2004). Changes in beverage intake between 1977 and 2001. *American Journal of Preventive Medicine*, 27(3), 205–210.
206. Critser, G. (2003). *Fat Land: How Americans Became the Fattest People in the World.* Boston: Mariner Books.
207. Brownell, K.D. and Horgen, K.B. (2004). *Food Fight.* Chicago: Contemporary Books.
208. Brody, J. (2006, July 11). Forget the second helpings. it's the first ones that count. *New York Times.*
209. Spencer, M. (2004, November 7). Let them eat cake. *The Guardian Weekly.*
210. Goode, E. (2003, July 22). The gorge-yourself environment. *New York Times*, p. F1
211. Winter, G. (2002, July 7). America rubs its stomach, and says bring it in. *New York Times*, p. 5.
212. Brody, J. (2006, July 11). Forget the second helpings. it's the first ones that count. *New York Times.*
213. Martin, A. (2007, March 25). Will diners still swallow this? *New York Times.*
214. Brownell, K.D. and Horgen, K.B. (2004). *Food Fight.* Chicago: Contemporary Books.
215. Young, L.R. and Nestle, M. (2002). The contribution of expanding portion sizes to the US obesity epidemic. *American Journal of Public Health*, 92(2), 246–249.
216. Brownell, K.D. and Horgen, K.B. (2004). *Food Fight.* Chicago: Contemporary Books.
217. Winter, G. (2002, July 7). America rubs its stomach, and says bring it in. *New York Times*, p. 5.

218. Pollan, M. (2003, October 26). The (agri)cultural contradictions of obesity. *New York Times Magazine,* p. 41.

219. Martin, A. (2007, March 25). Will diners still swallow this? *New York Times.*

220. Young, L.R. and Nestle, M. (2002). The contribution of expanding portion sizes to the US obesity epidemic. *American Journal of Public Health,* 92(2), 246–249.

221. McCrory, M.A., Suen, V.M.M., and Roberts, S.B. (2002). Biobehavioral influences on energy intake and adult weight gain. *Journal of Nutrition,* 132, S3830–S3836.

222. Critser, G. (2003). *Fat Land: How Americans Became the Fattest People in the World.* Boston: Mariner Books.

223. Rolls, B.J., Engell, D., and Birch, L.L. (2000). Serving portion size influences 5-year-old but not 3-year-old children's food intakes. *Journal of the American Dietetic Association,* 100(2), 232–234.

224. French, S.A., Story, M., and Jeffery, R.W. (2001). Environmental influences on eating and physical activity. *Annual Review of Public Health,* 22, 309–335.

225. Critser, G. (2003). *Fat Land: How Americans Became the Fattest People in the World.* Boston: Mariner Books.

226. *Ibid.*

227. Rolls, B.J., Engell, D., and Birch, L.L. (2000). Serving portion size influences 5-year-old but not 3-year-old children's food intakes. *Journal of the American Dietetic Association,* 100(2), 232–234.

228. Critser, G. (2003). *Fat Land: How Americans Became the Fattest People in the World.* Boston: Mariner Books.

229. Rolls, B.J., Morris, E., and Roe, L.S. (2002). Portion size of food affects energy intake in normal-weight and overweight men and women. *American Journal of Clinical Nutrition,* 76, 1207–1213.

230. *Ibid.*

231. *Ibid.*

232. Pollan, M. (2006). *The Omnivore's Dilemma: A Natural History of Four Meals.* New York: Penguin Press.

233. Brownell, K.D. and Horgen, K.B. (2004). *Food Fight.* Chicago: Contemporary Books.

234. Pollan, M. (2006). *The Omnivore's Dilemma: A Natural History of Four Meals.* New York: Penguin Press.

235. Senge, P.M. (1990). *The Fifth Discipline: The Art and Practice of the Learning Organization.* New York: Doubleday/Currency.

236. Sterman, J.D. (2000). *Business Dynamics: Systems Thinking and Modeling for a Complex World.* Boston: Irwin McGraw-Hill.

237. Senge, P.M. (1990). *The Fifth Discipline: The Art and Practice of the Learning Organization.* New York: Doubleday/Currency.

238. Sterman, J.D. (2000). *Business Dynamics: Systems Thinking and Modeling for a Complex World*. Boston: Irwin McGraw-Hill.

239. *Ibid.*

240. Bowers, D.E. (2000). Cooking trends echo changing roles of women. *Food Review*, 23(1), 23–29.

241. *Ibid.*

242. Foderaro, L.W. (2004, November 14). These days, the college bowl is filled with milk and cereal. *New York Times.*

243. Drewnowski, A. (2003). Fat and sugar: an economic analysis. *Journal of Nutrition*, 133, 838S-840S.

244. Shell, E.R. (2002). *The Hungry Gene: The Inside Story of the Obesity Industry*. New York: Grove Press.

245. Critser, G. (2003). *Fat Land: How Americans Became the Fattest People in the World*. Boston: Mariner Books.

246. French, S.A., Story, M., Jeffery, R.W. (2001). Environmental influences on eating and physical activity. *Annual Review of Public Health*. 22, 309–35.

247. French, S.A. (2003). Pricing effects on food choices. *Journal of Nutrition,* 133, 841S–843S.

248. Glanz, K., Rimer, B.K., Lewis, F.M. (Eds.). (2002). *Health Behavior and Health Education: Theory, Research, and Practice*. San Francisco: Jossey-Bass.

249. McCrory, M.A., Suen, V.M.M., and Roberts, S.B. (2002). Biobehavioral influences on energy intake and adult weight gain. *Journal of Nutrition*, 132, S3830–S3836.

250. Warner, M. (2005, May 15). Low-carbs? Who cares? Sugar is latest supermarket demon. *New York Times.*

251. Critser, G. (2003). *Fat Land: How Americans Became the Fattest People in the World*. Boston: Mariner Books.

252. Goode, E. (2003, July 22). The gorge-yourself environment. *New York Times*, p. F1

253. Critser, G. (2003). *Fat Land: How Americans Became the Fattest People in the World*. Boston: Mariner Books.

254. McCrory, M.A. et al., (1999). Dietary variety within food groups: association with energy intake and body fatness in men and women. *American Journal of Clinical Nutrition,* 69, 440–447.

255. Critser, G. (2003). *Fat Land: How Americans Became the Fattest People in the World*. Boston: Mariner Books.

256. Story, M., Neumark-Sztainer, D., and French, S. (2002). Individual and environmental influences on adolescent eating behaviors. *Supplement to the Journal of the American Dietetic Association*, 102(3), S40–S51.

257. Buckley, N. (2003, February 18). Unhealthy food is everywhere, 24 hours a day, and inexpensive. *Financial Times*, p. 13.
258. *Ibid.*
259. Goode, E. (2003, July 22). The gorge-yourself environment. *New York Times*, p. F1
260. Nestle, M. and Jacobson, M.F. (2000). Halting the obesity epidemic: a public health policy approach. *Public Health Reports*, 115, 12–24.
261. French, S.A., Story, M., and Jeffery, R.W. (2001). Environmental influences on eating and physical activity. *Annual Review of Public Health*, 22, 309–35.
262. Birch, L.L. and Fisher, J.O. (1998). Development of eating behaviors among children and adolescents. *Pediatrics*, 101(3 Suppl), 539–549.
263. Glanz, K., Rimer, B.K., Lewis, F.M. (Eds.). (2002). *Health Behavior and Health Education: Theory, Research, and Practice.* San Francisco: Jossey-Bass.
264. Stokols, D. (1992). Establishing and maintaining healthy environments. *American Psychologist*, 47(1), 6–22.
265. Sterman, J.D. (2006). Learning from evidence in a complex world. *American Journal of Public Health*, 96(3), 505–514.
266. Leonard, W.R. (2002). Food for thought: dietary change was a driving force in human evolution. *Scientific American,* 287(6):106–115.
267. Eaton, S.B., Eaton, S.B., Konner, M.J., and Shostak, M. (1996). An evolutionary perspective enhances understanding of human nutritional requirements. *Journal of Nutrition,* 126, 1732–1740.
268. Eaton, S. B., Eaton, S. B. III, and Cordain, L. (2002) Evolution, diet, and health. In: Ungar. P.S. and Teaford, M.F. (Eds.). *Human Diet: Its Origin and Evolution* (pp. 7–17). Westport, CT: Bergin and Garvey.
269. Philipson, T.J. and Posner, R.A. (2003). The long-run growth in obesity as a function of technological change. *Perspectives in Biology and Medicine,* 46(3), S87–S107.
270. Franklin, B.A. (2001). The downside of our technological revolution? An obesity-conducive environment. *American Journal of Cardiology*, 87, 1093–1095.
271. French, S.A., Story, M., and Jeffery, R.W. (2001). Environmental influences on eating and physical activity. *Annual Review of Public Health*, 22, 309–35.
272. Dunn, D. (1997). Introduction to the study of women and work. In: Dunn, D. (Ed.). *Workplace/Women's Place: An Anthology.* Los Angeles: Roxbury.
273. Nestle, M. and Jacobson, M.F. (2000). Halting the obesity epidemic: a public health policy approach. *Public Health Reports*, 115, 12–24.

274. French, S.A., Story, M., and Jeffery, R.W. (2001). Environmental influences on eating and physical activity. *Annual Review of Public Health*, 22, 309–35.
275. McArdle, W.D., Katch, F.I., and Katch, V.L. (1996). *Exercise Physiology: Energy, Nutrition, and Human Performance*. Baltimore: Williams & Wilkins.
276. French, S.A., Story, M., and Jeffery, R.W. (2001). Environmental influences on eating and physical activity. *Annual Review of Public Health*, 22, 309–35.
277. Brownell, K.D. and Horgen, K.B. (2004). *Food Fight*. Chicago: Contemporary Books.
278. Philipson, T.J. and Posner, R.A. (2003). The long-run growth in obesity as a function of technological change. *Perspectives in Biology and Medicine*, 46(3), S87–S107.
279. Brownell, K.D. and Horgen, K.B. (2004). *Food Fight*. Chicago: Contemporary Books.
280. Postrel, V. (2001, March 22). Americans' waistlines have become the victims of economic progress. *New York Times*, p. C2.
281. Franklin, B.A. (2001). The downside of our technological revolution? An obesity-conducive environment. *American Journal of Cardiology*, 87, 1093–1095.
282. Brownell, K.D. and Horgen, K.B. (2004). *Food Fight*. Chicago: Contemporary Books.
283. Shell, E.R. (2002). *The Hungry Gene: The Inside Story of the Obesity Industry*. New York: Grove Press.
284. *Ibid.*
285. Bray, G.A, Bouchard, C., and James, W.P.T. (Eds.). (1998). *Handbook of Obesity*. New York: Marcel Dekker.
286. Forrester, J.W. (1979). System Dynamics: Future Opportunities. Paper D-3108-1, The System Dynamics Group, Sloan School of Management, Massachusetts Institute of Technology.
287. Nestle, M. and Jacobson, M.F. (2000). Halting the obesity epidemic: a public health policy approach. *Public Health Reports*, 115, 12–24.
288. Shell, E.R. (2002). *The Hungry Gene: The Inside Story of the Obesity Industry*. New York: Grove Press.
289. French, S.A., Story, M., and Jeffery, R.W. (2001). Environmental influences on eating and physical activity. *Annual Review of Public Health*, 22, 309–35.
290. Cutler, D.M., Glaeser, E.L. and Shapiro, J.M. (2003). Why Have Americans Become More Obese? *Journal of Economic Perspectives*, 17(3), 93–118.
291. Koplan, J.P. and Dietz, W.H. (1999). Caloric Imbalance and public health policy. *JAMA*, 282(16), 1579–1581.

292. Hill, J.O., et al. (2003). Obesity and the environment: Where do we go from here? *Science*, 299, 853–855.
293. Shell, E.R. (2002). *The Hungry Gene: The Inside Story of the Obesity Industry*. New York: Grove Press.
294. French, S.A., Story, M., and Jeffery, R.W. (2001). Environmental influences on eating and physical activity. *Annual Review of Public Health*, 22, 309–35.
295. Liao, Y. (2002). Vehicle ownership patterns of American households. UTC-UIC Information Brief IB-10B-02, University of Illinois at Chicago, Urban Transportation Center.
296. Moore, M. (2003, April 23). City, suburban designs could be bad for your health. *USA Today*, p. 1.
297. Shell, E.R. (2002). *The Hungry Gene: The Inside Story of the Obesity Industry*. New York: Grove Press.
298. Spors, K. (2003, October 21). Don't just sit there. *Wall Street Journal*, p. R8.
299. Franklin, B.A. (2001). The downside of our technological revolution? An obesity-conducive environment. *American Journal of Cardiology*, 87, 1093–1095.
300. *Ibid.*
301. French, S.A., Story, M., and Jeffery, R.W. (2001). Environmental influences on eating and physical activity. *Annual Review of Public Health*, 22, 309–35.
302. Schlosser, E. (2002). *Fast Food Nation: The Dark Side of the All-American Meal*. New York: Perennial.
303. Brody, J. (2004, August 3). TV's toll on young minds and bodies. *New York Times*.
304. French, S.A., Story, M., and Jeffery, R.W. (2001). Environmental influences on eating and physical activity. *Annual Review of Public Health*, 22, 309–35.
305. Elias, M. (2005, March 9). Electronic world swallows up kids' time, study finds. *USA Today*.
306. Schlosser, E. (2002). *Fast Food Nation: The Dark Side of the All-American Meal*. New York: Perennial.
307. Dalton, S. ed. (1997). *Overweight and Weight Management: The Health Professional's Guide to Understanding and Practice*. Gaithersburg, MD: An Aspen Publication.
308. Brownell, K.D. and Horgen, K.B. (2004). *Food Fight*. Chicago: Contemporary Books.
309. McArdle, W.D., Katch, F.I., and Katch, V.L. (1996). *Exercise Physiology: Energy, Nutrition, and Human Performance*. Baltimore: Williams & Wilkins.

310. Wadden, T.A. and Stunkard, A.J. (Eds.). (2002). *Handbook of Obesity Treatment*. New York: Guilford Press.

311. McArdle, W.D., Katch, F.I., and Katch, V.L. (1996). *Exercise Physiology: Energy, Nutrition, and Human Performance*. Baltimore: Williams & Wilkins.

312. Markoff, J. (2004, December 30). Internet use said to cut into TV viewing and socializing. *New York Times*.

313. Hu, F.B. et al. (2003). Television watching and other sedentary behaviors in relation to risk of obesity and type 2 diabetes mellitus in women. *JAMA*, 289(14), 1785–1791.

314. French, S.A., Story, M., and Jeffery, R.W. (2001). Environmental influences on eating and physical activity. *Annual Review of Public Health*, 22, 309–35.

315. Racette, S.B., Deusinger, S.S., and Deusinger, R.H. (2003). Obesity: overview of prevalence, etiology, and treatment. *Physical Therapy*, 83(3), 276–288.

316. Nestle, M. (2002). *Food Politics: How the food industry influences nutrition and health*. Berkeley, CA: University of California Press.

317. Brody, J. (2004, January 20). The widening of America, or how size 4 became a size 0. *New York Times*, p. D7.

318. Nestle, M. and Jacobson, M.F. (2000). Halting the obesity epidemic: a public health policy approach. *Public Health Reports*, 115, 12–24.

319. Critser, G. (2003). *Fat Land: How Americans Became the Fattest People in the World*. Boston: Mariner Books.

320. McArdle, W.D., Katch, F.I., and Katch, V.L. (1996). *Exercise Physiology: Energy, Nutrition, and Human Performance*. Baltimore: Williams & Wilkins.

321. Pool, R. (2001). *Fat: Fighting the Obesity Epidemic*. Oxford: Oxford University Press.

322. Forrester, J.W. (1979). System Dynamics: Future Opportunities. Paper D-3108-1, The System Dynamics Group, Sloan School of Management, Massachusetts Institute of Technology.

323. Brownell, K.D. and Horgen, K.B. (2004). *Food Fight*. Chicago: Contemporary Books.

324. Shils, M.E., Olson, J.A., Shike, M., and Ross, A.C. (Eds.). (1999). *Modern Nutrition in Health and Disease*. Baltimore: Williams & Wilkins.

325. Mulvihill, M.L. (1995). *Human Diseases: A Systemic Approach*. Stamford, CT: Appleton and Lange.

326. Brown, G. (1999). *The Energy of Life: The Science of What Makes Our Minds and Bodies Work*. New York: Free Press.

327. Brooks, G.A., Fahey, T.D., White, T.P., and Baldwin K.M. (2000). *Exercise Physiology: Human Bioenergetics and Its Applications*. Mountain View, CA: Mayfield.

328. Bouchard, C. and Pérusse, L. (1993). Genetics of obesity. *Annual Review of Nutrition,* 13, 337–354.
329. Spirduso, W.W. (1995). *Physical Dimensions of Aging.* Champaign, IL: Human Kinetics.
330. Koplan, J.P. and Dietz, W.H. (1999). Caloric imbalance and public health policy. *JAMA,* 282(16), 1579–1581.
331. Diez-Roux, A.V. (1998). On genes, individuals, society, and epidemiology. *American Journal of Epidemiology,* 148(11), 1027–1032.
332. Franklin, B.A. (2001). The downside of our technological revolution? An obesity-conducive environment. *American Journal of Cardiology,* 87, 1093–1095.
333. Shell, E.R. (2002). *The Hungry Gene: The Inside Story of the Obesity Industry.* New York: Grove Press.
334. *Ibid.*
335. Racette, S.B., Deusinger, S.S., and Deusinger, R.H. (2003). Obesity: overview of prevalence, etiology, and treatment. *Physical Therapy,* 83(3), 276–288.
336. Murray, J.E. (1997). Standards of the present for people of the past: height, weight, and mortality among men of Amherst College, 1834–1949. *Journal of Economic History,* 57(3), 585–606; cited in Friedman, J.M. (2003). A war on obesity, not the obese. *Science,* 299, 856–863.
337. Wadden, T.A. and Stunkard, A.J. (Eds.). (2002). *Handbook of Obesity Treatment.* New York: Guilford Press.
338. Marx, J. (2003). Cellular warriors at the battle of the bulge. *Science,* 299, 846–849.
339. Shell, E.R. (2002). *The Hungry Gene: The Inside Story of the Obesity Industry.* New York: Grove Press.
340. American College of Sports Medicine. (1995). *ACSM's Guidelines for Exercise Testing and Prescription.* Baltimore: Williams & Wilkins.
341. Nuland, S.B. (2000). *The Mysteries Within: A Surgeon Reflects on Medical Myths.* New York: Simon and Schuster.
342. Bouchard, C. and Pérusse, L. (1993). Genetics of Obesity. *Annual Review of Nutrition,* 13, 337–354.
343. Stipanuk, M.H. (Ed.). (2000). *Biochemical and Physiological Aspects of Human Nutrition.* Philadelphia: W.B. Saunders.
344. Henig, R.M. (2006, August 13). Fat Factors. *New York Times.*
345. Oliver, J.E. (2006). *Fat Politics: The Real Story Behind America's Obesity Epidemic.* Oxford, UK: Oxford University Press.
346. Korner, J. and Leibel, R.L. (2003). To eat or not to eat: how the gut talks to the brain. *New England Journal of Medicine,* 349, 926–928.
347. Oliver, J.E. (2006). *Fat Politics: The Real Story Behind America's Obesity Epidemic.* Oxford, UK: Oxford University Press.

348. Kaufman, F.R. (2005). *Diabesity: The Obesity-Diabetes Epidemic that Threatens America—and What We Must Do to Stop It.* New York: Bantam Books.

349. Brownell, K.D. and Fairburn, C.G. (Eds.). (1995). *Eating Disorders and Obesity: A Comprehensive Handbook.* New York: Guilford Press.

350. Pool, R. (2001). *Fat: Fighting the Obesity Epidemic.* Oxford: Oxford University Press.

351. *Ibid.*

352. Bouchard, C. (1997). Human variation in body mass: evidence for a role of the genes. *Nutrition Reviews,* 55(1), S21–S30.

353. National Institutes of Health. (1998). *Clinical Guidelines on the Identification, Evaluation, and Treatment of Overweight and Obesity in Adults.* U.S. Department of Health and Human Services, NIH Publication No. 98–4083.

354. Pool, R. (2001). *Fat: Fighting the Obesity Epidemic.* Oxford: Oxford University Press.

355. Wadden, T.A. and Stunkard, A.J. (Eds.). (2002). *Handbook of Obesity Treatment.* New York: Guilford Press.

356. Whitney, E.N. and Rolfes, S.R. (1999). *Understanding Nutrition.* Belmont, CA: West/Wadsworth.

357. Pool, R. (2001). *Fat: Fighting the Obesity Epidemic.* Oxford: Oxford University Press.

358. Whitney, E.N. and Rolfes, S.R. (1999). *Understanding Nutrition.* Belmont, CA: West/Wadsworth.

359. Wadden, T.A. and Stunkard, A.J. (Eds.). (2002). *Handbook of Obesity Treatment.* New York: Guilford Press.

360. Pool, R. (2001). *Fat: Fighting the Obesity Epidemic.* Oxford: Oxford University Press.

361. Stubbs, J., Murgatroyd, P.R., Goldberg, G.R., and Prentice, A.M. (1993). Carbohydrate balance and the regulation of day-to-day food intake in humans. *American Journal of Clinical Nutrition,* 57, 897–903.

362. Stipanuk, M.H. (Ed.). (2000). *Biochemical and Physiological Aspects of Human Nutrition.* Philadelphia: W.B. Saunders.

363. Pool, R. (2001). *Fat: Fighting the Obesity Epidemic.* Oxford: Oxford University Press.

364. Stipanuk, M.H. (Ed.). (2000). *Biochemical and Physiological Aspects of Human Nutrition.* Philadelphia: W.B. Saunders.

365. Brown, G. (1999). *The Energy of Life: The Science of What Makes Our Minds and Bodies Work.* New York: Free Press.

366. Ravussin, E. and Tataranni, P.A. (1997). Dietary fat and human obesity. *Journal of the American Dietetic Association,* 97(7 Suppl), S42–S46.

367. Brownell, K.D. and Horgen, K.B. (2004). *Food Fight*. Chicago: Contemporary Books.

368. *Ibid.*

369. Ravussin, E. and Tataranni, P.A. (1997). Dietary fat and human obesity. *Journal of the American Dietetic Association*, 97(7 Suppl), S42–S46.

370. Brown, G. (1999). *The Energy of Life: The Science of What Makes Our Minds and Bodies Work*. New York: Free Press.

371. Brownell, K.D. and Horgen, K.B. (2004). *Food Fight*. Chicago: Contemporary Books.

372. Shell, E.R. (2002). *The Hungry Gene: The Inside Story of the Obesity Industry*. New York: Grove Press.

373. Pool, R. (2001). *Fat: Fighting the Obesity Epidemic*. Oxford: Oxford University Press.

374. Kleinfield, N.R. (2006, January 9). Diabetes and its awful toll quietly emerge as a crisis. *New York Times*.

375. Bray, G.A. (1998). *Contemporary Diagnosis and Management of Obesity*. Newton, PA: Handbooks in Health Care.

376. Capaldi, E.D. (Ed.). (1996). *Why We Eat What We Eat: The Psychology of Eating*. Washington, DC: American Psychological Association.

377. Pool, R. (2001). *Fat: Fighting the Obesity Epidemic*. Oxford: Oxford University Press.

378. Wadden, T.A. and Stunkard, A.J. (Eds.). (2002). *Handbook of Obesity Treatment*. New York: Guilford Press.

379. Eaton, S.B., Eaton, S.B., Konner, M.J., and Shostak, M. (1996). An evolutionary perspective enhances understanding of human nutritional requirements. *Journal of Nutrition*, 126, 1732–40.

380. Pool, R. (2001). *Fat: Fighting the Obesity Epidemic*. Oxford: Oxford University Press.

381. Brownell, K.D. and Horgen, K.B. (2004). *Food Fight*. Chicago: Contemporary Books.

382. Pool, R. (2001). *Fat: Fighting the Obesity Epidemic*. Oxford: Oxford University Press.

383. *Ibid.*

384. Lobstein, T. (2006). Comment: preventing child obesity-an art and a science. *Obesity Reviews*, 7(suppl 1), 1–5.

385. Kottke, T.E., et al. (2004). Obesity: another wolf at the door? *Clinical Obstetrics and Gynecology*, 47(4), 890–897.

386. Peters, J.C., Wyatt, H.R., Donahoo, W.T., and Hill, J.O. (2002). From instinct to intellect: the challenge of maintaining healthy weight in the modern world. *Obesity Reviews*, 3, 69–74.

387. Spake, A. (2003). The science of slimming: getting rid of all those unwanted pounds is as simple as calories in, calories out. *U.S. News and World Report*, 134(21), 34–38.

388. Boekaerts, M., Pintrich, P.R., and Zeidner, M. (Eds.). (2000). *Handbook of Self-Regulation*. San Diego: Academic Press.

389. Hill, J.O. and Billington, C.J. (2002). It's time to start treating obesity. *American Journal of Cardiology*, 89, 969–970.

390. Peters, J.C., Wyatt, H.R., Donahoo, W.T., and Hill, J.O. (2002). From instinct to intellect: the challenge of maintaining healthy weight in the modern world. *Obesity Reviews*, 3, 69–74.

391. Jairath, N. (1999). *Coronary Heart Disease and Risk Factor Management: A Nursing Perspective*. Philadelphia: W.B. Saunders.

392. Swinburn, B., Egger, G., and Raza, F. (1999). Dissecting obesogenic environments: the development and application of a framework for identifying and prioritizing environmental interventions for obesity. *Preventive Medicine*, 29, 563–570.

393. Larkin, M. (2003). Can cities be designed to fight obesity? *Lancet*, 362, 1046–1047.

394. Neel, J.V. (1999). The "thrift genotype" in 1998. *Nutrition Reviews*, 57(5), S2–S9.

395. Winter, G. (2000, October 29). Search for an easy solution fuels an industry rooted in gullibility. *New York Times*, p. 1.

396. *USA Today*, (2005, January 13). p. 1A.

397. Russell, S.A. (2005). *Hunger: An Unnatural History*. New York: Basic Books.

398. Kaufman, F.R. (2005). *Diabesity: The Obesity-Diabetes Epidemic that Threatens America—and What We Must Do to Stop It*. New York: Bantam Books.

399. Grady, D. (2004, June 17). Liposuction doesn't help health, study finds. *New York Times*.

400. Brooks, F.P. (1987). No silver bullet: essence and accidents of software engineering. *Computer*, 20(4), 10–19.

401. Bandura, A. (1997). *Self-Efficacy: The Exercise of Control*. New York: W.H. Freeman.

We Can't Manage What We Don't Understand

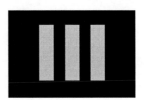

The Energy Balance Equation: Reigning Intellectual Paradigm or Straitjacket?

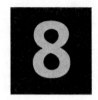

People approach any task, whether it is to manage their weight, their retirement account, or anything else, with mental models that reflect the world as they understand it. They create these models out of their prior experience and whatever knowledge they have (real or imaginary, naive or sophisticated). Once formed, mental models are all important because they determine not only how people make sense of the world, but also how they act and what strategies they use to achieve their goals.[1]

In searching for the perfect body, both the nature of the problem as well as its solution seem transparent enough on the surface. Figure 8.1 depicts the widely shared mental model of the problem and its solution.[2,3] Body weight is viewed as being dependent on the balance between energy intake (EI) and energy expenditure (EE), both of which are assumed to be under voluntary control. Unbalancing this *energy balance equation* in the direction of weight loss, therefore, would appear to be straightforward: reduce daily caloric intake below the daily energy requirements, increase energy expenditure (through increased physical activity for example), or do a little of both.

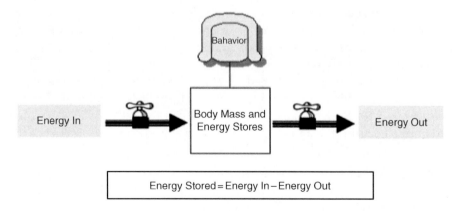

Figure 8.1

T.K.A. Hamid, *Thinking in Circles About Obesity*,
DOI 10.1007/978-0-387-09469-4_8, © Springer Science+Business Media, LLC 2009

As mentioned earlier, most overweight individuals attempt to lose weight on their own. For example, dieting, the mainstay of obesity treatment, is most often undertaken as a self-directed process with instruction from a book or often just by self-induced restraint. Indeed, one excellent indicator of the obesity trend is the number of diet books that are written and sold; more than 7,000 such books came up on a recent keyword search of Amazon.com.

The Magic Number

Instructions in self-help diet and weight-loss books go something like this: 1 pound (lb) of body fat contains 3,500 kilocalories (kcal). To shed a requisite number of pounds in a week or a month, one would simply use this magic number to figure out the size of the daily deficit in energy balance required. For example, here are typical instructions to shed 1 lb per week:

> Your weight is determined by your energy balance. . . . If you burn the same amount of calories as you eat, your weight stays the same. . . . If your goal is weight loss, subtracting 500 calories a day from this figure should promote losing about a pound a week, because 3,500 calories equal a pound [and 7 days × 500 calories per day = 3,500 calories per week].[4]

Translating the calculated daily energy deficit (of 500 kcal in the above example) into a more workable and personalized fixed-calorie diet plan requires just one additional calculation to estimate a person's normal level of energy intake, that is, to determine the level of caloric intake that is sustaining the person's current (undesired) weight. This is not difficult to do. In the many popular weight-loss books, one can choose from a plethora of strategies for either measuring or estimating this level. These strategies range from simple worksheets on which to record and count daily caloric intake, to more esoteric empirical formulas, such as energy is expended at the rate of about 1.875 kcal per minute for a man weighing 65 kilograms (kg) (1 kg = 2.2 lb) and 1.35 kcal per minute for a woman weighing 55 kg.[5]

Once this baseline is established, all the pieces are in place to engineer a fixed-calorie diet plan. So, for example, if the objective is to lose 2 lb per week (worth 2 × 3,5000 = 7,000 kcal), a caloric deficit of 1,000 kcal per day would be subtracted from the assessed current intake level to determine what the daily caloric input should be. Here is an example:

> If an obese woman who normally consumes 2,800 calories daily and maintains body mass at (175 lbs) wishes to lose weight by dieting, she would maintain her regular physical activity but reduce daily food intake to 1,800 calories to create a 1,000 calorie deficit. In 7 days, the accumulated caloric deficit would equal 7,000

calories, or the energy equivalent of (2 lbs) of fat.... To reduce body fat an additional (3 lbs), the reduced caloric intake of 1,800 calories would have to be maintained for another 10.5 days; at this point, body fat theoretically would be reduced at a rate of 1 lb per every 3.5 days.[6]

As was briefly noted in Chapter 1, this model for assessing energy balance is linear. It is also static and unbounded—and just plain wrong. For example, it takes weight-loss projections to absurd values; a negative energy balance of 1,000 calories per day would result in a loss of about 8 lb in a month and an unlikely 100 lb in a year!

Using such a simplistic energy balance equation may help sell more diet books, but this open-loop model and the calculations derived from it, as will be explained in more detail in the next few chapters, does not adequately capture the complexity (or accurately predict the dynamics) of human weight and energy regulation. It is not the first time (nor will it be the last) that conventional wisdom has been proven wrong.

John Kenneth Galbraith, the man who coined the phrase "conventional wisdom," did not consider it a compliment. Conventional wisdom, Galbraith often lamented, reflects our tendency to associate truth with convenience. Because comprehending the true character of a complex system or problem can be mentally tiring, he argued, people all too often cling to simplified conceptualizations, as though to a raft, because they are easier to understand. In Galbraith's view, conventional wisdom is simple, convenient, comfortable, and comforting, but not necessarily true.[7]

The next few chapters provide a more detailed and systematic critique of the energy balance equation in order to clarify its many limitations. But first, let's reflect on just how the energy balance equation became the reigning intellectual paradigm in the diet industry.

From the Experts' Mouths to the Journalists' Ears to the Public's Mind

The energy balance equation originated in the academic literature to provide a simplified framework for studying and understanding laboratory observations of human energy regulation.[8] Its primary purpose, thus, was not to predict how human weight and energy regulation change over time, but to give researchers a way to make sense of and account for their observations of energy intake, energy expenditure, and energy stores (not unlike the accountant's balance sheet, which summarizes and accounts for a corporation's revenues and costs over the past year). From there, it diffused quickly and widely into the popular literature to become the mental model that most dieters (as well as many health care professionals) use to explain weight gain and predict diet outcomes. How and why this unfolded is a classic example of the process by which ideas and innovations diffuse in human society.

More than 40 years ago, Everett M. Rogers developed his theory on the diffusion of innovations to explain how new ideas spread. He published it in his 1962 book titled *Diffusion of Innovations,* which is currently in its fifth edition. Rogers argued that three types of knowledge facilitate society's adoption of a new idea or innovation: *awareness*, or knowledge that the innovation exists; *procedural knowledge* about how to use the innovation; and *principles knowledge,* or understanding how the innovation works.[9]

In the case of the energy balance equation, all three types of knowledge were in place and, as Rogers would have predicted, helped promote its diffusion and widespread adoption.

To most people, the principles of the energy balance equation are not only easy to understand but also almost self-evident. The equation is a simple statement of the intuitive notion of the conservation of energy—that changes in stored energy equals energy intake minus energy expenditure. It is also simple-to-use procedural knowledge. The energy balance equation gives us just two parameters to examine: total energy intake and total energy output. With the magic number 3,500 kcal/lb in hand, an energy deficit/surplus of any size can be easily translated into a loss/gain of body weight.

With a growing and desperate public need for answers, the energy balance equations proved, in Galbraith's words, a seductive "raft." Not only did it have academic credibility, but, unlike most academic material, it was also quite accessible. This accessibility helped promote *awareness knowledge*, as it was easy to explain and easy to sell, and, unfortunately, also easy to misuse by the growing number of self-described diet gurus, authors of self-help books, journalists writing in newspapers and magazines, and eventually by anyone and everyone on the Internet. As the self-help industry universally embraced it, so did legions of dieters, as well as many health care professionals.

However, merely repeating something, whether in writing, on the Internet, or in conversation, does not make it true.

Like the accountant's balance sheet, the energy balance equation is a static backward-looking instrument. Because it does not capture the involuntary adaptive processes of human energy regulation, it cannot faithfully project how body weight will or will not change in response to some intervention, just as using a balance sheet would be inappropriate for predicting a corporation's future financial performance.

As we will see in Chapters 10 and 11, the reality of human energy regulation is far more complex and far more dynamic than the open-loop model of Figure 8.1 implies, primarily because, unlike the figure, the two limbs of energy balance are not independent, but instead are physiologically linked, interacting in complex ways and often compensating for each other in the face of interventions.[10] This means that we cannot voluntarily change one factor—decrease energy input, for example—and assume that the other (energy expenditure) will hold constant. (For example, recall from Chapter 1 that when a person goes on a diet, the body compensates for the induced energy deficit by, among other things, dropping its maintenance energy requirements.) Figuring out the net effect of our voluntary actions and the body's involuntary compensatory reactions is necessarily a messier picture than the one painted in Figure 8.1. The real picture is difficult to see for two reasons: first, because the interactions are not directly visible; and second, because we are part of the lacework ourselves (not independent observers, observing at a distance). Thus, it is doubly hard for us to see the whole pattern of interactions.[11]

But, perhaps most of all, we do not see it because it simply does not fit what we believe or like to believe about ourselves.

We Like to Believe that We Are in Full Control

> Now as a rule when people find one particular intuition so wildly intriguing that they regularly stand by it and forsake lots of information that is technically more correct, they do so because the intuition *fits*. It is somehow part of a bigger scheme of things that they simply can't discard. So, for example, people once held tight to the Ptolemaic idea that the sun revolves around the earth, in part because this notion fit their larger religious conception of the central place of the earth in God's universe.[12]

A great deal of research in behavioral decision making has revealed that what and how we think is not just a matter of logic and information processing, but that human cognition is also very much affected by needs and emotions. Prior beliefs and self-serving interpretations weigh heavily into the social judgment process, and people's expectations often correspond closely with what they would like to see happen or to what is socially desirable rather than to what is objectively likely.[13]

One area in which most individuals' perceptions appear to be more self-serving than realistic concerns beliefs about personal control. Many theorists have maintained that a sense of personal control is integral to one's self-concept and self-esteem. We all need to feel that we have some control over our environments, which helps us have the confidence that we can handle potential threats and exercise some control over them. So we convince ourselves that we do.[14]

Research evidence, however, suggests that people's beliefs in their personal control are often greater than can be justified.[15,16] Dr. Ellen Langer, a professor of psychology at Harvard, coined the phrase "illusion of control" to refer to people's systematic tendency to exaggerate their perceptions of personal control. (In her laboratory studies on gamblers, Langer and her associates demonstrated how people believe and act as if they have control in situations that are actually determined by random events.) In health, the degree to which people exaggerate the control they perceive they have over their future well-being and their bodies is striking.[17] For example, studies have shown that many cancer patients professed a high degree of control over the future course of their cancer, even when their prognoses were poor and recurrence was a virtual certainty.[18]

How much control a person has over weight is one of the most pressing questions about weight control. The notion that we are in complete control of our bodies is enormously seductive—and it sells.

Notice that the energy balance equation only includes variables we control. In the open-loop structure of the energy balance equation (Figure 8.1), both energy intake (EI) and energy expenditure (EE) are assumed to be under voluntary control. So, it should not surprise us that most individuals (as well as the culture in general) assume more control than they actually have, that most people believe that every overweight person can achieve slenderness and should pursue that goal, and that obese people are stereotyped as lacking self-control.[19]

One consequence of the misperception about control is that people may set unrealistically high goals that will increase the likelihood or costliness of failure. Excessive persistence in futile endeavors increases the costs (e.g., time, effort, and money) that accompany the failure. The end result is often increased frustration and other emotional costs. In the health domain, exaggerated perceptions of control create an atmosphere in which people can see their bad health as a personal or moral failing. Thus, the burden of illness is joined by the burden of guilt.[20]

The message of the next few chapters is this: Control over our bodies must be considered within the context of biological realities—realities that the energy balance equation fails to capture. Because, as mentioned, the equation is a static backward-looking instrument, much like the accountant's balance sheet, it does not capture the involuntary adaptive processes of human energy regulation. Therefore, it cannot faithfully project how body weight will or will not change in response to some intervention. The energy balance equation is truly a legacy of earlier times, when we were computationally poor.

People need to manage their bodies like CEOs, not like accountants, and they need forward-looking *dynamic* tools to do it effectively.

What We Know that Ain't So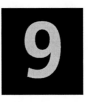

It's not what we don't know that causes trouble. It's what we know that ain't so.
—Will Rogers

Looking Back Versus Looking Forward

Human reasoning usually involves two different kinds of cognitive processes: looking backward to understand the past, and looking forward to predict the future. While the two modes of thinking are interdependent, they are conceptually different.[21] For example, while one may be able to explain how the eclipse of the sun occurs, most of us would not be able to predict when the next eclipse will occur. On the other hand, drivers may accurately predict the rattling sound that occurs every time they depress their car's gas pedal, but may not be able to explain it.

Although we use both types of thinking all the time, we are often unaware of the subtle but crucial differences, and that we need different models to understand or explain versus to predict. This misunderstanding, I believe, is why the energy balance equation provides both insight and confusion when it comes to managing energy balance in humans.

As mentioned earlier, the energy balance equation arose in the academic literature as a framework to account for and understand changes in energy intake, expenditure, and stores in experimental observations. Its view of the human body as a transformer of energy—an "engine," if you will, that transforms the food we eat and the air we breath into heat and fuel for the mechanical work performed by muscles and the biological work necessary to maintain the body's structure and functions—is actually quite old.[22] Because humans and animals are "warm," and body heat has long been perceived as the essence of being alive, the nature of our "innate fire" has intrigued

T.K.A. Hamid, *Thinking in Circles About Obesity*,
DOI 10.1007/978-0-387-09469-4_9, © Springer Science+Business Media, LLC 2009

scientists and philosophers for millennia. The Greek philosophers Plato, Aristotle, and Hippocrates and the Roman physician Galen thought, for example, that the innate fire was in the heart and reckoned it was somehow related to food.[23] But the truly scientific answer to this question came much later, in the latter half of the 18th century, from the experimental work of Lavoisier in France. Lavoisier was interested in heat production in living things and concocted the first-ever animal calorimeter to measure it experimentally. His experiments sowed the seeds for the later development of the principles of thermodynamics and their eventual applicability to biological systems, which ultimately led to the conception of the energy balance equation.[24,25]

As a physics equation for capturing the conservation of energy, the energy balance equation is obviously true: body weight can increase only if energy intake exceeds expenditure. As a bookkeeping tool, it can provide us with the framework to account for (or "book") any and all changes among the body's three energy "accounts." As such, it would be perfectly appropriate as a tool to track any imbalances between energy intake and energy expenditure over a day or a week, and ensure they are faithfully reflected in the body's energy stores.

But, again, it is a backward-looking instrument that aims to capture the results of past decisions, not predict future performance. The distinction between a model that helps us look back to explain past behavior and one that helps us look forward to predict future performance is a crucial distinction and a subtle one. While some models can both look backward and predict future performance—Newton's equations of motion are one (rare) example—most models do not. As more and more of us become consumers of models, not only professionally but also in running our private lives, it is increasingly important that we are aware of the differences so as not to misuse the models we rely on.

A good example of how a model can be very useful in one role (explaining) but not in the other (predicting) is Darwin's principle of natural selection. Darwin's principle has allowed us to explain the appearance and disappearance of many types of living species (and their characteristics). However, when it comes to predicting the emergence or disappearance of a species of organism, Darwin's principle of natural selection remains silent (Figure 9.1).[26]

It is fairly obvious in the case of evolution that the model's value is in explaining what has been observed about a species, not to predict its future evolution. But the distinction for many models is not as clear, especially for abstract models such as mathematical and financial models. The energy balance equation and the corporate balance sheet are just two examples.

While the energy balance equation per se is not faulty, its application to weight loss is. Specifically, its misapplication by the self-help industry and

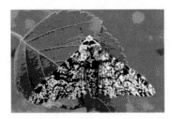

Figure **9.1** A model like the Principle of Natural Selection, although of great utility for explaining what has already happened, is almost totally useless when it comes to telling us what will happen next. There is nothing in natural selection that would say that *Biston betularia* (the peppered moth, with its pepper-and-salt camouflage pattern) would develop the camouflage of darkly-pigmented wings to stave off extinction, as opposed, say, to developing the ability to hurrow underground or secrete a poisonousfluid as an adaptation enhancing its chances of survival. So when it comes to prediction, the Principle of Natural Selection is as useless. . . it addresses explanation (but is not intended or useful to answer the question of prediction)". (*Source:* Casti, J.L. (1997). *Would-Be Worlds: How Simulation Is Changing the Frontiers of Science*. New York: John Wiley. (Image courtesy of Bernard Fransen.)

the public at large to *predicting* change in human weight and energy balance over time is a real problem that drags us into two kinds of traps—two kinds of miscalculations relating to both the quantity and quality of weight loss.

The First Trap: Linear Thinking

Let's consider some of the assumptions made when applying the energy balance equation, as well as the implications for predicting treatment outcome. One explicit assumption is that the there is a fixed energy cost of 3,500 calories per pound of lost tissue. Another, less obvious, assumption is that the body's energy requirements remain steady as body size decreases.[27]

The many discussions in the literature—the quotation below is a typical example—imply that maintaining an energy deficit on some fixed-calorie diet regimen will cause body weight to drop in direct proportion to the size and duration of the diet's energy deficit. This implication is widely accepted.

> [C]ut your daily calorie intake by 500 to lose 1 pound a week (3,500 ÷ 7 = 500). To lose 1.5 pounds, you need to cut 750 calories a day. A 2-pound-a-week loss means eliminating 1,000 calories a day.[28]

For the obese woman on a 1,800-calorie diet (in Chapter 8), the drop in body weight would look like this:

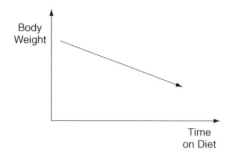

Figure 9.2 Linear drop in body weight as would be predicted by the energy balance equation

The relationship is linear. It is also unbounded, which, as already explained, can result in absurd weight-loss projections. The absurdity, by the way, applies equally in the other direction, that is, in the case of gaining weight. For example, as Ravussin and Swinburn[29] explain, "[I]f a small increase in energy intake, such as a (l00 kcal) from an extra piece of toast, is sustained over a long period (say, 40 years) then the weight gain predicted by the static (linear) equation is an unlikely (400 lbs)."

In reality, the rate of weight loss (or gain) is far from linear. It tends to decline over time, even if the prescribed diet is maintained.[30]

Of course, the overly simplified assumption of linearity is not peculiar to energy balance (or the overweight). It is a common bias (some have called it a trap) in how we tend to view the world.

What does linear thinking mean, and why do we engage in it? The word *linear* comes from the Latin word *linearis*, which means *created by lines*. To think linearly is to think that effect is always proportional to cause, for example, that a 3,500-kcal energy deficit per week causes a loss of 1 lb per week, 2 lb in 2 weeks, and so on for a month of dieting, a year, forever. In its simplest form, a linear model or formula is a straight-line relationship. For example, if we assume a pound of body fat is worth 3,500 kcal, then the formula for the monthly caloric deficit *(D)* to shed a number of pounds *(W)* is $D = 3,500 * W$. This formula's graph is a straight line, as shown in Figure 9.3; hence the term *linear*.

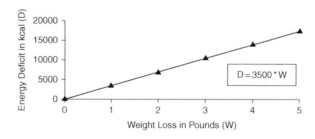

Figure 9.3 Weight loss as a *linear* function of an energy deficit

Psychologists have found that we have a tendency to think in this linear fashion about many things, probably because it is both intuitive and cognitively convenient. For example, when thinking about change in some system, what can be more intuitive than to think that change in system output is proportional to change in input; that is, small inputs have small effects and large inputs have large effects. Similarly, when extrapolating a trend into the future, whether involving growth (something going up) or decline (something going down), it is easiest to project linearly, that is, to assume that the quantity increases or decreases by the same absolute amount per time period.[31]

While such thinking is convenient (and, in some cases, may serve as a "good-enough approximation"), in reality, it is almost always invalid.[32] Changes in system outputs are not always proportional to changes in input, and things rarely happen in straight lines.[33] Our world is highly nonlinear, and our bodies are no exception.

What makes a bias like the linearity bias potentially problematic is its invisibility. Like all cognitive biases, it seems to be hardwired into our thinking processes, making it hard to recognize, even as we fall right into it.[34] With linear blinders on, it is no wonder that behavior (or misbehavior) in many of our systems often takes us by surprises and can frustrate us, because doing the obvious thing (quite often) does not produce the obvious desired outcome.[35] Even experts are not immune to the linearity trap, although they often seem to fall into it by choice!

Science has recognized for centuries that effect in complex systems is not always proportional to cause. But because nonlinear systems were usually too complex to solve mathematically, necessity imposed a tradition of ignoring nonlinearity.[36] "Whenever nonlinear equations appeared, they were immediately 'linearized'—in other words, replaced by linear approximations."[37]

> In fairness, [though,] the reliance on linear theory and the avoidance of nonlinear systems was justifiable prior to the development of computer simulation because analytical solutions to nonlinear dynamic systems cannot in general be found. Early theorists of dynamic systems made the assumption of linearity because it was the only way to make progress.[38]

The problem, however, is that the tradition of linear thinking took hold. Today, even after the advent of modern computers and the availability of inexpensive simulation techniques, too many scientists continue to be wedded to a linear worldview, reluctant to give up their linear mathematical procedures. It is a costly tradition, hampering the development of realistic and faithful models of real-world systems and unnecessarily undermining our ability to manage our overwhelmingly nonlinear systems (whether it is our economy or our bodies).[39]

This must change, and a necessary step toward doing that is to understand what causes systems to behave nonlinearly. Research has suggested that, in many systems, an important source of nonlinearity—and surprising behavior— is feedback.

We saw examples of this in Chapter 4 when we discussed reinforcing processes and how they can lead to escalation. For example, we saw that when growth is driven by positive feedback (as in the process of compounding interest in a bank deposit or the spread of an epidemic), the rate of increase (of money in the bank or infected people) grows much faster than linearly—it grows exponentially.

Nonlinearity can also arise out of *negative* feedback. In human energy regulation, the homeostatic mechanisms between body mass and energy stores and energy expenditure (depicted in Figure 9.4) is one example of negative feedback. This one feedback mechanism (missing in the model of Figure 8.1) is an important reason why the energy balance equation gets it so wrong. The simple plumbing analogy below demonstrates how such a negative feedback process induces nonlinearity in our system of energy and weight regulation and why seeing this is terribly important to properly figure out the outcome of prolonged energy imbalance.

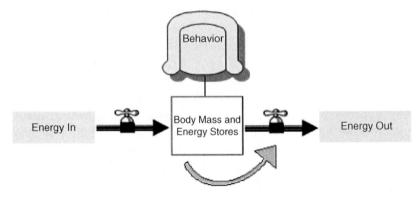

Figure 9.4 Feedback mechanism between body mass/energy stores and energy expenditure

A Plumbing Analogy

While the determinants of human energy regulation are quite complex (as we shall soon see), at some basic level, the process resembles that of filling and draining a bathtub (Figure 9.5).

Like the level of energy stores in the human body, the quantity of water in a tub changes as a function of the rates of water flowing in and draining out. To illustrate, assume that we start with the tub containing, say, 200 liters (L) of water, and that both the inflow and outflow rates are constant, with water flowing in at the rate of 80 liters/second (L/s), and draining out (by gravity) at the constant rate of 100 L/s. Since the outflow exceeds the inflow, the water

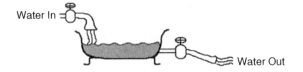

Water In

Water Out

Figure 9.5 Plumbing analogy of human energy regulation

level in the bathtub will drop. More precisely, the net loss rate equals 100 – 80 = 20 L/s. Since this net outflow (loss) is *constant,* the volume of water will drop in a straight line, as shown in Figure 9.6.

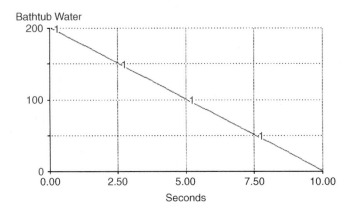

Figure 9.6 Linear drop of water level

There is one problem, though, with this scenario: it is not quite realistic. In a real system, water draining by gravity would not drain at a constant rate, because as the water level in the tub falls, the magnitude of water pressure at the drain will decrease, and that will slow the rate at which the water drains out. In other words, the outflow rate will not remain steady at 100 L/s, the initial draining rate when the tub contained 200 L of water. As the level of water starts to drop, the concomitant drop in water pressure at the drain will cause the outflow rate to also drop to 99 L/s, then to 98, 97, and so on. That is, the drop in water level causes an ever-decreasing magnitude of net outflow. Eventually, this "hydraulic adaptation" will cause the outflow rate to decrease from 100 L/s to 80 L/s, that is, to a level that matches the water inflow rate. At that point, the system will reach a state of equilibrium because what is draining out (at 80 L/s) would be exactly equal to what is pouring in. Once there, the water in the tub settles at this equilibrium level, as shown in Figure 9.7.

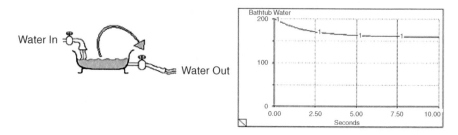

Figure 9.7 Water level affects flow rate, just as body weight affects energy expenditure

Notice how, in Figure 9.7, the rate at which the system drops to its new equilibrium diminishes over time. The adjustment rate is rapid at first, but then tapers over time (a pattern called exponential decay). Notice, also, that the water level settles at a level that is substantially higher than what was (linearly) expected (which was a completely empty tub).

The above dynamic undoubtedly looks familiar to most dieters. The pattern of weight loss experienced by many a dieter indeed exhibits a striking similarity to the behavior of the bathtub: an initial phase of gratifying weight loss followed by a second (asymptote) phase in which weight loss slows and then stops. In a manner analogous to the plumbing example above, when body weight drops during food energy deprivation (dieting), the loss of body tissue (like the loss of water in the bathtub) induces an involuntary decrease in the body's maintenance energy requirements. This decreases total energy expenditure and effectively shrinks the diet's energy deficit, which, in turn, and unfortunately for the dieter, dampens the rate of weight loss. If the energy deficit persists, body weight will decrease to the point where the body's diminished total energy expenditure matches the diet's diminished energy intake. At that point, weight loss ceases, and the new lower steady-state weight is maintained.[40]

Like our filling and emptying a tub, weight loss during prolonged underfeeding is not linear but rather curvilinear, and, as in our plumbing analogy, it is not unbounded. Rather, it declines with time, even if the prescribed diet is maintained. Those who rely on the linear and unbounded energy balance equation for making treatment recommendations rarely understand these limitations of the model, much less are prepared to communicate such information to the public.[41]

A Second Trap: Energy as a Single Currency

A second failing of the simplistic energy balance equation is that it does not provide the dieter with enough discriminatory power to contrast treatment options. The model suggests (and it is widely held) that a decline in body weight is determined solely by the size of the energy deficit, irrespective of how the energy deficit is induced. A daily energy deficit of 1,000 kcal can be induced, for example, by eliminating beer (four cans) and dessert (cheese cake) from a daily diet or by jogging for 7 miles. Statically, since both these strategies would create the same caloric deficit, they are treated in both the academic literature and the media as though they were perfectly interchangeable, that is, as if energy were a single "currency."

Consider three examples appearing in three different media: a newspaper article, an academic journal, and an Internet item. From *USA Today:*

> You have to burn 3,500 calories more than you consume to lose a pound. If you usually eat 2,200 calories a day to maintain your weight, you need to cut back by 500 calories or increase exercise by that much to create the 500-calorie deficit to lose 1 pound a week.[42]

In an academic journal:

> Losing one pound requires burning 3,500 more calories than you eat. There are three ways to accomplish this:
>
> - Cut 3,500 calories from your diet.
> - Burn 3,500 extra calories through increased activity.
> - Eat less and exercise more for a combined total deficit of 3,500 calories.[43]

On the Internet:

> To lose one pound, a person must burn 3,500 calories more than are consumed (500 calories per day over the course of a week). For example, reducing calories by 300 per day and increasing daily activity to burn off an additional 200 calories should result in a weight loss of one pound per week.[44]

In reality, how an energy deficit is created does matter, because whenever significant amounts of body weight are lost, both fat mass (FM) and fat-free mass (FFM) participate, with their relative contributions depending on how the energy deficit was created (as well as on a person's initial body composition). What this relative contribution is matters a great deal because different body tissues have different metabolic rates (different fuel-burning requirements). For example, creating a desired energy deficit through exercise can protect against the loss in fat-free mass.[45,46] By conserving and even increasing the fat-free body mass (the principal metabolically active component of total body mass), exercise partially blunts the aforementioned drop in metabolic activity (the drop of water pressure at the bathtub drain) that accompanies diet-based weight loss.[47] That, in turn, can significantly impact the time course (and ultimate size) of weight loss. (Part IV presents experiments that quantify this impact precisely, and Chapter 10 explains the feedback mechanisms that regulate it.)

Contrary to popular belief, then, how an energy deficit is created does matter. A 1,000-kcal caloric deficit from a diet can be quiet different from a 1,000-kcal caloric deficit from exercise. Energy, in other words, is *not* a single currency.

We Need a Better "Map"

Like a good roadmap, our mental models help us get about in the world. Indeed, it is through our mental models that we "see" the world—not in terms of our visual sense of sight, but in terms of perceiving, understanding, interpreting[48]:

> Suppose you wanted to arrive at a specific location in central Chicago. A street map of the city would be a great help to you in reaching your destination. But suppose you were given the wrong map. Through a printing error, the map labeled "Chicago" was actually a map of Detroit. Can you imagine the frustration, the ineffectiveness of trying to reach your destination? You might work on your *behavior*—you could try harder, be more diligent, double your speed. But your efforts would only succeed in getting you to the wrong place faster.... The point is, you'd still be lost. The fundamental problem has nothing to do with your behavior or your attitude. It has everything to do with having a wrong map. If you have the right map of Chicago, then diligence becomes important, and when you encounter frustrating obstacles along the way, then attitude can make a real difference. But the first and most important requirement is the accuracy of the map.

The lesson is a simple one. We cannot expect to effectively manage what we do not understand. We have spent the better part of the obesity epidemic wedded to an inadequate energy balance equation model. We can do better.

We took a first step in this chapter. The goal here was to turn the mirror inward, to examine the assumptions inherent in our reigning mental model—the energy balance model—and to highlight their deficiencies. We started to see that the regulation of energy balance is far from being a simple conversation between two key players—energy input (EI) and energy expenditure (EE)—as suggested by the open-loop model of Figure 8.1.

This chapter highlighted a missing loop in the energy balance equation (energy expenditure → energy stores → energy expenditure). The next two chapters extend this discussion further. As we close more loops, we will see how the system begins to get more realistic and more complex: how weight reflects activity levels and activity levels reflect weight; that appetite shapes body weight, and body weight, in turn, regulates appetite; and how these factors are all interconnected, pushing on each other and being pushed on in return. Although perhaps not obvious to us, it will become clear why these circular mechanisms and their interactions account for much of what happens to our bodies over the long term.

Closing the Loops on Energy Balance: Energy Output Side

10

Tip of a Physiological Iceberg!

In the simplistic energy balance model, cause and effect run one-way (Figure 10.1). The two limbs of energy balance—energy intake (EI) and energy expenditure (EE)—are considered independent (exogenous) variables under our *voluntary control,* and body weight is the outcome of the balance between the two.

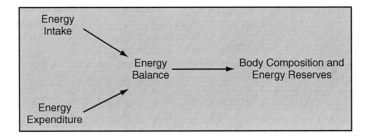

Figure 10.1 Simplistic one-way model of energy balance

In reality, as already explained, the cause-and-effect relationships in human weight and energy regulation are not one-way, and energy balance is not entirely under our voluntary control. Rather, the regulation of energy balance in the human body is significantly influenced by involuntary homeostatic adaptations that regulate both energy expenditure and energy intake. Furthermore, these hard-wired adaptations, such as the metabolic downshifting during energy deprivation that limits tissue depletion, are substantial enough to often overwhelm the impact of our voluntary actions (10.2).

This chapter and the next highlight important mechanisms of human energy regulation that the energy balance model misses. The aim is to

T.K.A. Hamid, *Thinking in Circles About Obesity,*
DOI 10.1007/978-0-387-09469-4_10, © Springer Science+Business Media, LLC 2009

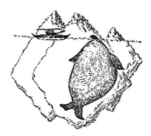

Figure 10.2 The energy balance equation shows only the tip of a physiological iceberg

demonstrate that ignoring these under-the-surface (or, in this case, under-the-skin) processes seriously limits our understanding of disease causation and distorts our expectations about treatment outcomes.

Let's start by examining the energy-expenditure side of the equation.

"Under-the-Surface" Determinants of Energy Expenditure

To stay alive, we must expend energy continuously, literally every second of every day. An adult male expends, on average, between 2,700 and 3,000 kcal per day, whereas his female counterpart expends between 2,000 and 2,100 kcal.[49] Where is all this energy going?

The total amount of energy we expend can be divided conceptually into three components: resting (also referred to as maintenance) energy, physical activity, and food processing (Figure 10.3). The largest component is the resting energy expenditure (REE), defined as the energy expended to sustain the basic metabolic functions of an awake individual at rest. It is the amount of energy required to maintain the basic internal housekeeping functions of

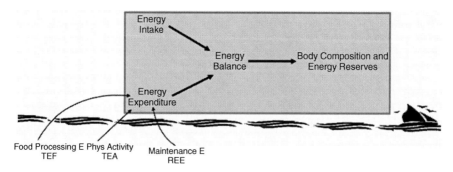

Figure 10.3 The three components of energy (E) expenditure: REE, resting energy expenditure; TEA, thermic effect of activity; TEF, thermic effect of food

the body—to keep our heart beating, our lungs breathing, and our nerves transmitting.[50] In the typical 21st-century sedentary adult, the REE makes up much more than it used to (and was supposed to), as much as 60 to 70 percent of total energy expenditure.

Going a step deeper, we see in Figure 10.4 that the REE level is determined by two factors: body composition and energy balance. The body's composition establishes its *nominal* REE level—a baseline level—that is then adjusted upward or downward as a function of a person's energy balance (i.e., as a function of what the person does with his or her body).

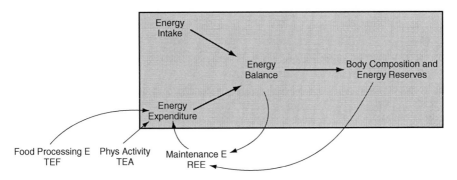

Figure 10.4 Two factors regulate the REE level

Let's consider first the body-composition–REE link. Body composition is a player in the energy expenditure game because the various tissues of the body have very different qualitative and quantitative fuel requirements. Clinically, human body composition can be viewed as being composed of two compartments: fat-free mass (FFM) and fat mass (FM). Fat-free mass constitutes the skeleton, muscles, connective tissue, organ tissues, skin, bone, and water. The second compartment, body fat, is composed of two types: (1) *essential fat*, which is the fat associated with bone marrow, the central nervous system, viscera (internal organs), and cell membranes; and (2) *storage fat*, which is fat stored in adipose tissue.[51] Although the percent distribution of the FM-FFM compartments can vary quite significantly over a wide range among people as a result of physical and behavioral differences, a major determinant is a person's gender. "A normal-weight man, for example, has from 12 to 20 percent body fat; a woman, because of her greater quantity of essential fat (in mammary glands and the pelvic region) 20 to 30 percent."[52]

Fat mass and FFM have very different qualitative and quantitative fuel requirements. Fat tissue, which is composed primarily of inert triglyceride is less metabolically active than FFM and, thus, has a lower rate of fuel consumption per unit mass.[53] As a result, a person's *nominal* resting energy expenditure (REE) is determined *not* by his or her *absolute* body mass, but rather by the so-called metabolic mass, which is defined by the person's body composition in terms of FM versus FFM.

We can see from Figure 10.4 that there is a second factor affecting REE, namely, energy balance. As already explained, during caloric deprivation, the body adapts physiologically to the negative energy balance by decreasing the metabolic activity of the tissue mass at the cellular level in order to conserve energy and restrain the rate of weight loss. In the event of overconsumption and weight gain, there is, conversely, an increase in REE per unit mass; that is, there is an "exaggerated" increase in daily REE beyond that effectuated by the increase in tissue mass.[54] The REE per unit of metabolic mass, in other words, increases with positive energy balance and decreases with negative energy balance. These up/down adjustments in REE, experimental research has found, can increase or decrease a person's daily REE by as much as 20 percent.[55–57]

The second-largest component of daily energy expenditure is the energy expended for muscular work, known as the thermic effect of activity (TEA). This is the energy we expend in moving around as we work and play. For today's typical urban dweller, who increasingly is not engaged in heavy labor in making a living, TEA accounts for 15 to 20 percent of daily energy expenditure.

The expenditure of energy on physical activity also varies considerably among people, from the very minimal activity of the bed-ridden patient, to the strenuous toil of a Mexican Pima farmer, to the professional athlete who trains 6 hours a day with high intensity.[58] Generally speaking, though, in our modern environment, the individual differences in TEA tend to arise not so much from the nature of the work people do, but from the type of leisure activities they pursue.[59] People involved in sports and who exercise regularly and heavily, for example, can easily double or even triple their daily expenditure.[60]

Notice, in Figure 10.5, that there is a link from body composition to TEA, because the amount of energy expended when we exercise depends not only on the type of activity, its intensity, and its duration, but also on the person's body weight and composition. This link captures two types of effects that body composition has on TEA. Because most physical activities involve contracting the muscles to move the body (or its parts), a person's body weight affects the amount of energy needed to do that moving.[61] Thus, when two people with different weights do the exact same exercise routine side by side, the person moving a smaller body will expend less energy.[62]

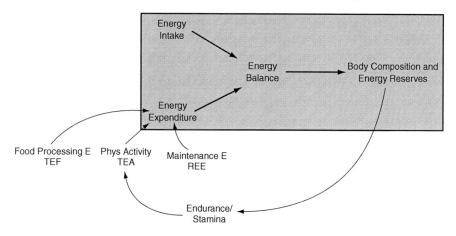

Figure 10.5 The link from body composition to TEA

Body composition (which is shaped partly by a person's history of physical activity or lack of it) also reflects the amount and quality of energy stores a person has. The size and composition of people's energy stores determine the total fuel that is available for physical activity, as well as the fuel mix (fat versus glucose) their muscles use. Obviously, the size of our fuel "tanks" is an important determinant of how much activity (especially intense activity) a person can sustain. But fuel mix is also an important factor. Because of the huge disparity between our fat and glucose stores—our fat stores are almost fifty times larger—the more fat (and the less glucose) our muscles use, the further and longer we can go.[63]

How is that fuel mix regulated? The fuel-mix the muscles use depends on an interplay among several factors: the fuels available, the intensity and duration of the activity, and the degree to which the body is conditioned to perform that activity. For much of our day-to-day activities and during low-to moderate-intensity physical activity, the muscles can derive their energy from both glucose and fatty acids. But when we engage in intense activity (running for the bus, escaping a charging rhino, or winning a squash game), our bodies expend energy at a rate that exceeds the capacity of the heart and lungs to supply oxygen to the muscles. In this case, to fuel the work, the muscles draw more heavily on glucose, which is the only fuel that can be used anaerobically; that is, it can be metabolized to produce energy without the simultaneous use of oxygen.[64]

Differences in body composition affect the size and utilization rate of our very *limited* glucose reserves, and this translates into significant variability among individuals in terms of the level of intensity and the duration of activity that can be sustained.

Muscle cells that repeatedly deplete their glycogen through hard work adapt to store greater amounts of glycogen to support that work. Conditioned muscles also rely less on glycogen and more on fat for energy, so glycogen breakdown and glucose use occur more slowly in trained than in untrained individuals at a given work intensity.... Oxygen delivery to the muscles by the heart and lungs plays a role, but equally importantly, trained muscles are better equipped to use the oxygen because their cells contain more mitochondria.[65] Untrained muscles depend more heavily on anaerobic glucose breakdown, even when physical activity is just moderate.[66]

How much exercising a particular person's glycogen reserves will sustain depends on the intensity and duration of effort, as well as on the fitness and nutritional status of the exerciser. An overweight, sedentary person embarking on a new exercise regimen to treat obesity not only starts with more limited glycogen stores, but also tends to use his reserves at a faster rate than, for example, a trained athlete.

The third component of energy expenditure is the thermic effect of food (TEF), which constitutes the various metabolic costs associated with processing a meal, such as the costs of digestion, absorption, transport, and storage of nutrients within the body. (It is referred to as the *thermic* effect of food because the acceleration of activity that occurs when we eat produces heat as the gastrointestinal (GI) tract muscles speed up their rhythmic contractions, and the cells that manufacture and secrete digestive juices begin their tasks.) The TEF accounts for approximately 10 percent of total daily energy expenditure in moderately active individuals, but obviously can increase or decrease depending on the amount and the composition of a person's diet (Figure 10.6).[67]

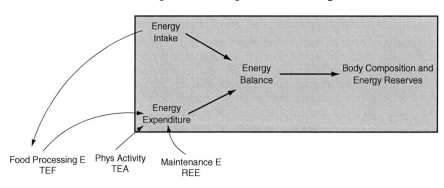

Figure 10.6 What and how much we eat affect TEF

When more energy than needed is consumed, the composition of the meal also affects how much of the *excess* energy gets stored. Of the three macronutrients, fat is stored most efficiently by the body, meaning the pathways from excess fat input to body fat require the fewest metabolic steps, burning off just 5 percent of the ingested calories in the process of storing it. By contrast, to store excess protein and carbohydrates, the body "wastes" as much as 25 percent of the ingested calories, because additional energy is required to convert protein and carbohydrates to appropriate storage form, that is, converting excess glucose to glycogen or fat and excess amino acids to fat storage. That is why fat, when consumed in excess, is more fattening than carbohydrate or protein.[68]

The System in Action: "Under the Surface" Responses to Energy Imbalance

Thus, we can see that, contrary to the energy balance equation, energy intake (EI) and energy expenditure (EE) are not independent, exogenous, and entirely voluntary variables, and human energy and weight regulation is far from the open loop system depicted in Figure 10.1. Energy balance regulates body weight and is simultaneously regulated by it. Weight loss/gain is not only the consequence of energy imbalance; it is also the mechanism by which energy balance is eventually restored.[69] The relationships are circular, not one-way.

We see the dynamic implications of these circular relationships whenever the system is nudged off-balance, as when we voluntarily induce a negative energy balance when dieting. Any weight loss we achieve then triggers *involuntary* declines in all three components of energy expenditure: TEF, REE, and TEA. These declines, in turn, affect the trajectory of subsequent weight loss (if any).

Since TEF constitutes the metabolic costs of processing a meal, eating less while on a diet would naturally lower the TEF. That effect is depicted as link 1 in Figure 10.7. Because TEF accounts for only 10 percent of the daily energy expenditure, the drop is typically not large in absolute terms, however.

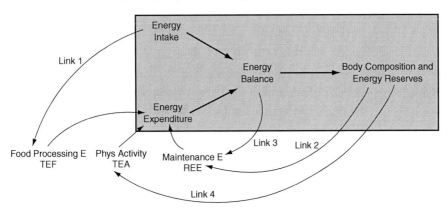

Figure 10.7 Integrating the multiple links

The impact of weight loss on resting energy expenditure, on the other hand, can be substantial. When body mass is lost during energy restriction, both FM and FFM participate (approximately 60 to 70 percent FM and 30 to 40 percent FFM). As lean body tissue, the metabolically active component of total body mass, is shed during weight loss, REE falls accordingly. This is captured by link 2 in Figure 10.7 from body composition and energy reserves to REE. As REE drops, the size of the body's energy deficit effectively shrinks, which, in turn, slows subsequent losses in body weight. Because resting energy expenditure accounts for a sizable chunk of total energy expenditure, this drop in REE can significantly alter the body's energy balance (decreasing it) and dampen the dieter's weight reduction effort.[70]

Unfortunately for the dieter, additional homeostatic adaptations occur during food energy restriction that cause REE to decline by amounts that exceed that which is associated with the loss in lean body tissue.[71] To restrain the rate of tissue loss even more, the body conserves additional energy by decreasing REE per unit mass. This metabolic adaptation (captured by link 3 in Figure 10.7) is achieved chiefly through hormonal mechanisms that operate to decrease the metabolic activity at the cellular level. In essence, the body enhances the tissues' metabolic efficiency, a process I likened in Part II to changing incandescent light bulbs to fluorescent bulbs to save energy.[72] The survival value of such an energy-conserving adaptation that aims to limit tissue depletion during food scarcity is obvious.

Results from experimentation on human subjects have demonstrated just how swift these body defenses against tissue loss are. In a classic experiment to quantify the adaptation in REE in response to negative energy balances, Jebb et al.[73] tracked changes in REE in three healthy male subjects (average weight 73.67 kg). Their experiment was conducted in two phases. The first was a maintenance phase in which the three subjects lived in a metabolic suite for 7 days and were fed a balanced diet to maintain energy balance. After the maintenance week, and while still living in the metabolic suite, the three subjects were underfed for 12 days (phase 2). The diet was set at 833 kcal/day, approximately two thirds below the subjects' maintenance diet.

The substantial energy deficit imposed on the subjects caused, as would be expected, a progressive drop in their body weights. The real revelations, however, were the magnitude and swiftness of the drop in their resting energy expenditure. The REE responded almost immediately and progressively, so that by the end of the 12-day period, the drop in REE was, in percentage terms, twice as much as the drop in the subjects' body weight—an 8.3% drop in REE versus a 4.3% drop in weight.

For any dieter, these energy-sparing adaptations cause the diet to become progressively less effective. The result is much earlier weight-loss plateaus than the static energy equation would predict. The depression in REE also explains why it is often so difficult for obese subjects who lose weight to maintain their newly reduced weight, and why weight regain (recidivism) is so common. It is hard, in part, because to maintain their new lower weight, formerly obese people must consume 10 to 20 percent fewer calories than people of the same weight who have never been obese, and who therefore would not be experiencing a diet-induced depression in REE.[74,75]

Finally, as body mass declines, the energy expended in weight-bearing physical activity also declines, since less energy would be needed to move a lighter body.[76] The size of that drop depends on the types of activities. Consider, for example, walking: in a 1-mile walk, a 90-kg person (198 lb) burns about 105 kcal, but a 70-kg person (154 lb) walking the same distance burns only 80 kcal[77]—almost a 25 percent difference.

The impact of body weight on energy expenditure during physical activity is captured by link 4 in Figure 10.7. As with the other links, this determinant of energy expenditure is not *static*. Its effect on energy expenditure is *dynamic*, meaning that it changes over time as a person's weight changes. For example, an overweight person on an exercise program can lose a substantial amount of weight early on, but then, as weight drops, he or she loses progressively smaller amounts over time.[78]

The cumulative effect of all this is that, in response to an induced energy deficit and initial weight loss, all components of energy expenditure will decline. The thermic effect of feeding decreases with a decreased energy intake; resting metabolic rate decreases as body weight decreases and metabolic efficiency increases, and less energy is expended in moving the lighter body. As a result, a given decrease in energy intake causes a negative energy balance—and weight loss—of ever-decreasing magnitude.[79] Ultimately, the body's diminished total energy expenditure drops to where it matches the diet's diminished energy intake. At that point, weight loss ceases and the new lower steady-state weight is maintained.[80]

Implications for Treatment

Another serious limitation of the simplistic energy balance equation is that it does not provide the patient—the decision maker—with enough discriminatory power to contrast treatment options. It does not, for example, explain why the same treatment strategy can produce different results for different people, or why different strategies (e.g., dieting versus exercising) that induce the same caloric imbalance can produce different results in the same person.

Let's consider each issue in turn.

Failure to Account for Individual Differences

The energy balance equation is a one-size-fits-all model that does not, and cannot, capture individual differences.

Yet, we all know that there is much variability in how different people respond to life's health challenges, and that some individuals gain or lose more weight than others on comparable energy imbalances. Genetic differences obviously play a role in such individual differences, but so do differences in body composition (i.e., FM versus FFM). Body composition has practical implications for treatment because it is an attribute over which we do have some control. Unlike our genes, body composition is not a done deal.

Our body composition changes, voluntarily or involuntarily, whenever our body weight changes, voluntarily or involuntarily. Whenever a significant amount of body weight is lost or gained, both FFM and FM participate in the process, albeit in varying proportions.[81] As FM and FFM are added or shed in different proportions, body composition must change. The cause-and-effect relationship is not unilateral, however; it is mutual.

A person's initial body fat content at the start of a diet has a lot to say about the composition of the tissue that he or she will end up losing. Gilbert B. Forbes demonstrated this in a series of seminal experiments he conducted in the 1980s to study human body composition and how it changes with weight loss or gain. Based on a series of body-composition studies of individuals of varying body fat content, Forbes[82] derived empirical relationships that predict the relative changes in body composition when body weight is gained or lost. Essentially, what he found was that during weight loss, obese people lose more weight as fat than do lean people, and the fatter a person is, the higher will be his or her FM loss as a percentage of total weight loss. Conversely, during weight gain, obese people add more weight as fat than do lean people, who add more lean tissue. (There are, of course, situations in which this does not occur. For example, exercising makes it possible to lose some weight without sacrificing FFM.[83])

A person's initial body composition, thus, affects the composition of tissue lost during energy deprivation, and this, in turn, affects the trajectory and magnitude of the ultimate weight loss. Because FFM is the principal metabolically active component of total body mass, an individual who loses proportionally more lean mass shows greater declines in energy expenditure than someone (on the *same* diet) who loses more fat. This, in turn, affects the person's energy balance and subsequent weight loss.

In addition, since "the energetic equivalent of a given amount of body mass either gained or lost depends on its composition,"[84] by affecting the *composition* of the tissue lost or gained, initial body composition also directly affects the *quantity* of tissue lost or gained. To see how, consider the situation of a male dieter who has just endured a *net* energy deficit of 1,000 kcal in a 24-hour period. (Assume that this 1,000-kcal deficit is the *net* result after we account for the dietary deficit and the body's metabolic adjustments.) How much weight he will actually lose depends on the composition of the lost tissue, which will, in turn, be affected by his initial body composition. To demonstrate the magnitudes involved, let's consider three extreme cases: losing only FM, losing only FFM, or losing a 50:50 mixture of the two.

To be able to figure out those differences, we need first to determine the energetic equivalents of the different tissue types:

> Lean tissue such as muscle is about 73% water, with the remaining 27% being largely protein with smaller amounts of fat and carbohydrate. In contrast, adipose tissue is only about 15% water, the remainder (85%) being storage lipid with a very small amount of protein contributing to the cell structure and intracellular enzymes. Given these differences in the composition of body tissues, the amount of energy represented by a [pound] of body weight will differ accordingly. For example, the body energy lost when a [pound] of muscle is lost would be roughly 500 kcal [0.27 * 1,844 kcal/lb for protein].... Loss of a [pound] of adipose tissue (85% lipid) represents a body energy loss of about 3,500 kcal [0.85 × 4,100 kcal/lb for fat].... Thus, a [pound] of body fat represents nearly [seven] times the energy for fuel represented by a pound of lean tissue.[85]

Thus, if our dieter loses only FM, he would lose 0.3 lb; if he loses only FFM, he would lose 2 lb; and if he loses a 50:50 mixture of the two, he would lose half a pound.

How an Energy Deficit Is Induced Also Matters

The energy balance equation implies (and it is a widely held view) that a decline in body weight is determined solely by the size of the energy deficit, irrespective of how that deficit is induced. In reality, however, how a caloric deficit is created does matter. The patterns of weight change that result from strategies aimed at decreasing the energy input (EI) side of the equation (i.e., dieting) can be very different from those aimed at increasing the energy expenditure (EE) side (i.e., exercising), *even when the strategies are calorically equivalent.*

Two factors cause the divergence. First, the (under-the-surface) TEF will be higher in the exercising scenario since more food energy will be consumed (link 1 from energy intake to TEF in Figure 10.7). Second, and of greater significance, the two strategies will have different impacts on the *composition* of weight loss (the FM and FFM components), which, in turn, will result in different impacts on the body's REE. For example, when exercise is used to create a desired energy deficit, it can protect against the loss in FM (muscle mass) and may even increase it.[86] By conserving and even increasing FFM, exercise may temper the drop in resting metabolism that frequently accompanies diet-based weight loss.[87] (This effect is captured by link 4 in Figure 10.7.)

So, our version of the "$64,000 question" becomes: Which would cause us to lose more pounds—exercise or a calorically equivalent diet?

Our analysis above would suggest that the answer to this is not at all clear-cut. On the one hand, exercising may help us lose more weight because REE does not drop as much. On the other hand, because the composition of lost tissue will be more fat and less lean tissue, exercise could cause us to lose less.

Whether the *net* effect favors exercising or dieting is essentially a book-keeping (computational) issue. It is, however, an issue we are not yet ready to tackle here, but one that we will address in Part IV.

Seeing Through the Complexity

While the preceding discussion is still far from a complete picture, as we looked only at the energy output side of the equation, it already illustrates how the regulation of energy balance involves a far more complex network of dynamic interrelationships and mutual interactions. Furthermore, our peek beneath the surface revealed that energy balance is not entirely under our control, but is significantly influenced by involuntary physiological adaptations that regulate both energy expenditure and (as we shall see in the next chapter) energy intake. It is precisely these involuntary "defenses" that render attempts at appetite control and weight reduction so difficult. However, most people (and many health care workers) do not see this. Instead, people readily cling to the myth that they have absolute control over weight loss.

This emerging picture of human energy and weight regulation is admittedly a far more complex picture than the open-loop energy balance equation. While seeing this picture increases our understanding, it comes at a price. Having to contend with many interdependencies instead of two independent and controllable variables is a much more difficult task, one that can easily undermine confidence and responsibility, "as in the frequent refrain, 'It's all too complex for me,' or 'There's nothing I can do. It's the system.'"[88]

But remember this: complexity is not a purely objective attribute of a problem or a system. The level of complexity or messiness we perceive is in large part a subjective matter. Like beauty, in other words, complexity is in the eye of the beholder.

> Take, for example, the everyday activity of driving a car. For a beginner, this is a complex business. He must attend to many variables at once, and that makes driving in a busy city a hair-raising experience for him. For an experienced driver, on the other hand, this situation poses no problem at all. The main difference between these two individuals is that the experienced driver reacts to many "super-signals." For her, a traffic situation is not made up of a multitude of elements that must be interpreted individually. It is a "gestalt."... Super-signals/(structures) reduce complexity, collapsing a number of features into one.[89]

Seeing through the complexity in systems—whether that system is our body, a nuclear reactor, or the U.S. economy—to the underlying structures ("super-signals") that drive system behavior is the raison d'être of the discipline of systems thinking this book advocates.[90] Indeed, one of the most important, and potentially most empowering, insights to come from the young field of systems thinking is that certain patterns of structure recur again and again in many systems, whether physical, biological, or social. "Just as in literature there are common themes and recurring plot lines that get recast with different characters and settings,... these [system structures] are common to a very large variety of [complex] situations,... [revealing] an elegant simplicity underlying the complexity of [systems]."[91]

Learning to recognize these recurring structures—the "super-signals"—is a powerful leverage that allows us to see through complexity to the deeper patterns that lie behind the events and the details.[92]

Revisiting the Bathtub Analogy

[M]ost complex behaviors usually arise from the interactions (feedbacks) among the components of the system, not from the complexities of the components themselves.[93]

Systems science has revealed that there are only a few basic component types that serve as the building blocks of all types of systems, whether physical, biological, or social.[94] We have already examined two of the key building blocks that underlie many complex phenomena: positive and negative feedback loops. Now, we look at how the latter underlies the behavior in two systems that, on the surface, appear to be quite different: the human energy regulation system and the bathtub.

The feedback structures underlying the two systems are depicted in Figure 10.8.

As we saw in our first tub encounter, the level of water in a bathtub rises or falls as a function of the rates of water flowing in and draining out. If the outflow exceeds the inflow, water level falls, but it will not fall at a constant rate and it will not continue to fall forever. As water level in the tub falls, the magnitude of water pressure at the tub's drain decreases, which causes the outflow rate to slow. It is a circular negative feedback loop that can be followed on the diagram: a net outflow at the drain → a drop in water level → drop in water pressure at the drain → less water outflow. The net result of this adapting system is that the water level drops at a continually decreasing rate. Eventually, the outflow rate decreases to a level that matches the water inflow, causing the water level in the tub to level off.

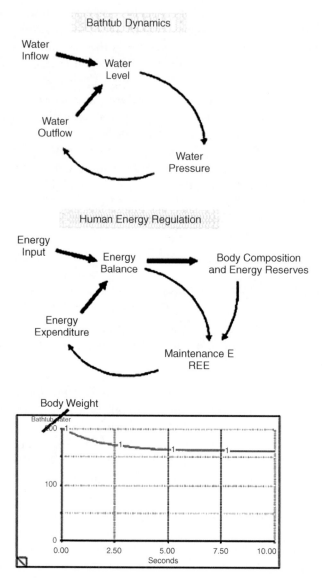

Figure 10.8 Similar feedback structures underlie water draining from a tub and the body's energy regulation

Just like water draining from a tub, negative feedback structures underlie the homeostatic adaptations to negative energy balance that cause weight loss in humans to exhibit a similar pattern. However, in human energy expenditure, rather than having a single drain, we have three. Of the three, REE is by far the largest drain (accounting for 60 to 70 percent of the total energy budget for most sedentary individuals), and, thus, the REE-related adaptations (loops) are often the most consequential.

Figure 10.8 shows the two energy-conserving adaptations to REE. Both are negative feedback processes that resemble the one regulating water flow in the bathtub. It is easy to trace the following two interrelated loops in the figure:

1. A negative energy balance → a drop in REE (as a result of increased metabolic efficiency and the concomitant drop in REE per unit mass) → a drop in daily energy expenditure → shrinking of the deficit in energy balance. (It is link 3 in Figure 10.7.)
2. A negative energy balance → a loss in body weight → a drop in REE (as a result of the loss in lean tissue) → a drop in daily energy expenditure → shrinking of the deficit in energy balance. (It is link 2 in Figure 10.7.)

In a dieting scenario, these two feedback loops work in concert to defend against tissue loss, causing the rate at which weight is lost to decline with time. Eventually, as with the tub, these metabolic adaptations cause total energy expenditure to decrease to a level that matches energy intake. At that point, "the individual will then once again be in energy balance, but with a lower energy intake, lower energy expenditure, and lower energy stores."[95]

Failure to appreciate the full range of the body's compensatory feedback mechanisms leads to confusion and misattribution. For example, it leads to exaggerated weight-loss goals that people fail to meet. Misattributing that failure to insufficient will rather than to the intransigence of the body creates an atmosphere in which unmet goals can be perceived of as a personal or moral failing, and the burden of illness is compounded by the burden of guilt.[96]

Learning to "Squint"

It is no fluke that the energy balance equation—our reigning intellectual paradigm—is an open-loop model.

Studies of human judgment, causal attribution, and problem solving in many domains show that people generally ignore feedback processes in their cognitive maps and adopt an event-based, open-loop view of causality.[97] Examples of open-loop thinking are everywhere, such as when thinking that appetite affects weight, exercise affects body composition, stimuli affect responses, ends affect means, and desires affect actions. All those assertions are incomplete, however, because each of them demonstrably also operates in the opposite direction: weight affects appetite, body composition affects exercise, responses affect stimuli, means affect ends, and actions affect desires. In every one of these examples causation is circular, not linear.[98] But we do not see that.

Why do we see straight lines when reality works in circles? For two primary reasons: visibility (what we see when we open our eyes) and time delays.

When we look with our eyes, we see "stuff." We see material things like people, food, tubs, and buildings. Feedback processes, on the other hand, are not physical objects, they are causal *relationships* between objects. To see them takes some training and requires more effort—more effort than simply opening our eyes and letting the appropriate chemical receptors be simulated. We have to squint *with our mind* to see feedback relationships.[99]

To illustrate, consider our simple bathtub system, and assume you are observing someone filling the bathtub with water—say in preparation for taking a bath (Figure 10.9). If you observe the process, what you will see is this: faucet opening → water flowing → water level rising. These observed processes, however, do not tell the whole tub-filling story. Most notably, they miss the essence of how the tub-filling *goal* regulates the tub-filling process until that goal is attained.

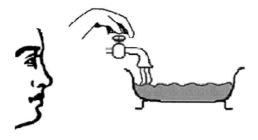

Figure 10.9 Things we see when observing a person filling a bathtub

When we take a bath, we have a desired water level in mind; that's our goal. We plug the drain, turn on the faucet, and watch the water level rise. As the water level rises, we adjust the faucet position to slow the flow of water and then turn it off when the water reaches our desired level (Figure 10.10).[100]

Notice that the goal—our desired water level—and the feedback connections are not visible in the system. "If you were an extraterrestrial trying to figure out why the tub fills and empties, it would take awhile to figure out that there's an invisible goal and a discrepancy-measuring process going on in the head of the creature manipulating the faucets. But if you watched long enough, you could figure that out."[101]

When we observe this process in daily life, we see Figure 10.9 (without the connections), and we naturally think of the faucet controlling the amount water in the tub, but do not think that at the same time the faucet is being controlled through our sight and action by the water in the bathtub.[102] That is, we think of unidirectional cause-and-effect linkages rather than the feedback loop structure that actually exists.

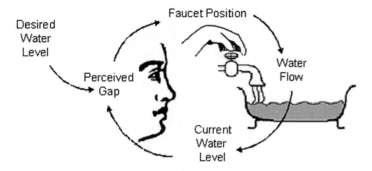

Figure 10.10 Goal-seeking feedback loop regulating the filling of a bathtub to a desired level

In the case of human energy and weight regulation, the feedback relationships are even harder to see, because many aspects of that physical system are even more opaque. The rise and fall of our energy stores, for example, are not as visible as the rising and falling water level in a tub. Further, because with energy and weight regulation we are part of all the lacework ourselves, it is doubly hard to see the patterns of interactions.[103]

In addition to the lack of visibility, another important reason we often fail to see the loops is the asymmetry in the delays associated with cause and effect (e.g., as when the effect of X on Y is immediate and directly apparent, but the feedback effect of Y on X is delayed by days or months). In many of the things we do, the consequences of our actions are not evident in the moment the action is being taken (as when smoking today leads to lung cancer many years in the future). Because we are conditioned to use cues such as temporal and spatial proximity of cause and effect to judge causal relationships, we often fail to "close the causal loop."[104]

The misperception of feedback, however, comes at a price. Misperceiving feedback often results in actions that generate unanticipated (often undesired) surprises,[105] and when this happens, we are quick to claim these to be unfortunate side effects. But do not fool yourself. "Side effects are not a feature of reality but a sign that our understanding of the system is narrow and flawed."[106]

> To avoid [side effects] ... requires us to expand the boundaries of our mental models so that we become aware of and understand the implications of the feedbacks created by the decisions we make. That is, we must learn about the structure ... of the increasingly complex systems [which we are managing].[107]

That is precisely what we have tried to do in this chapter.

Closing the Loops on Energy Balance: Energy Input Side

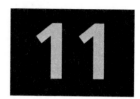

Body Defenses on the Second Energy Front

While failure to attain desired levels of weight loss is a common disappointment for many dieters, what to many is even more discouraging is the difficulty of *maintaining* those subpar weight losses. The record shows that a majority of dieters who succeed in losing weight eventually regain it, typically regaining one third to two thirds of lost weight within a year and almost all of it within 5 years.[108–110] So, it is not surprising that the growing consensus in the field is that the real challenge in obesity treatment is not losing the weight, but keeping it off.[111]

It is difficult to maintain weight loss because our bodies fight back. When any significant weight is lost (e.g., as a result of dieting), the body interprets the loss as a deprivation "crisis" that needs to be contained, and so it sets out to do that. That the body appears to have a mind of its own may seem diabolical to frustrated dieters, but in truth, the body's resistance is neither mysterious nor capricious. Let's not forget that, throughout human history, food deprivation has ordinarily been the result of ecological scarcity. Hence, our built-in physiological defenses in response to food deprivation are the body's attempt to survive in the face of food scarcity; there is nothing diabolical about that. There was simply no evolutionary reason for our bodies to anticipate (or be designed for) self-imposed deprivation in an ecology of plenty—that is, dieting.

In the previous chapter, we discussed the reduction in metabolic rate on the energy expenditure (EE) side of the energy balance equation as one compensatory mechanism to conserve energy and limit tissue loss during caloric deprivation. It is not the sole defense. Because of the importance of ensuring that sufficient energy reserves are maintained for survival and reproduction, complementary physiological adaptations evolved on the energy intake (EI) side to simultaneously boost caloric intake and replenish the body's depleted energy reserves.[112] What this means is that food intake is a behavior that is

T.K.A. Hamid, *Thinking in Circles About Obesity*,
DOI 10.1007/978-0-387-09469-4_11, © Springer Science+Business Media, LLC 2009

not, as we like to think, entirely under voluntary control. Rather, as we shall see, it is an activity that is regulated, in part, by the body's fat depot.

Together, the body's complementary defenses on both the input and output "fronts" are what render attempts at weight maintenance so difficult.

Two-Tier System: Short-Term and Long-Term

When most of us think about our food intake or appetite, we tend to focus on the short-term: meal to meal or day to day. Because cultural and social conventions are often major determinants not only of the food we choose to eat, but also of the size of a meal, its timing, and its composition, food intake naturally appears to be a behavior that is under voluntary control, and there is some truth in that. It is, however, far from the whole story. Metabolic and physiological mechanisms play a major, albeit (to us) less visible, role in regulating our energy intake.

During the past half-century, scientific data have shown that the initiation and termination of feeding are very complex processes that are part reflective and part reflexive. They also have shown that, like other forms of human behavior, food intake is an activity that is mediated by the brain.[113] Specifically, a small region at the base of the brain, the hypothalamus, has been shown to play a major role in controlling food intake and energy homeostasis. (In animal studies, for example, placing tiny lesions in this area causes obesity or leanness, depending on where the lesions are placed.[114])

The emerging conception of human food intake is that it is regulated not by one but by two regulatory subsystems, one short-term and the other long-term, as is depicted in Figure 11.1. The short-term component regulates *satiation*—the feeling of fullness or (nutritional) satisfaction during a meal

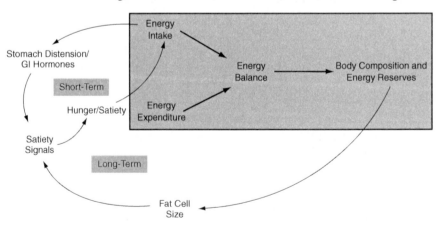

Figure 11.1 Short- and long-term subsystems for regualting food-intake

that brings a period of eating to an end. The other, long-term component influences inter-meal *satiety*—the inhibition of hunger as a consequence of food ingestion and assimilation. Satiation affects a single meal's size, while satiety determines the frequency of meals.[115,116]

The brain plays critical roles in both the short-term (regulating appetite) and the long-term (monitoring the body's energy reserves). In recent years, considerable research has focused on decoding the signals that continually shuttle between the brain and the stomach. Now, scientists believe that they have a pretty good understanding of how (1) incoming signals from diverse sources within the body are integrated in the brain to produce a real-time picture of the body's energy status; and (2) how the brain, in response, orchestrates output messages to trigger or suppress appetite.[117]

Short-Term Component

The *short-term* component controls the onset and cessation of feeding on a meal-related basis. As a meal is consumed, the ingested food interacts with an extensive array of chemo- and mechanoreceptors along the gastrointestinal (GI) tract that relay information about the ingested food to the hypothalamus (mainly via the vagus nerve).[118]

As we all know from personal experience,

> a full belly is a simple but sure sign that the body has recently taken in energy as food, and [is often the cause] to reduce appetite. One way that this physical state is communicated to the brain is via distension-sensitive nerve fibers that carry signals from the stomach and intestine, ultimately reaching appetite-control centers.[119]

In addition to gastric distension, gut peptides, such as cholecystokinin (CCK) and ghrelin, provide added signals to the brain about the amount of food eaten and the kinds of nutrients received.

In a part of the hypothalamus called the arcuate nucleus (ARC), indicators of energy and feeding status that are coming from these diverse sources act upon groups of neurons associated with appetite or satiety. It is the stimulation of these neurons that induces in us feelings of hunger or fullness and, ultimately, causes us to start or stop eating. For example, when the appetite-related neurons are stimulated by an empty stomach, the ARC cells release appetite-stimulating peptides (such as the neuropeptide Y [NPY]), which act to induce appetite and promote eating.[120] Conversely, as we consume food, signals from the stomach and intestine to the brain activate the second type of neurons (the satiety-related group), producing the opposite, anorexigenic effect—or loss of appetite.[121]

Humans do not eat pure energy, of course; we eat nutrients that are oxidized by the body to provide energy. The amount of daily energy a person consumes is determined by the amount of food consumed, together with the diet's composition. The predominant energy-yielding nutrients in the human diet are the three macronutrients: protein, carbohydrate, and fat.[122] Interestingly, the three macronutrients differ not only in their energy content but also in the extent to which they produce satiation and sustain satiety.

> Of the three energy-yielding nutrients, protein is the most satiating. Foods rich in carbohydrates and fibers also effectively extend the duration of satiety by filling the stomach and delaying the absorption of nutrients. In contrast, fat has a weak satiating effect; consequently, eating high-fat foods leads to passive overconsumption.[123]

Long-Term Component

It is not enough that our bodies muster enough energy resources to fuel our immediate metabolic and physical activities. To enhance survival in a food-scarce environment and in the inevitable periods of energy deprivation, the human energy regulation system, like that of the many other species that do not have constant access to food, evolved to maintain the body's long-term energy reserves. In this two-tier system, energy-yielding nutrients in a meal are used to fuel the body's immediate metabolic and physical activities, and any excess is rearranged into long-term storage, primarily in the form of fat reserves, to be used between meals and overnight, when fresh energy supplies run low. The long-term regulatory component monitors the depletion/repletion of these fat reserves.

The choice of fat as the body's primary storage medium was no evolutionary accident. "Fat contains twice the energy-per-unit weight of protein or carbohydrate—nine kilocalories per gram of fat as compared with four kilocalories per gram of protein or carbohydrate."[124] Thus, for a given tissue mass, a person can store several times as much energy in the form of fat as in the form of carbohydrate. That would have been exceedingly important to our ancestors, who had to be highly motile to survive.[125] But even for 21st-century humans, fat's higher energy density means that carrying enough "fuel" is not too burdensome for us, which is a good thing.

> The average young woman carries on her body about one month's worth of energy as fat, which of course would be a very good thing were she, like her ancient ancestors, well out of supermarket range and foraging daily for roots and berries . . .
> If this same young woman were reduced to storing in her body all that energy as carbohydrate, she would probably be too bulky to walk.[126]

The capacity of the human body to adjust to excess calorie intake by adding body fat is impressive (Figure 11.2).[127] Over a lifetime, an extremely obese person may accumulate 300 or even 400 lb, enough to supply his or her energy requirements for a year or more. ("Medical journals tell of one 450-lb man who fasted under medical supervision for a year and two weeks, taking nothing but zero-calorie liquids, and lost nearly 280 lb without any ill effects."[128]) For any individual, the level of body fat is the cumulative sum of the differences between energy intake and energy expenditure, and faithfully reflects the balance (over time) between the two.

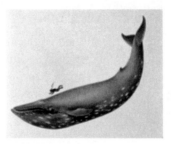

Figure 11.2 Pound for pound, humans are fatter than whales. The great blue whale, the largest mammal on earth, packs enough blubber on its carcass to stuff a typical bedroom from floor to ceiling. Yet fat accounts for only about 12 percent of its body weight. The fattest human on record, Jon Minnoch of Bainbridge Island, Washington, died in 1983 at age forty-two, dragging an estimated fourteen hundred pounds of flesh to his grave. Minnoch was about 80 percent fat. The average middle-aged American lies somewhere between minnoch and the whale. Blue whales are the biggest mammals on earth, but, pound for pound, humans are by far the fattest "(Shell, 2002, p. 49)". (*Source*: Shell, E.R. (2002). *The Hungry Gene: The Inside Story of the Obesity Industry*. New York: Grove Press)

To be able to maintain the body's energy reserves long-term, the regulatory system must be able to sense the status of the body's energy stores and adjust feeding accordingly, that is, adjust the frequency or size of meals. Thus, the system can be seen as having two key components: (1) the adiposity signals that report the status of the body's fat stores to the brain; and (2) the brain centers that receive and decode the signals to influence feeding behavior.[129] The system's first limb, the adiposity signaling mechanism, consists of hormones that are secreted by the body in proportion to the size of its aggregate fat mass. One key hormone in this signaling system is leptin, the product of the *ob* gene.[130] The cloning of the *ob* gene in 1994 and the discovery of leptin and the brain's leptin receptors were major breakthroughs in deciphering the signaling mechanism between the body's fat stores and the brain centers that control eating.[131]

Leptin is synthesized in fat cells and secreted into the bloodstream in concentrations that are proportional to total fat stores. In this way, changes in leptin's plasma level concentration indicate to the brain alterations in the state of the body's aggregate energy reserves. That is, increased levels of leptin signal increased body fat, and, conversely, a drop in leptin reflects a depletion of fat stores.[132]

For the leptin adiposity signals to influence energy balance, they need to directly influence the regulatory centers in the brain that produce the basic drive to eat. That is, the adiposity signals must somehow be transduced within the brain into hunger/satiety signals, thereby influencing the frequency or size of meals. Recent leptin-related discoveries have helped reveal just how elegantly this is accomplished. As the adipocyte's hormonal signals cross into the brain's hypothalamus, which, as mentioned, is the area of the brain that plays a major role in controlling food intake and energy homeostasis, stimulation of the brain's leptin receptors serves to enhance or decrease the potency of the brain's endogenous hunger/satiety signals. That is, the sensitivity of the brain to the (short-term) meal-initiating and meal-terminating signals is modulated, in part, by the size of the adipose mass, so that

> an individual who has recently eaten insufficient food to maintain its weight will be less sensitive to meal-ending signals and, given the opportunity, will consume larger meals on the average. Analogously, an individual who has recently overeaten and gained excess weight will, over time, become more sensitive to gastrointestinal meal-terminating signals [and tend to eat smaller meals over time].[133]

In this way, the brain's short-term signals that control the size or frequency of individual meals are adjusted in proportion to changes in body adiposity.[134,135]

The functions of the long- and short-term subsystems thus overlap, with clear cross-talk between the adiposity-regulatory centers in the brain and the brain regions that produce the basic drive to eat.[136] Any change in short-term energy balance sufficient enough to alter fuel stores (e.g., during prolonged dieting) elicits compensatory changes in the long-term regulatory system. These changes, in turn, induce pressures (via the short-term subsystem) to reverse the underfeeding and replenish the depleted energy stores.[137]

It turns out, then, that the adipose mass is not the passive reservoir of body energy it was once thought. It is a bodily asset that is actively monitored and regulated. Changes in its size are communicated to the brain and directly impact feeding and energy regulation as the body seeks to maintain its stores at desired levels. The system is asymmetric, however.

Two Asymmetries, Not One

> Since survival is more acutely threatened by starvation than obesity, it should come as no surprise that this system is more robustly organized to galvanize in response to deficient energy intake and stores than to excess energy.[138]

Asymmetry in the system is achieved by the fact that the neuronal and endocrine factors generated to stimulate feeding when fat stores decrease (as a result of a negative energy balance) are more potent than are the inhibitory signals generated when fat stores increase (as a result of overfeeding).

This, as was briefly discussed in Chapter 2, was demonstrated by the series of experiments conducted by Mattes et al.[139] to show how humans compensate for increases or decreases in the energy content of their diet. Those results suggest that humans seem to be "hard-wired" to compensate fully for any caloric dilution in their diet, but not the reverse—that is, we are more tolerant to increases in caloric intake.

Leptin's discovery is helping to shed light on the biological underpinnings of this asymmetry. For example, it has been shown experimentally that when a person's fat stores shrink, the drop in leptin production leads to an increase in appetite and a decrease in metabolism.[140–143] By contrast, when a person's fat stores grow upon gaining weight, experimental results show that "beyond a certain point, increased leptin production does little to inhibit appetite."[144]

The much more limited role that leptin plays in preventing weight gain is thought to be caused by increases in cellular resistance to the leptin signal, perhaps another evolutionary adaptation to promote fat storage.[145] Leptin resistance (like insulin resistance in the development of diabetes) would explain why obese people sustain their high body weights, even though they have higher-than-normal levels of leptin in their bodies.[146,147] Over time, as body fat increases, their brains lose the ability to respond to leptin's signal. "The fatter they get, and the more leptin they make, the more insensitive the hypothalamus becomes. Eventually the hypothalamus interprets the elevated level as normal."[148]

Thus, leptin's main role, many obesity researchers now think, "is not to keep us from getting fat, ... but to keep us from getting too thin."[149]

There is a second asymmetry in the regulation of energy and body weight in humans: When body fat is shed during weight loss, fat cells dwindle in size but not in number.[150] Recall that the primary form in which excess food energy is stored in the body is fat in the fat tissue. The amount of fat in a person's body reflects both the *number* and the *size* of the fat cells. Through childhood and adolescence, the number of fat cells increases gradually and continuously as the body naturally grows in size (increasing in number approximately fivefold between the ages of 1 and 20 for a nonobese individual).[151,152] After reaching adulthood, a person's fat cell number may continue to increase as a result of weight gain.

During an extended period of positive energy balance, fat cells expand in size to accommodate excess energy surplus, until they reach their biological upper limit (about 1.0 µg of fat).[153,154] When the cells approach maximal or "peak" size, a process of fat cell proliferation is initiated, ultimately increasing the body's total fat cell number. Thus, obesity develops when a person's fat cells increase in number, in size, or, quite often, both. Once fat cells are formed, however, the number seems to remain fixed, even if weight is lost. That is, with weight loss, cells reduce in size, but no cells are lost.[155–157]

This was demonstrated experimentally in a study that tracked the change in adipose tissue characteristics of 19 obese adults as they reduced their body masses from an average of 149 kg (328 lb) to 103 kg (227 lb) during a weight-loss program (Figure 11.3). The average number of fat cells before weight reduction was 75 billion; this remained unchanged, even after the 46-kg (101-lb) reduction. Fat cell size, on the other hand, was reduced from 0.9 to 0.6 µg of lipid per cell, a decrease of 33 percent. Thus, "a shrinkage of adipocytes with no change in cell number is the major change in adipose cellularity following weight loss in adults."[158,159]

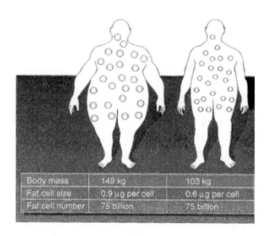

Figure 11.3 Changes in adipose cellularity with weight reduction in obese subjects

The picture of the fat cell's lifecycle, thus, is a depressing one for the obese. Each time body weight increases, new fat cells may be formed, and they are next to impossible to dispose of.[160] It is a biological trap, and one with important implications for energy and weight regulation.

A Homeostatic System with a Difference

At the heart of any homeostatic system, a control process acts to bring the state of the system being controlled in line with some goal or target. This is true whether the target is the speed of an automobile, the temperature of a room, or the body's core temperature. If the controller—the car's cruise control, the room's thermostat, or the brain, respectively—senses a discrepancy between the desired and actual states, it initiates corrective action to bring the state of the system back in line with the goal. In the human body, a multitude of hormonal-based control processes maintain the body's internal stability in just this fashion. In most cases, the homeostatic process strives to maintain some body variable within a set (and invariant) normal level. For example, the human body seeks to maintain core temperature at around 98.6° Fahrenheit in the face of variable (sometimes extreme) ambient temperatures and/or activity levels.[161] If the body's state deviates from normal, the body initiates corrective actions to return itself to the desired state. For example, if body temperature should rise, sweating is induced through the simulation of the sweat glands, and the evaporation of the sweat cools the body down to 98.6° Fahrenheit. Conversely, if body core temperature drops, the heartbeat increases and shivering is induced. The resultant heat-producing muscle contractions raise the body's temperature back to normal.

The regulation of the body's energy stores, however, is different in a very significant way: its target is not static (like desired body temperature). Instead, the set point in energy store regulation is a moving target that can ratchet up over time. In this case, a dynamic control scheme was necessary to allow for the natural growth in body weight from childhood through adulthood. In addition, such an adaptive control scheme would have conferred a survival advantage throughout human prehistory, allowing for the buildup of energy reserves in times of plenty. A key regulator in setting and resetting this moving target is fat-cell size.[162]

Here is a hypothetical example to explain how this adaptive scheme works. Consider the case of an average man, Mr. Average. He is 6 feet tall and weighs 180 lb, which would translate into a body mass index (BMI) of 24. A fat-tissue analysis indicates that fat cells in his body number 25 billion and are of an average size, 0.5 μg. Mr. A.'s weight has remained relatively steady over the last few years. Like most of us, he has experienced occasional, modest fluctuations, sometimes gaining, sometimes losing a few pounds, but always managing to revert back to what he justifiably considered his normal weight. But then some change in lifestyle, perhaps a move from the city to the suburbs, or a change of jobs or family status, embarks him on an extended period of positive energy balance (e.g., persisting nutritional excess and/or diminished physical activity). When we revisit him a year later, we find that he has gained 40 lb.

To accommodate his expanded fat mass, his fat cells would have grown in size and increased in number. This would not occur uniformly throughout his body because newly acquired fat is never deposited uniformly among the body's distributed fat stores. Fat deposits are modulated by body enzymes, such as the enzyme lipoprotein lipase (LPL), which is mounted on fat cell membranes, and whose activity is partially regulated by sex-specific hormones: estrogen in women and testosterone in men. In men, for example, fat cells in the abdomen produce abundant LPL, and, as a result, men tend to store fat there and develop central obesity.[163]

Unhappy with his new state of affairs, Mr. A. decides to go on a diet to lose weight—and he does. His target, not surprisingly, is to drop back down to 180 lb, the weight he considered normal before his recent (temporary, he hopes) weight gain. Unfortunately for Mr. A., the escalation in his weight and the changes to his body (at the cellular level) that accompanied it are neither completely temporary nor completely reversible. As some of his fat cells grew and divided (particularly in those areas that experience larger increases), his fat cell number would have increased, say, to 28 billion. As a result, as he starts losing the weight, the "I am at target level" signal from the body's energy stores to the brain will come at an elevated body weight, the one associated with 28 billion cells at an average size of 0.5 µg. This will happen at a body weight around 200 lb. A drop in weight below this newly elevated target level, say to his original 180 lb, will necessarily cause his 28 billion fat cells to shrink to an average size that is below 0.5 µg. This will be interpreted as a depletion of energy reserves below "desired," and so would trigger his hormones to scream to the hypothalamus, "Eat, eat, eat!"[164]

Gaining a significant amount of weight thus produces some irreversible anatomical and physiological changes that cause body energy reserves to be regulated at a higher set point. Specifically, fat-cell theory maintains that the body's dynamic set point for energy regulation may be determined by the size of fat cells, and the weight at which this occurs depends on the number of cells. Weight loss beyond the point at which cells reach normal size would signal a depletion of energy reserves below "desired," and so induce overeating to refill fat cells.[165,166]

Research in fat-tissue cellularity is also starting to shed light on precisely how fat cells signal the brain the status of their size. The mechanism is believed to be analogous to how mechanoreceptors lining the gastrointestinal tract sense gastric distension and relay information about the stomach's nutrient content to the brain. As fat cells fill with fat and increase in size, the stretching of the fat-cell membrane (and the associated increase in the cell-membrane tension) signals the brain as to the size of fat cells. Both hormonal and enzymic mechanisms mounted on fat-cell membranes appear to be involved in this signaling process.[167,168]

Thus, fat-cell size and number together modulate eating so as to maintain aggregate fat stores while striving to maintain fat-cell size at some normal level. This creates a dynamic mechanism that sets (and resets) the set point for the human energy regulation system. Because the body strives to achieve and maintain normal fat-cell size, the increased number of fat cells that invariably accompanies excessive weight gain results not only in an elevation of body weight, but also in the defense of that body weight. The significance of this for obesity treatment and prevention is clear: It is crucial to reach the overweight patient before fat-cell proliferation sets in. This, as Buckmaster and Brownell explain, can make all the difference:

For example, consider two men each weighing 250 lb, one with a normal number of fat cells, which are enlarged (enlarged fat cells are said to be *hypertrophic*), the other with an excessive number of fat cells (*hyperplasticity* refers to an increased number of fat cells), which are normal sized. For the hypertrophically obese man, weight loss and maintenance are possible [easier] since he can reduce his fat cell size and still sustain adequate lipid volume. However, the hyperplastic man already has normal-sized fat cells, and weight loss results in adipose cell depletion to below normal levels. Even if extraordinary motivation enables the hyperplastic man to overcome his set point, he will be physiologically prone to regain the weight later.[169]

Obese people, thus, do not get any help from their adipose tissue to reduce their appetites. Quite the opposite. The obese appear to suffer from a homeostatic balance that has settled at an elevated level due to the increase in the number of fat cells. Losing a significant amount of weight drops them below what their bodies consider to be the proper weight (because it would replete their fat cells and reduce them in size below normal), and triggers compensatory adjustments, such as increased hunger and caloric intake, which lead to weight regain. Hence the biological trap: The obese often become fat from eating too much and (continue to) eat too much because they are fat—because their bodies are seeking to maintain the higher weight associated with their elevated number of fat cells. Appetite shapes body weight, and body weight influences appetite.[170]

Beyond Physiology: Closing the Behavior–Physiology Loop

12

Not Only Do We Eat Food, We Also Think About It

The eating behavior of humans is unique because it is, on the one hand, controlled by biological states of need (short- and long-term) and, on the other hand, cognitively mediated—that is, we make reasoned decisions about what and what not to eat. We are the only species on the planet "in which hungry individuals will voluntarily refuse to consume readily available, appealing food"[171] in order to meet some particular objective—from achieving aesthetic or health goals to demonstrating a moral conviction (e.g., as in a political hunger strike).[172]

Dieting is a perfect case in point. When individuals reduce food intake to diet, they do so not because their physiology requests it. They do it for personal reasons usually at variance with physiological drives—reasons that are cognitive and deliberate rather than physiological and automatic. Indeed, successful dieting entails overriding the body's built-in homeostatic physiological controls with cognitive controls aimed at achieving an individual's personal aspirations for what his or her weight should be.[173] In a sense, we can say that the success or failure of a diet depends on how well—or poorly—the individual's cognitions control eating behavior.

For many dieters, one question that continues to cry for answers (perhaps louder than most) is this: Why is it that, short-term, people seem quite capable of slashing off sometimes significant amounts of weight by reducing food intake (or simply not eating), but that this success is often short-lived, and eventually the urge to eat wins out?[174] Why is it so difficult for most people to maintain weight loss long-term?

The simplistic energy balance equation, with its one-dimensional view of eating as a biological process of fuel intake, is, not surprisingly, silent on this issue.

T.K.A. Hamid, *Thinking in Circles About Obesity*,
DOI 10.1007/978-0-387-09469-4_12, © Springer Science+Business Media, LLC 2009

Which Requires More Effort: To Do or Not to Do?

In principle, performing almost any behavior should require more exertion than not performing it. Eating a piece of pie, for example, requires various muscular movements of arm, fingers, and jaw. Yet most dieters can attest that refraining from such behaviors can seem more difficult and draining than performing them. In such cases, refraining from the desired behavior involves more than mere passive inaction: Refraining from behaving requires an act of self-control by which the self alters its own behavioral patterns so as to prevent or inhibit its dominant response. A hungry person would normally respond to desirable food by eating it, and so a dieter requires some internal process to prevent that response. That internal process may require a form of exertion that seems more difficult and strenuous than eating.[175]

Dieting to lose weight or trying to keep it off is an act of self-control, not unlike resisting temptations, persevering to finish tiring tasks, breaking bad habits, and the like.[176] In all such cases, *self-control is the process of the self exerting control over the self.* We do it any time we inhibit immediate desires or gratification, and when we prevent ourselves from carrying out a strong but undesirable impulse.[177] In exercising self-control, people exert cognitive control over their body's impulses rather than allowing them to proceed automatically, often because they see that to be in their best long-term interest.

But, as we all know, self-control is no leisurely stroll in the park. It can be (and often is) a challenge, and people are often frustrated by their failures to keep promises and resolutions, to resist temptations so as to control their diet and maintain a desired weight. All too often, we give in and indulge in the "forbidden" behaviors because we lack the self-control to restrain ourselves.[178]

In dieting, as with many other cases of self-regulation, the feeling is that of an inner conflict going on in which we are pulled in opposite directions. That conflict is between the cognitive and the biologic, between one's desire to keep to a strict diet and the urge to "gobble down that doughnut that someone has placed on the table in front of you (Figure 12.1)."[179]

It is important to realize, however, that in self-regulatory challenges—dieting being as good an example as any—this contest of strengths between one's cognitive and biological drives is not a static, discrete event that abruptly arises and is instantaneously resolved one way or the other. All too often, the process is a drawn-out, dynamic affair with ebbs and flows along the way, and where early "wins" may be followed by "defeats," and vice versa.[180] Understanding how this faculty develops and functions and, equally importantly, being able to explain the common dysfunctions (defeats) in

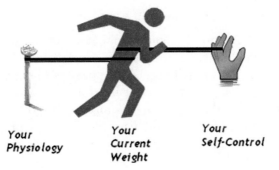

Your Physiology   *Your Current Weight*   *Your Self-Control*

Figure 12.1 Dieting involves a contest of strengths. (*Source:* Adapted from Senge, P.M. (1990). *The Fifth Discipline: The Art and Practice of the Learning Organization* (p. 157). New York: Doubleday/Currency.)

self-regulatory performance, has been a major thrust of social cognitive theory and research,[181] and for good reason.

The capacity to self-regulate is one of the most dramatic and impressive human functions.[182] "It has provided us with an adaptive edge that enabled our ancestors to survive and even flourish when changing conditions led other species to extinction."[183] On the personal level, our regulatory skill, or lack of it, lies at the core of our sense of self and is a key determinant of success in many spheres of life—whether family, school, or business.[184–186] This certainly applies to successful self-regulation of health behavior, and particularly to the maintenance of healthy body weight.

In recent years, there has been an increasing appreciation of the self-regulatory process—both its theoretical importance and great practical utility—and its role in obesity treatment. Thus, the next few sections provide a brief overview of the influential self-control strength model and explain its important implications for the regulation of human body weight.

Strength (and Weakness) Model of Human Self-Regulation

Roy F. Baumeister, Dianne Tice, and Mark Muraven (all of Case Western Reserve University), together with Todd Heatherton (of Harvard), are accredited with formulating the *strength model of human self-regulation*.[187,188] The model helps explain self-control performance, not only statically, in terms of individual or task differences, but also dynamically, as a function of the persistence and duration of the self-control effort over time.

There are three key ingredients to the model:

1. The act of self-regulation is an effortful process that requires strength to override impulses and resist temptations.[189]
2. The human capacity for self-regulation operates like a muscle, and is a limited resource that is partially consumed in the process of self-control. Acts of self-control, thus, not only require the use of strength, but also reduce the amount of strength available for subsequent self-control efforts. As with muscular strength, after exertion self-control strength is replenished with rest.[190]
3. Self-control performance is a product of an individual's level of self-control strength—availability of the resource—and his or her motivation to exert self-control—its mobilization.[191] That is, the motivation for exerting self-control and the level of self-control strength jointly determine the amount of self-control exerted.[192]

That exertion leads to depletion, which, in turn, can lead to lingering self-control exhaustion and reduced performance, is an important distinction between a limited- strength model and a limited-capacity model (as in attentional-focus or working memory).

> [In the self-control strength model,] the depletion of regulatory capacity is not just concurrent [with exertion] but rather continues for a period of time. The resource is limited in such a way that expending it is followed by a period of scarcity, until it builds up again. This is roughly the difference between attention and muscular strength: Both may be limited, but one's quantity of available attention returns to full as soon as current demands on it cease, whereas muscular exertion is followed by a period of reduced capacity. Hence after self-regulation ... [on a difficult task, subsequent] self-regulation ... may not be as effective, because regulatory capacity is reduced. Eventually, with sufficient rest, regulatory strength should return to its previous level, but in the short term the person should have a reduced capacity for self-regulation.[193]

Thus, self-control strength is conceptualized as a reservoir or stock that is consumed and replenished over time, with self-control exertion and rest. Such a stock-and-flow structure would be identical to that of the plumbing analogy used to clarify the dynamics of energy balance (Figure 12.2). That is not just a happy coincidence. It is a perfect example of the important systems-thinking insight that systems across diverse domains—whether biological, engineering, or social—*share common patterns of structure.*

In particular, the stock-and-flow structure shown in Figure 12.2 is a common building block in a wide range of familiar systems. One example is a firm's inventory, in which inventory (the stock) increases by the inflow of production and decreases by the outflow of shipments. Your bank balance is

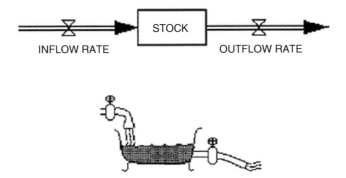

Figure 12.2 Top: Stock-and-flow structure. Bottom: Hydraulic metaphor

a stock that increases with deposits (the inflow) and decreases by withdrawals (the outflow). Human memory is an example of a cognitive stock that accumulates the difference between learning and forgetting.[194]

Recognizing these generic structures and understanding their associated behavior patterns (across diverse domains) provides a powerful conceptual leverage in the study and understanding of complex systems. In this case, the stock-and-flow conceptualization can be very handy in helping us sort out checkbook-balancing–like issues that are of great practical significance: When would exertion lead to temporary depletion of self-control capacity? And does that (necessarily) lead to a deterioration in subsequent regulatory performance?

A First Course in Managing Stocks and Flows

For any stock-and-flow system, the fundamental laws of conservation and accumulation mean that the rates of flow into and out of the stock govern how the quantity of the stock varies over time. For example, if outflow is higher than inflow, the stock level must gradually decrease and, given enough time, may completely deplete. If, and how fast, total depletion of a stock occurs will depend on the initial size of the stock and the magnitude of the imbalance between the inflow and outflow. The larger the *net* outflow and the smaller the stock's size, the faster total depletion occurs. Of course, once a stock is depleted, its outflow will necessarily dry up. In that sense, we can say that there is mutual interdependence between a stock and its flows: the net outflow rate (if positive) depletes the stock, and a depleted stock constrains its own outflow.

Managing the relative strengths of the two opposing rates—the inflow and outflow—is critical to managing a stock's level. This is perhaps easier to see in a *physical* stock-and-flow system, such as that of water flowing into and draining out of a bathtub or of exerting muscular energy. Consider, first, the case of the bathtub shown in Figure 12.2 (bottom). Note that the tub's drain is unplugged, with water flowing out. Unplugging the drain, however, is not in itself enough to cause the tub to empty out. That would depend on whether the rate with which the water drains exceeds the rate of water flowing in, that is, on whether the rate at which water is pouring in *compensates for* the rate at which it is being drained out.

The relative strengths of inflow-versus-outflow rates, together with the size of the stock, also explain why muscular exertion, in the case of physical activity, may or may not deplete muscular capacity and diminish physical performance. For a person living a sedentary lifestyle, for example, muscular exertion on daily activities such as eating, driving, working at the office, shopping, and so on, is always modest, so that the drain on energy reserves (mostly the fat stores in this case) is slow enough that it is adequately compensated for by daily food intake. As a result, there would be no deterioration in the person's performance. Such a state of relative stability, however, changes whenever a person engages in intense physical activity. As mentioned earlier, when a person exercises at high intensity, the muscles must draw on the body's limited glycogen reserves to obtain the glucose needed to fuel the work. The higher the intensity of physical activity, the higher the drain rate on the glycogen energy stock. Because glycogen reserves in the human body are relatively limited (a few hundred grams amounting to about 2,500 kcal), our glycogen stock can sustain only 1 to 2 hours of intense activity before it depletes.[195] Once depleted, the muscles fatigue, thus diminishing our capacity to continue exercising.

Just as humans are able to sustain low-intensity muscular exertion in daily activity, they also are capable of exerting modest levels of self-control and sustaining the effort day in and day out. This suggests that the amount of self-control needed for our daily social functioning, such as stopping at a stop sign or standing in line even when in a hurry, or holding our tempers, is low enough that normal periods of rest can compensate for the slow depletion rate. Indeed, many have proposed that the human capacity to inhibit anti-social impulses, and to do it continuously, has been a key facilitator and even a necessary condition of civilized life.[196,197]

But what about when we have to (or choose to) exert *more-than-modest* levels of self-control? Resisting stronger impulses, such as not eating even when persistently hungry, obviously requires more self-control than resisting less appealing temptations or weaker impulses (say, speeding on the highway).[198,199] Would normal rest be enough, then, to compensate for the faster depletion rate? Or is the human capacity for self-regulation, like our glycogen stores, a limited resource that intense exertion depletes relatively quickly?

To self-control researchers, the theoretical question that needed to be answered was whether the human capacity (stock) for self-control is large enough to sustain intense and, if necessary, extended exertion without deteriorating. It is a question that required an empirical resolution.

The Evidence: To Use It Is to Lose It, at Least Temporarily

Over the last 20 years or so, a wide range of studies have been conducted using many different techniques and measurements to assess self-regulatory depletion in humans. These studies have assessed human performance in controlled laboratory settings, and have analyzed people's autobiographical accounts of self-regulatory experiences—both successes and failures.[200]

Many of these studies were conducted at Case Western Reserve University by Baumeister's group.[201] A major thrust of their laboratory experiments was to assess how human subjects perform when they engage in a series of self-regulatory tasks. In their typical experiment, the researchers had experimental subjects exert self-control on some initial task and then measured their self-control performance on a subsequent (often different) task.[202] The experiments covered a wide range of tasks, including traditional forms of self-control, such as tasks involving delayed gratification and resisting temptations (e.g., eating, smoking, and drinking alcohol), as well as tasks involving persistence in performing frustrating mental exercises (in this case, anagrams) and endurance of physical discomfort (athletic or manual-labor tasks in which the subjects needed to continue performing despite physical fatigue).[203]

The results were consistent across the wide range of studies and generally point toward the following conclusions: The capacity for self-regulation, just like muscular strength, is a limited resource that is subject to temporary depletion.[204] As people exert self-control, subsequent self-control capability degrades over time.[205] As Baumeister's group succinctly put it, "To use it is to lose it, at least temporarily."[206]

The researchers expected and found individual differences in both innate capacity and the motivation to mobilize one's reserves. Some people, we know from personal observation, are much better able than others to hold their tempers, maintain their diets, limit their drinking, save money, persevere at work, and so forth.[207] The experiments not only confirmed such impressions, but also empirically demonstrated that the differences in individuals' degrees of self-regulation can be substantial. In other words, when it comes to self-control strength, some people have a much larger stock than others.[208,209]

The researchers also found that incentives for exerting self-control influenced the degree of deterioration in self-regulatory performance. Participants who were given greater incentives to exert self-control exhibited less deterioration and performed better. In particular, tasks with more attractive outcomes and in which success seemed more likely increased the subjects' motivation to exert self-control, and that, in turn, improved their performance. That is, self-control performance was found to be the product of individuals' motivation to exert self-control and their prior exertions of self-control.[210]

Furthermore, the experimental results also showed (again akin to muscular exertion) that self-regulation in one area reduced the subsequent ability to self-regulate in another area.[211] This suggests that different self-regulation tasks draw on the same resource. In other words, it appears that a single capacity underlies the wide variety of self-regulatory functions and that "any and all attempts at self-control require the use of this resource."[212] The good news is that the degradation in self-control strength is not permanent. With rest (sleep also plays a role, the research indicates), people normally regain their lost strength.

Since the same resource is used for many (or conceivably all) acts of self-control, we would hope that the resource is large. Apparently, it is not. The present findings reveal that (for most people) this resource is rather limited. Acts of self-regulation in many of these experiments were relatively brief, and yet performance was significantly degraded on subsequent tasks.[213]

A Challenge for the Self: How to Accomplish a Lot with a Little

An important and obvious implication of these results is that people's capacity for self-regulation needs to be managed like any other limited resource, and must not be squandered.[214] It is a challenge not unlike, say, managing one's energy consumption while driving a vehicle on a route where there are few refueling stops. Making the trip depends on not running out of fuel between fill-ups, and that will depend not only on how much fuel is in the tank, but also on how we manage our consumption of it (how fast we burn it). Driving at a high speed increases the rate at which fuel will be burned, decreasing the maximum travel distance. On the other hand, when driving at moderate speeds, fuel consumption would be higher, increasing our range (Figure 12.3).

To reiterate, performance in many self-control challenges is determined not only by the size of our tank (stock), which we typically have little control

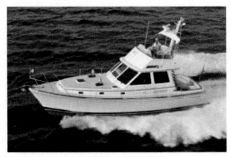

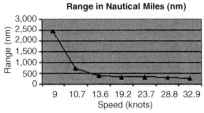

Figure 12.3 Range depends on fuel capacity and on speed. Consider this sexy Alden 44 Fly Bridge. It comes with two 600 horsepower engines, and afuel capacity of 600 gallons. Could it take us from San Francisco to Los Angeles? As with self-control, reaching our destination will depend on what resources we have and how effectivelywe manage those resources. If (because we are in a hurry) we drive the boat hard at 33 knots (its top speed), fuel consumptionwould rise and miles per gallon (mpg) would fall-to a low of 0.48 mpg. At that rate, the yacht'srange would be 290 nautical miles (nm)—not enough to make it. On the other hand, at a cruise speed of 9 knots, fuel consumption would be4.52 mpg, extending our range to 2,700 nautical miles

over, but also, and equally importantly, by what we do with what we have—a choice we *do* control.

How effective are dieters at managing their limited capacity for self-regulation? The research indicates some good news and a lot of bad news. First, the good news: Recent findings indicate that more and more people are getting better at losing weight, at achieving levels of weight loss that are substantial enough to improve their health, and at maintaining weight loss for extended periods. Of the estimated 55 million Americans who will go on a diet this year, we can expect that between 5 and 20 percent of them will succeed in losing 5 to 10 percent of their initial body weight and will keep it off for at least a year.[215–218]

The bad news, however, is that dieters who successfully sustain a long-term weight loss remain a minority. For the vast majority of dieters, long-term success remains elusive. The research continues to show that most dieters are trapped in a recurring cycle of weight loss and regain. "*Yo-yo dieting* became the colloquial term for this process."[219] The cycle typically starts with lofty weight-loss goals, followed by short-lived losses, and invariably ending with a regain of the weight.[220,221]

Why?

Most overweight individuals tend to set weight-loss goals that reflect their image of what their ideal body weight should be, based, perhaps, on personal notions of aesthetics, advertised "poster" success stories, or standard height/

weight charts read in a book or magazine article.[222,223] In one revealing study, a group of overweight women participating in a weight-loss program were asked to identify their desired weights before beginning the program. Their goal weights amounted to a whopping 32 percent reduction from their initial weight, which far exceeds the 5 to 10 percent reduction commonly recommended by experts and reported by the most successful weight-loss studies.[224,225] Particularly interesting was the fact that the women's weight-loss targets were nearly three times the amount that they themselves had typically lost in previous efforts, suggesting that personal experience did not dampen their "irrational exuberance."

The unrealistic goals that people set not only virtually guarantees that they cannot be fulfilled, but in fact contribute to relapse, not unlike the hurried skipper in the example above, who drives his boat too hard and runs out of fuel as a direct result (Figure 12.3). The two phenomena are related.

Why Goals Matter, and How More May Be Less

If, as most people tend to assume, the only risk of setting an unrealistic weight loss goal is failure to attain it, then setting such a goal would appear to have no serious downside. Dieters who shoot for their dream body weight, no matter how unreasonable, would nevertheless always settle for what is achievable. That is the scenario shown in Figure 12.4 depicting the dieter as he or she struggles to attain the "ideal" weight goal, falling short (of the "dream goal" level), but ending up no worse than someone who had started with a more modest goal.

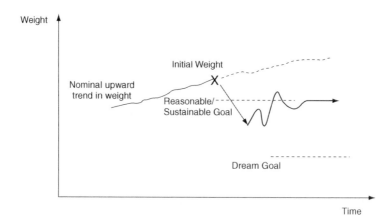

Figure 12.4 The mental model: no downward risk for aggressive goals

In reality, though, setting an unrealistic goal poses a more serious risk: the risk of relapse. That's the scenario shown in Figure 12.5 and the one most commonly encountered in practice. In this familiar pattern, dieters seeking lofty weight-loss goals are able to slash off large amounts of weight by eating very little or even starving themselves, but then run out of regulatory gas and end up, after a period of short-lived success, regaining the weight, often with "interest."[226] For these dieters, who are, by far, the majority, the end result leaves them worse off than if they had begun with and maintained a more modest weight-loss goal.

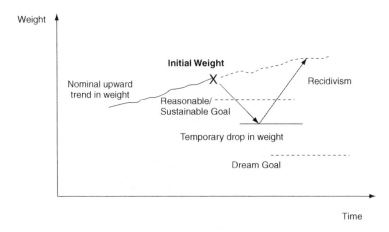

Figure 12.5 The real downward risk

Whether we are managing body weight, personal finances, or fuel consumption, the goal we set not only defines the *end* to a purposeful task, but also shapes the *means* to achieving it. Therefore, establishing a *different* goal can and does *create* an altogether very different endeavor and, quite possibly, a very different outcome.

In the case of dieting, the greater the weight-loss goal, the greater the caloric deficit must be. For example, rather than pursue a moderate-deficit diet (MDD), which typically is in the range of 1,200 to 2,000 kcal/day, the dieter may opt for a low-calorie diet (LCD) providing 800 to 1,200 kcal/day, or even a very-low-calorie diet (VLCD) providing fewer than 800 kcal/day. The greater the caloric deficit, the more acute the person's hunger, and the greater the self-control needed to override the deprivation and sustain the diet,[227,228] the greater the drain rate the dieter imposes on his or her self-control capacity (stock). That is obvious. But what is often less obvious is how much harder that effort becomes.

People can seriously underestimate the escalation in hardship because, as psychologists have found (and as we have already noted), people intuitively view causality in linear terms, expecting effect always to be proportional to cause. That is to say, we to tend to think that if *A* causes *B* to happen, then 2*A* must cause 2*B* to happen.

But the escalation in effort needed to accomplish a task often increases exponentially, not linearly, as task difficulty increases. This principle is not unique to dieting, but applies to many tasks, both cognitive and physical. It is, perhaps, easier to grasp in physical tasks such as, say, muscular exertion. Consider, for example, walking, which is, for most people, their major physical activity outside their sedentary lifestyles. Figure 12.6 portrays how energy expenditure escalates as walking speed increases, at speeds ranging from 1 to 10 kilometers (km) per hour (equivalent to 0.62 to 6.2 mph). Clearly, as speed increases, energy expenditure rises, not in a linear fashion, but exponentially.[229] (By the way, if we were to plot the relationship between the speed of the powerboat in the earlier example and its fuel consumption, we would get a similar-looking curve.)

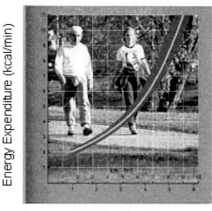

Speed (mph)

Figure 12.6 Energy expenditure escalates as walking speed increases. (*Source:* McArdle, W.D., Katch, F.I., and Katch, V.L. (1996). *Exercise Physiology: Energy, Nutrition, and Human Performance* (p 169). Baltimore: Williams & Wilkins.)

At low walking speeds, such as at the 1- to 2-mph pace of normal daily activities, the exertion of muscular energy (the stock's outflow rate) is modest enough that the drain on energy reserves can be adequately compensated for by daily rest and food intake (the inflow rate). It is, in other words, a level of exertion that is sustainable, meaning that if we chose to, we could sustain this level of physical activity for extended periods of time without depleting our muscular energy stock. In fact, we can sustain it for very extended periods, as in the case of Deborah De Williams, who, on Friday, October 15, 2004, arrived back in her hometown of Melbourne after having set a world walk record as the first woman to walk around Australia, walking in a clockwise direction along Australia's National Highway 1 (Figure 12.7). She completed the 9,715-mile walk in 343 days (which also earned her a second world record for the longest walk in the shortest time). De Williams had walked close to 30 miles per day, at a speed of 2 miles per hour, which translates into walking 14 hours every day for almost a year. That is a *sustained stock*, if there ever was one.[230]

As the above speed-versus-energy-expenditure plot shows, walking faster can quickly increase the rate of energy expenditure. Once our rate of energy expenditure exceeds our ability to replace it, our energy reserves must

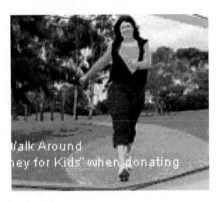

Figure 12.7 Deborah De Williams on her walk around Australia. (*Source:* www.walkaroundoz. org.au.)

deplete over time. How fast? Consider what it takes to run a marathon. The human energy "stock" (even the best stocked) is barely large enough to sustain the 26-mile marathon run. (That is quite a bit less than De Williams's 9,715 miles.) Those runners resilient enough to endure it will most certainly arrive with empty tanks (Figure 12.8).

Not unlike walking or running, the self-regulatory effort in weight loss escalates not linearly, but exponentially, with the difficulty of the goal. Our body's weight set point "seems to have a certain give to it, so that a person can stay a bit below it with relatively little effort."[231] Larger weight losses, on the other hand, are difficult to tolerate. Fat-cell theory provides one possible

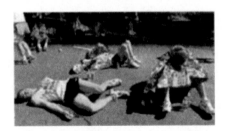

Figure 12.8 New York marathon

mechanism for this physiological nonlinearity. As the enlarged fat cells of an overweight dieter (which had expanded in size during weight gain to accommodate excess energy storage) shrink back to their normal size (or slightly below it) subsequent to modest weight loss, the physiological signals to overeat and regain the weight are often easy to override. But if the weight loss effort persists and the fat cells deplete to below-normal levels, the "volume" of the physiological message to the brain's appetite-control center increases, eventually becoming a scream: "EAT, EAT, EAT!"[232]

Experimental studies show just how "deafening" this message can become. In acute-dieting experiments, obese people who lost large amounts of weight developed a psychiatric syndrome called semi-starvation neurosis, a condition that had been noticed before in people of normal weight who had been starved. These experimental subjects continuously fantasized about food or about breaking their diet; they dreamed of food, and they became anxious and depressed (some even had thoughts of suicide).[233]

In previous chapters, we discussed several of the many other nonlinearities inherent in the complex adaptive system of human energy regulation. Recall, for example, the discussion on how, even if one maintains a constant caloric deficit, weight loss tends to decline with time because decreases in body weight are accompanied by drops in the body's maintenance energy requirements, as well as by drops in the energy cost of weight-bearing physical activity (because of moving a lighter body).[234] This downward adaptation in energy expenditure as weight is lost causes dieting to become more difficult as it progresses. The same effort that produces noticeable weight loss in the early first phases may produce less or no weight loss in the later phases. (This is why weight loss during prolonged underfeeding is *curvilinear*, not linear.)

The stock-and-flow concept, with the aid of basic "spoon" arithmetic, can also help us understand why hardship escalates more than proportionally with escalating caloric restriction. To illustrate, I will use myself as an example. Let's say that my normal and steady body weight is W lb, and that my steady-state daily diet to maintain that weight is four "spoons" of foodstuff (let's assume that a spoon packs the equivalent of 1,000 kcal of dietary energy). As a stock and flow, I would look like this (Figure 12.9):

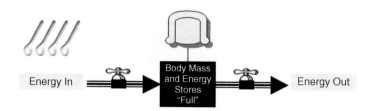

Figure 12.9 Four spoons of food-stuff keep in energy balance

Now consider two dieting scenarios: (a) decreasing caloric intake by 25 percent (to three spoons per day); and (b) doubling the caloric deficit to 50 percent (i.e., to only two spoons per day). What kind of condition would I be in, say, 2 weeks into the diet?

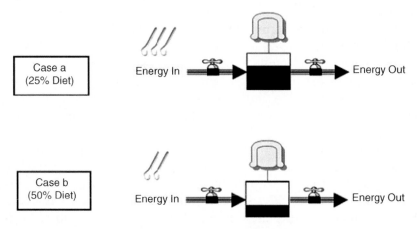

Figure 12.10 Greater depletion of my energy reserves in case "b"

You would find, first, that I had lost weight in both cases and, second, that my struggle to keep it off is much higher in case b than in case a. To bring me back to my normal body weight, my physiological regulatory system will, in both cases, be signaling me to eat more, but not just one spoon more in case a and two in case b. In the immediate term, I would need to consume more than my four-spoon steady-state diet to rebuild my depleted reserves (as depicted in Figure 12.10). The amount I must eat will be significantly more in case b than in case a because of the larger cumulative loss to my energy stock (Figure 12.11).

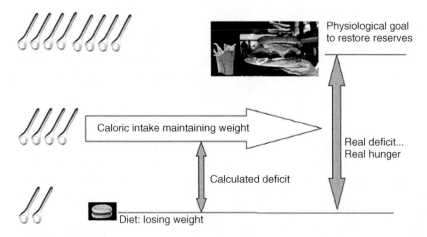

Figure 12.11 To make up for the deficit, I'll need more than four spoons of food-stuff—possibly much more

The elevated drive to overconsume after weight loss (relative, that is, to pre-diet levels) is a phenomenon that has been demonstrated experimentally. In feeding experiments on humans, food intake was found to markedly increase above pre-diet levels—by more than 50 percent in one study—once dietary control was relaxed after a period of food restriction (and the experimental human subjects were allowed to eat freely). Furthermore, researchers found that this hyperphagic response persisted several weeks after body weight had reached the pre-diet level.[235,236] "The experiences of semi-starved explorers over-indulging in food for weeks and months on their return from expeditions also document particularly well this phenomenon of energy over-consumption."[237,238]

The bottom line is that the harder we push, the harder the body pushes back. The greater the weight loss, the greater the sensation of hunger and the drive to eat and, hence, the greater the exertion of self-control and the higher the risk of self-control depletion.[239] As deprivation accumulates or escalates, many dieters would, no doubt, attest, hunger can end up consuming us, and food becomes the focal point of every thought and action.[240]

Weight Cycling: Not Once, Not Twice

While most dieters undoubtedly understand that they would succeed more often if their diet goals were more realistic, dieters' personal agendas rarely include such modest goals.

> Losing less weight, taking longer to lose it, and abandoning one's hopes that weight loss will produce a complete social and personal makeover are not the sort of things that dieters are eager to do. Nor are they encouraged to. The diet industry [at least large segments of it] thrives for two reasons—big promises and repeat customers. These two reasons are interrelated: The big promises attract the customers in the first place, and the magnitude of the promises virtually guarantees that they cannot be fulfilled.[241]

It makes for a very attractive business model.

Recall that the goal set by the group of women cited above, a 32 percent reduction in weight, was not only high in theoretical terms; it was unreasonable even relative to the women's own past performance, being, on average, three times as large as what this group of women had typically lost in past efforts. And that is not all that is shocking. Research studies consistently find that people are perennially overly optimistic when it comes to predicting favorable outcomes for themselves.[242] Even when people fail to meet their overly optimistic expectations, they can be quite adept at concocting self-serving interpretations to justify maintaining their unrealistic beliefs.[243] Furthermore, because of the complexities and ambiguities in real-life experiences, weight-loss and loss-maintenance failures do not necessarily cause people to reassess their underlying beliefs. Instead of questioning their own expectations, they commonly react "[by blaming] the failure on not having had enough willpower, with a simultaneous commitment to starting the diet again, but this time promising to try harder."[244]

Such a common attribution is enhanced by various circumstances:

> First and foremost, testimonials provided by others who have allegedly succeeded using the same diet imply that the fault in one's own case must lie in oneself rather than in the diet.... [Second,] the promoters of the diet in question have a vested interest in blaming the dieter rather than the diet. If the dieter consults the diet promoter—be it her doctor, her friend, the clinic where the diet program was obtained—she is likely to be told that she is at fault, in what amounts to classic instance of blaming the victim. The victim, who has supposedly failed to make the full effort required for success, has before her the opportunity to redeem herself by trying harder next time. Failure is due to an attributionally unstable characteristic [effort] and is therefore correctable.[245]

By maintaining their unrealistic expectations, people become trapped in weight cycling, the endless repeating rounds of weight loss and regain.[246] It is a dynamic that the self-control strength model predicts.

Understanding How Cycles Happen

Cycles are interesting and very common modes of behavior. We encounter them in our physical world (as with the cycles of the seasons, night and day, and the oceans' tides), in our social and economic systems (such as the boom and bust cycles in the economy), and in our own bodies and well-being (which rely on wake-sleep cycles and circulatory and cardiac cycles).

In a wide variety of social, biological, and physical systems, cyclic behavior arises from a very simple and common structure: a system in which two resources (stocks) interact with one another such that the rise in one drains the other, and vice versa. In nature, we see this in predator–prey situations; in business, in inventory–labor interactions; and in human weight regulation, in the contest of strength between the cognitive and the biological. Let's see how.

We have already seen two sets of stocks and flows in the human psychobiological system for feeding regulation. One is the body's energy stock, with food intake as its inflow rate and energy expenditure as its outflow rate. The other is this chapter's discussion of the stock of human self-control, with its replenishment and exertion rates. Up to this point, these two sets have been described separately. In reality, of course, these two sets of processes are not isolated phenomena, but are interacting components of a psychobiological system for human feeding regulation. Indeed, it is the interaction between these two stock-and-flow systems that gives rise to the weight cycling phenomenon.

In Figure 12.12, we take the extra step of combining the two stock-and-flow processes into an integrated whole. What we end up with is one of the classic archetypes for oscillatory behavior: that of two stock-and-flow systems locked together in a negative feedback embrace.

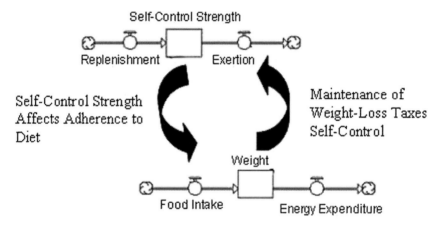

Figure 12.12 Combining self-control and energy-regulation stock-and-flow processes

Specifically, in this now integrated psychobiological system for human feeding regulation, self-control strength (which we can designate as stock 1) affects adherence to the diet and, hence, the regulation of the food intake rate into stock 2 (body weight). This regulatory function is not a free lunch; constraining food intake to decrease or maintain the weight stock at a low level is an effortful process that consumes self-control strength. This means that the state of the body-weight stock (stock 2) regulates the exertion rate (the outflow rate) of the self-control stock. Stock 1 acts as a catalyst for the *inflow* rate to stock 2, and, likewise, stock 2 returns the favor and acts as a catalyst for the *outflow* from stock 1. The dynamic interdependence of these two stock-and-flow processes is what generates a cyclic pattern of weight loss and relapse.

In Figure 12.13, by following the numbered arrows down from top to bottom, we can walk through one such cycle. At the start of a diet cycle,

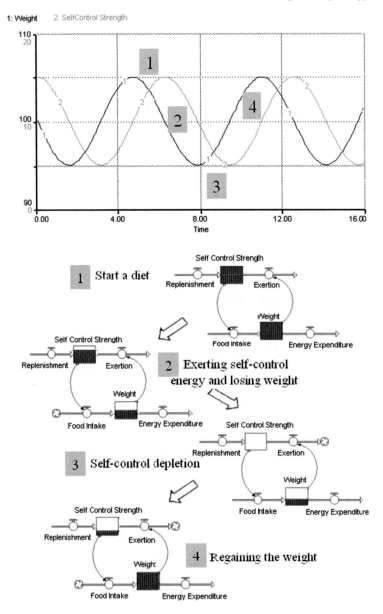

Figure 12.13 A cycle of weight loss and regain

both stocks would typically be relatively full (such as at point 1). Voluntary restriction of one's food intake when starting a diet causes weight—stock 2— to gradually drop. Because the dieting process consumes self-control energy, the dieter drops to point 2 in the figure, with both stocks partially depleted.

But this particular dieter does not stop there. Her futile persistence to shed an unrealistic amount of weight causes her to keep going, depleting both stocks further. When that process ultimately depletes her self-control strength, she hits bottom—at point 3 in the cycle. While, from a weight-loss standpoint, reaching that juncture may be cause for celebration, unfortunately for her, she will not stay at that point. With a depleted stock 1, the dieter's grip on the feeding inflow "spigot" loosens, and with adherence to the diet progressively weakening as a result, the weight stock invariably refills, propelling her back to the top of the cycle, at point 4.

This two-stock feedback structure, while admittedly far too simplified to capture the complexity and idiosyncrasies of human weight regulation, does, in fact, capture the essential elements that drive human weight-cycling behavior. Interestingly, this particular two-stock structure is fundamentally the same structure that underlies cyclic behavior in many other familiar systems. For example, a similar two-stock feedback structure drives such common items (systems) as the pendulum clock and a child's Slinky toy. (If we were to mathematically represent the variables in these systems and their interrelationships, the variables would assume different names; rather than body weight, feeding, and energy expenditure, we would have, for example, pendulum or spring mass, force, and momentum, but the differential equations that capture their dynamic interactions will have similar forms.)

A major difference, though, is that a pendulum clock is a simple man-made system whose components are carefully isolated from the environment so as to generate a regular motion. The human system for feeding behavior, however, is far from isolated. It interacts in complex ways with a multitude of other systems (physiological, social, environmental) and is continuously bombarded by all sorts of random effects from an unanticipated illness to the occasional feast or famine. Thus, the cyclic behavior of a complex system, such as weight regulation, assumes a less regular, less symmetric shape than the pendulum-like form of oscillation shown in Figure 12.13.[247]

For example, in real-life scenarios the cyclic behavior of weight loss and regain is often superimposed upon a longer-term upward drift in weight. Figure 12.14 (from one of the few studies that tracked variations in patterns of body weight in free-living subjects over prolonged periods) shows the average weights of 31 women over a 25-year period. Over that extended period, this group of women (whose average age was 40 years) dieted an average of five times.[248] Notice that as the women's weights cycled between weight loss and regain, their weights also trended upward over time.

There are at least two mechanisms through which yo-yo dieting could lead to such an upward drift in weight. First, when dieters fall off their unrealistic regimens, they tend to go on eating binges.[249,250] The urge to overeat,

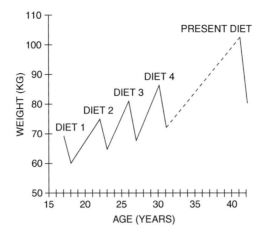

Figure 12.14 Weight and dieting histories of 31 women, all of whom had engaged in a minimum of four diets

especially after a period of acute dieting, may be driven by the psychological pressures—the frustrations and deprivation—that accumulate during weight suppression.[251,252] Second, some investigators found that repeated cycles of weight loss and regain are associated with increased metabolic efficiency, which makes subsequent dieting more difficult and predisposes people to gaining weight.[253]

Longer-Term Risks

Although weight cycling is surely a source of frustration to many dieters, the risks associated with repeated cycles of weight loss and regain far exceed mere disappointment. A substantial body of epidemiological research shows that repeated cycles of weight loss and regain increase the risks of chronic diseases (particularly coronary heart disease) and even premature death, independent of obesity itself.[254,255]

Weight cycling also has been found to have serious "psychic costs," such as loss of self-esteem, depressive mood states, and life dissatisfaction.[256,257] Of particular concern is that repeated failures to attain expected weight-loss targets often leads to loss of *self-efficacy*—that all important feeling of confidence in one's ability to accomplish some goal or perform a particular activity, including confidence in overcoming the barriers that may arise.[258–261]

Less Is More

Like any other limited (and exhaustible) resource, self-regulatory capacity needs to be managed and must not be squandered. But squandering it, not managing it, is what most dieters habitually do.

Thankfully, however, things may be changing. A growing understanding of the biological factors that regulate body weight and of the cognitive difficulty of maintaining large weight losses is prompting a redefinition of the "successful" goals of obesity treatment. Slowly but surely, moderation is becoming the overriding theme in weight-loss efforts.[262]

A major impetus for this has been the growing evidence that moderate weight losses of only 10 to 15 percent of initial weight, even among substantially overweight individuals, is associated with a significant improvement in nearly all parameters of health, including blood pressure, heart morphology and functioning, lipid profile, glucose tolerance (among diabetics), sleep disorders, and respiratory functioning.[263] This has prompted a growing number of federal agencies and health organizations to call for setting more realistic weight goals rather than striving for an "ideal" weight. For example, the federal guidelines on the identification, evaluation, and treatment of overweight now recommend "an initial weight loss of about 10% of body weight over a 6-month period at a rate of 1–2 pounds per week."[264] Even more modest, the Institute of Medicine of the National Academy of Sciences defines successful long-term weight loss "as a 5% reduction in body weight that is maintained for at least 1 year."[265]

Establishing goals based on reasonable rather than ideal weights is, no doubt, "a dramatic paradigm shift with implications for how treatment is selected, delivered, and evaluated."[266] It is a shift, however, that we must carefully tread. The risk here is to be lulled into thinking that this suddenly transforms treatment into a quick-and-easy task. Unfortunately, that is not the case.

The evidence on this is unambiguously clear: maintaining moderate weight loss, even many years after the initial weight loss, requires, for most people, a great deal of effort. It is a message that emerges loud and clear from the "live" experiences of successful long-term weight loss maintainers in the ongoing National Weight Control Registry (NWCR) study. (The NWCR consists of approximately five thousand individuals who have, on average, maintained weight loss for more than 5 years, and counting.[267]) In a recent study of these very "successful losers," a significant number of them reported that they still have to work hard to keep weight off, 5, 10, and even 15 years after losing the weight.[268–270]

The practical (and hopeful) lesson to take away from this chapter is this: When reasonable goals are set and are achieved or exceeded, there will be rewards instead of disappointments. This, research studies have recently shown, can turn the mutual interdependence of self-efficacy and weight-loss effort into a self-reinforcing process. In one study, pretreatment weight-control self-efficacy facilitated weight loss, and the achievement of reasonable weight-loss goals, in turn, reinforced the subjects' (all were women) belief structure and led to better outcomes in maintaining the weight loss.[271]

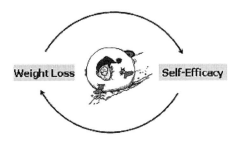

Figure 12.15 Self-efficacy facilitates weight loss efforts, and successful weight loss strengthens self-efficacy

It is a great example of turning a self-reinforcing feedback process to work for us instead of against us. (And in an area—self control— where we can use and help we can get). Learning to recognize and harness the power of positive feedback to one's advantage is a powerful conceptual leverage one gains from applying the systems approach.

All of this further underscores the lessons of the self-regulation strength model. Self-control performance is the product not only of self-control strength—how much an individual has in the tank—but also of the motivation to mobilize one's resources and exert the self-control effort. Therefore, adopting reasonable goals helps in two ways: dieters do not run out of regulatory gas, and they maintain the necessary fortitude to go the distance.

Looking Back and Looking Forward

13

Looking Back

The focus of Part III has been on understanding how the reality of human energy regulation is far more complex and far more dynamic than the static, open-loop model of the simplistic energy balance equation, in part because the two limbs of energy balance are not independent, but instead are physiologically linked, interacting in complex ways and often compensating for each other in the face of interventions.[272] Part III has also addressed how nonlinear feedback processes underlie many of the interactions and mutual independences in human energy regulation; how some of these interactions induce positive feedback effects, while others are negative; and how feedback processes operate at multiple overlapping levels (as homeostatic processes at the physiological level, between the physiological and the behavioral, and between people and their external environment).

Though not directly visible to us, these circular mechanisms and their interactions account for much of what happens to our bodies over the long term; they are what make attempts at appetite control and weight reduction so difficult. As we closed the loops, the system became more realistic, but also much more complex, which is why, as is often stated, the very same traits that make the feedback-systems approach attractive—putting things back together and recognizing the feedback interactions among them—also make it somewhat slippery and elusive[273]—or it *used* to.

T.K.A. Hamid, *Thinking in Circles About Obesity*,
DOI 10.1007/978-0-387-09469-4_13, © Springer Science+Business Media, LLC 2009

Understanding Is a First Step, But Far from Sufficient

Understanding is an important and necessary step toward better management of any complex system, such as our body, but it is not sufficient. As was argued earlier, effective control of a dynamic system, whether it is the energy regulation of our bodies or the energy regulation of an atomic reactor, requires two essential skills: understanding and prediction. Without a capability to predict the system's behavior, perfect understanding is of little practical utility. The ability to infer system behavior is essential if we are to know how our actions influence the system. Thus, prediction is as essential as understanding in devising appropriate interventions for change. The two skills are needed together.

The two modes of reasoning are interdependent, but are conceptually different. Furthermore, experience from working with human subjects in many domains indicates that even when people learn to comprehend the detailed relationships and interactions in complex systems, they are usually unable to accurately predict the dynamic behavior these relationships imply. That is, being able to mentally "run" the model to figure out the dynamic implications over time is a much more difficult task.[274] In the words of Jay Forrester, the father of system dynamics: "[T]he human mind [can] grasp pictures, maps, and static relations in a wonderfully effective way. But with respect to systems of interacting components that change through time, the human mind is a poor [predictor] of behavior."[275] The more complex the system, the harder prediction becomes.

Our discussions in previous chapters suggest that human bioenergetics belong to the class of *multiloop nonlinear feedback systems,* which is the same class that defines some of our most complex technological systems, including chemical refineries, autopilots, and communication networks. Engineers have long appreciated that the complex feedback structures of such systems is often a source of puzzling behavior and that intuition alone is unreliable in estimating how these systems change over time. Human bioenergetics is no exception.

As with many multiloop systems, discerning the dynamic behavior of any one of the system's individual loops in isolation can be reasonably easy, but figuring out the behavior of a dense network of interconnected feedback loops is often extremely tricky. To illustrate, consider two interrelated loops we have discussed before (Figure 13.1):

1. A negative energy balance → a drop in resting energy requirements (REE) (as a result of increased metabolic efficiency and the concomitant drop in REE per unit mass) → a drop in daily energy expenditure → shrinking of the deficit in energy balance.

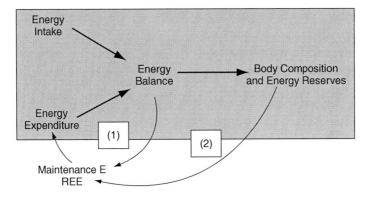

Figure 13.1 Two loops regulating the REE level

2. A negative energy balance → a loss in body weight → a drop in REE (as a result of the loss in lean tissue) → a drop in daily energy expenditure → shrinking of the deficit in energy balance.

In a dieting scenario, these two feedback loops work in concert, reinforcing one another to defend against tissue loss. As a result, the rate at which weight is lost on a diet declines with time (even if the prescribed diet is maintained) until a new equilibrium body weight is reached, typically, at a level that is significantly above that expected from the apparent caloric deficit.

These feedback adaptations complicate the predictive task for the dieter. In Figure 13.2, the left graph shows how a simplistic linear system (without feedback compensation) would be straightforward to predict, in which a pound of weight is lost at the fixed energy cost of 3,500 calories. As depicted by the graph on the right, weight loss is far more complex in reality. Not only is the weight loss achieved by food restriction invariably less than that expected from the simplistic linear model, but the feedback effects between the body's energy reserves and energy expenditure mean that the *same*

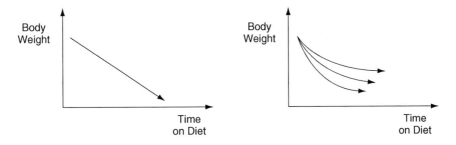

Figure 13.2 Left: Linear model: one scenario. Right: Multiple loops: multiple scenarios

energy deficit can lead to multiple possible scenarios. The outcome depends on the many differences that exist among individual dieters, such as a dieter's initial body composition, because the composition of tissue lost during weight reduction depends on the initial body fat content of the subject. Obese people, for example, lose more weight as fat than do lean people, who lose more lean tissue. Because fat and nonfat tissue types have different energy densities, such differences translate into differences in the amount of weight lost/gained.

But there is more. The outcome of a weight-loss intervention also depends on the way in which the energy deficit is engineered (e.g., dieting versus exercising). For example, if the energy deficit were to be induced by an exercise treatment rather than by dieting, such an intervention would induce an increase in muscle (fat-free mass [FFM]), which could, in turn, elevate rather than lower maintenance energy requirements (REE). Such an adaptive response, shown in Figure 13.3 as loop 3, adds an additional wrinkle to the prediction task. In this case, the new loop counteracts rather than reinforces loops 1 and 2. By conserving and even increasing the FFM (the principal metabolically active component of total body mass), exercise partially blunts the drop in maintenance energy expenditure that accompanies diet-based weight loss.[276]

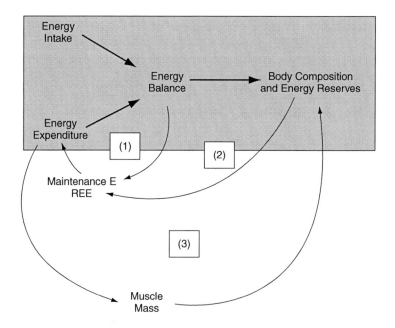

Figure 13.3 As we add loops, the model becomes more realistic... and more complex

From this simple example, we can see that even though the behavior of each of the loops discussed above may be reasonably obvious in isolation, assessing the resulting *net effect* of their interactions, and being able to do it accurately and reliably, is not. Indeed, many experimental studies have shown that the ability to trace the behavior generated by a system of only three nonlinear feedback loops (such as we have here) is already beyond the capacity of human intuition.[277] (In Chapter 14, we will have the opportunity to "experience" that first-hand.)

Looking Forward

Engineers turn to computer simulations to learn about the behavior of complex engineering systems. Biological systems, it is becoming increasingly clear, are far more complex and harder to understand than many of our technological systems.[278] Why, then, don't we use the same approach and make models of physiological systems, such as of our bodies, and use the models to predict behavior? We can, and we should.

A key takeaway message from the book is this: We cannot and should not rely on intuition alone in managing our bodies. With its many interrelated subsystems and processes (some counteracting, some reinforcing) the human body is simply too complex to effectively manage by human intuition alone. The long time delays and the many interactions between many of the body's parts and processes mean that interventions (diets) can have a multitude of consequences, some obvious and many not so obvious, some immediate and others distant in time and space (as when intervention in one part of the body affects another). To effectively manage a system as complex as the human body requires a bookkeeping tool that is more reliable (and efficient) than human intuition. The digital computer, a complementary innovation to systems thinking, provides us with that tool.

In Part IV, I argue for and aim to demonstrate (in laymen's terms) the feasibility and value of a new generation of dynamic tools that support interaction and customization for personal health and wellness management. We are in a position to do this because of the great advances in systems sciences, medicine, and computer technology over the last few decades.

Thanks to the availability of affordable, high-quality computing capabilities and increasingly user-friendly software, ordinary people are today in a position, for the first time in history, to have access to and to effectively employ models of systems as complex as their own bodies. The dieter, like the engineer, can now have a tool kit with which to learn answers that would seldom be obtainable by intuition alone, and to do so quickly and at little cost.

This is not to suggest that we all need to become model builders. What I am suggesting is that we all need to become capable model *consumers.* As computers continue to proliferate, more and more of the decisions we make, whether at home, in business, or in government, will involve the results of models. Indeed, the ability to understand and evaluate computer models is fast becoming a prerequisite for the scientist, policymaker, and citizen alike.[279]

Nowhere is this more essential, and potentially more rewarding, than in managing our health and well-being.

Notes

1. Senge, P.M. (1990). *The Fifth Discipline: The Art and Practice of the Learning Organization*. New York: Doubleday/Currency.
2. McArdle, W.D., Katch, F.I., and Katch, V.L. (1996). *Exercise Physiology: Energy, Nutrition, and Human Performance*. Baltimore: Williams and Wilkins.
3. Whitney, E.N. and Rolfes, S.R. (1999). *Understanding Nutrition*. Belmont, CA: West/Wadsworth.
4. Hensrud, D. (2000). *Mayo Clinic on Healthy Weight*. Rochester, MN: Mayo Clinic Health Information.
5. Encyclopedia Britannica Online. (1999). Nutrition, Human.
6. McArdle, W.D., Katch, F.I., and Katch, V.L. (1996). *Exercise Physiology: Energy, Nutrition, and Human Performance*. Baltimore: Williams and Wilkins.
7. Levitt, S.D. and Dubner, S.J. (2005). *Freakonomics: A Rogue Economist Explores the Hidden Side of Everything*. New York: William Morrow.
8. Brownell, K.D. and Fairburn, C.G. (Eds.). (1995). *Eating Disorders and Obesity: A Comprehensive Handbook*. New York: Guilford Press.
9. Rogers, E.M. (1983). *Diffusion of Innovations*. New York: Free Press.
10. Vasselli, J.R. and Maggio, C.A. (1997). Mechanisms of appetite and body weight regulation. In: Dalton, A. (Ed.). *Overweight and Weight Management: The Health Professional's Guide to Understanding and Practice*. Gaithersburg, MD: Aspen.
11. Senge, P.M. (1990). *The Fifth Discipline: The Art and Practice of the Learning Organization*. New York: Doubleday/Currency.
12. Wegner, D.M. (2002). *The Illusions of Conscious Will*. Cambridge, MA: Bradford Books.
13. Taylor, S.E. and Brown, J.D. (1988). Illusion and well-being: a social psychological perspective on mental health. *Psychological Bulletin*, 103, 193–210.

14. Russo, E. (1990). *Decision Traps: The Ten Barriers to Decision-Making and How to Overcome Them.* New York: Fireside.
15. Langer, E.J. (1975). The illusion of control. *Journal of Personality and Social Psychology,* 32, 311–328.
16. Taylor, S.E. and Brown, J.D. (1988). Illusion and well-being: a social psychological perspective on mental health. *Psychological Bulletin,* 103, 193–210.
17. Haidt, J. and Rodin, J. (1999). Control and efficacy as interdisciplinary bridges. *Review of General Psychology,* 3, 317–337.
18. Taylor, S.E., Wayment, H.A., Collins, M.A. (1993). Positive illusions and affect regulation. In: Wegner, D.M. and Pennebaker, J.W. (Eds.), *Handbook of Mental Control.* Englewood Cliffs, NJ: Prentice Hall.
19. Brownell, K.D. (1991). Personal responsibility and control over our bodies: when expectation exceeds reality. *Health Psychology,* 10, 303–310.
20. *Ibid.*
21. Einhorn, H. J. and Hogarth, R. M. (1987). Decision making: going forward in reverse. *Harvard Business Review,* 65(1): 66–70.
22. Encyclopedia Britannica Online. (1999). Nutrition, Human.
23. Buchholz, A.C. and Schoeller, D.A. (2004). Is a calorie a calorie? *American Journal of Clinical Nutrition.* 79(5), 899S–906S.
24. *Ibid.*
25. Burniat, W., et al. (Eds.) (2002). *Child and Adolescent Obesity: Causes and Consequences, Prevention and Management.* Cambridge, UK: Cambridge University Press.
26. Brownell, K.D. and Fairburn, C.G. (Eds.). (1995). *Eating Disorders and Obesity: A Comprehensive Handbook.* New York: Guilford Press.
27. Weinsier, R.L., Bracco, D., and Schultz, Y. (1993). Predicted effects of small decreases in energy expenditure on weight gain in adult women. *International Journal of Obesity,* 17, 693–699.
28. Kirby, J. (1998). *Dieting for Dummies.* New York: Hungry Minds.
29. Ravussin, E. and Swinburn, B.A. (1992). Energy metabolism. In: Sunkard, A.J. and Wadden, T.A. (Eds.). *Obesity: Theory and Therapy* (pp. 97–123). New York: Raven Press.
30. Weinsier, R.L., Bracco, D., and Schutz, Y. (1993). Predicted effects of small decreases in energy expenditure on weight gain in adult women. *International Journal of Obesity,* 17, 693–699.
31. Sterman, J.D. (2000). *Business Dynamics: Systems Thinking and Modeling for a Complex World.* Boston: Irwin McGraw-Hill.
32. Sterman, J. D. (1991). A skeptic's guide to computer models. In: Barney, G.O., Kreutzer, W.B., and Garrett, M.J. (Eds.). *Managing a Nation,* 2nd ed. Boulder, CO: Westview Press.

33. Zimmerman, B., Lindberg, C., and Plsek, P. (1998). *Edgeware: Insights from Complexity Science for Health Care Leaders.* Irving, TX: VHA.

34. Hammond, J.S, Keeney, R.L., and Raiffa, H. (1998). The hidden traps in decision making. *Harvard Business Review*, 76(5), 47–58.

35. Casti, J.L. (1994). *Complexification: Explaining a Paradoxical World through the Science of Surprise.* New York: Harper Collins.

36. Sterman, J.D. (2000). *Business Dynamics: Systems Thinking and Modeling for a Complex World.* Boston: Irwin McGraw-Hill.

37. Capra, F. (1996). *The Web of Life: A New Scientific Understanding of Living Systems.* New York: Anchor.

38. Sterman, J.D. (2000). *Business Dynamics: Systems Thinking and Modeling for a Complex World.* Boston: Irwin McGraw-Hill.

39. *Ibid.*

40. Polivy, J. and Herman, C.P. (2002). If at first you don't succeed: false hopes of self-change. *American Psychologist*, 57(9), 677–689.

41. Pilkey, O.H. and Pilkey-Jarvis, L. (2007). *Useless Arithmetic: Why Environmental Scientists Can't Predict the Future.* New York: Columbia University Press.

42. Hallmich, N. (2005, January 5). 20 tips to lose 20 pounds.*USA Today*, p. 8D.

43. Roberts, S.S. (2004). Weight-loss scams: what to watch out for. *Diabetes Forecast*, 57(2), 46–48.

44. Calorie Control Council. http://www.caloriecontrol.org.

45. Ballor, D.L. and Poehlman, E.T. (1994). Exercise-training enhances fat-free mass preservation during diet-induced weight loss: a meta-analytical finding. *International Journal of Obesity*, 18, 35–40.

46. McArdle, W.D., Katch, F.I., and Katch, V.L. (1996). *Exercise Physiology: Energy, Nutrition, and Human Performance.* Baltimore: Williams & Wilkins.

47. *Ibid.*

48. Covey, S.R. (1989). *The 7 Habits of Highly Effective People.* New York: Fireside.

49. *Ibid.*

50. Kaufman, F.R. (2005). *Diabesity: The Obesity-Diabetes Epidemic that Threatens America—And What We Must Do to Stop It.* New York: Bantam.

51. Spirduso, W.W. (1995). *Physical Dimensions of Aging.* Champaign, IL: Human Kinetics.

52. Whitney, E.N. and Rolfes, S.R. (1999). *Understanding Nutrition.* Belmont, CA: West/Wadsworth.

53. Wadden, T.A. and Stunkard, A.J. (Eds.). (2002). *Handbook of Obesity Treatment.* New York: Guilford Press.

54. Leibel, R.L., Rosenbaum, M., and Hirsch, J. (1995). Changes in energy expenditure resulting from altered body weight. *New England Journal of Medicine*, 332, 621–628.

55. Dullo, A.G. and Jacquet, J. (1998). Adaptive reduction in basal metabolic rate in response to food deprivation in humans: a role for feedback signals from fat stores. *American Journal of Clinical Nutrition*, 68, 599–606.

56. Heshka, S. Yang, M., Wang, J., Burt, P. and Pi-Sunyer, F.X. (1990). Weight loss and change in resting metabolic rate. *American Journal of Clinical Nutrition*, 52, 981–986.

57. Saltzman, E. and Roberts, S.B. (1995). The role of energy expenditure in energy regulation: findings from a decade of research. *Nutrition Reviews* 53, 209–220.

58. Wilmore, J.H. (2001). Physical energy: fuel metabolism. *Nutrition Reviews*, 59(1), S13–S16.

59. Encyclopedia Britannica Online. (1999). Nutrition, Human.

60. Whitney, E.N. and Rolfes, S.R. (1999). *Understanding Nutrition*. Belmont, CA: West/Wadsworth.

61. Encyclopedia Britannica Online. (1999). Nutrition, Human.

62. Hill, J.O., Thompson, H., and Wyatt, H. (2005). Weight maintenance: what's missing? *Supplement to the Journal of the American Dietetic Association*, 105(5), S63–S69.

63. Roizen, M.F. and Oz, M.C. (2006). *You on a Diet: The Owner's Manual for Waist Management*. New York: Free Press.

64. Whitney, E.N. and Rolfes, S.R. (1999). *Understanding Nutrition*. Belmont, CA: West/Wadsworth.

65. Mitochondria are structures within a cell responsible for producing a high-energy compound (called ATP) aerobically.

66. Whitney, E.N. and Rolfes, S.R. (1999). *Understanding Nutrition*. Belmont, CA: West/Wadsworth.

67. *Ibid*

68. Danforth, E. (1985). Diet and obesity. *American Journal of Clinical Nutrition*, 41, 1132–1145.

69. Wadden, T.A. and Stunkard, A.J. (Eds.). (2002). *Handbook of Obesity Treatment*. New York: Guilford Press.

70. Novotny, J.A. and Rumpler, W.V. (1998). Modeling of energy expenditure and resting metabolic rate during weight loss in humans. In: Clifford, A.J. and Muller, H.G. (Eds.). *Mathematical Modeling in Experimental Nutrition*. New York: Plenum Press.

71. Dullo, A.G. and Jacquet, J. (1998). Adaptive reduction in basal metabolic rate in response to food deprivation in humans: a role for feedback signals from fat stores. *American Journal of Clinical Nutrition*, 68, 599–606.

72. Shetty, P.S. (1990). Physiological mechanisms in the adaptive response of metabolic rates to energy restriction. *Nutrition Research Reviews* 3, 49–74.

73. Jebb, S.A., et al. (1996). Changes in macronutrient balance during over- and underfeeding assessed by 12-d continuous whole-body calorimetry. *American Journal of Clinical Nutrition*, 64, 259–66.

74. *Ibid.*

75. Rosenbaum, M., et al. (1997). Obesity. *New England Journal of Medicine*, 337(6), 396–407.

76. Stipanuk, M.H. (Ed.). (2000). *Biochemical and Physiological Aspects of Human Nutrition*. Philadelphia: W.B. Saunders.

77. Wier, L.T. et al. (2001). Determining the amount of physical activity needed for long-term weight control. *International Journal of Obesity*, 25, 613–621.

78. *Ibid.*

79. Brownell, K.D. and Fairburn, C.G. (Eds.). (1995). *Eating Disorders and Obesity: A Comprehensive Handbook*. New York: Guilford Press.

80. Polivy, J. and Herman, C.P. (2002). If at first you don't succeed: false hopes of self-change. *American Psychologist*, 57(9), 677–689.

81. Forbes, G.B. (1987). *Human Body Composition: Growth, Aging, Nutrition, and Activity*. Berlin, Heidelberg: Springer-Verlag.

82. *Ibid.*

83. Ballor, D.L. and Poehlman, E.T. (1994). Exercise-training enhances fat-free mass preservation during diet-induced weight loss: a meta-analytical finding. *International Journal of Obesity*, 18, 35–40.

84. Stipanuk, M.H. (Ed.). (2000). *Biochemical and Physiological Aspects of Human Nutrition*. Philadelphia: W.B. Saunders.

85. *Ibid.*

86. Ballor, D.L. and Poehlman, E.T. (1994). Exercise-training enhances fat-free mass preservation during diet-induced weight loss: a meta-analytical finding. *International Journal of Obesity*, 18, 35–40.

87. McArdle, W.D., Katch, F.I., and Katch, V.L. (1996). *Exercise Physiology: Energy, Nutrition, and Human Performance*. Baltimore: Williams & Wilkins.

88. Senge, P.M. (1990). *The Fifth Discipline: The Art and Practice of the Learning Organization*. New York: Doubleday/Currency.

89. Dörner, D. (1989). *The Logic of Failure*. New York: Metropolitan Books.

90. Senge, P.M. (1990). *The Fifth Discipline: The Art and Practice of the Learning Organization*. New York: Doubleday/Currency.

91. *Ibid.*

92. *Ibid.*

93. Sterman, J.D. (2000). *Business Dynamics: Systems Thinking and Modeling for a Complex World*. Boston: Irwin McGraw-Hill.

94. *Ibid.*

95. Wadden, T.A. and Stunkard, A.J. (Eds.). (2002). *Handbook of Obesity Treatment.* New York: Guilford Press.

96. Brownell, K.D. (1991). Personal responsibility and control over our bodies: when expectation exceeds reality. *Health Psychology,* 10, 303–310.

97. Sterman, J.D. (2000). *Business Dynamics: Systems Thinking and Modeling for a Complex World.* Boston: Irwin McGraw-Hill.

98. Weick, K. (1979). *The Social Psychology of Organizing.* New York: Addison-Wesley.

99. Richmond, B. (1991). *Systems Thinking: Four Key Questions.* Hanover, NH: High Performance Systems.

100. Senge, P.M. (1990). *The Fifth Discipline: The Art and Practice of the Learning Organization.* New York: Doubleday/Currency.

101. Meadows, D. (1999). Leverage Points: Places to Intervene in a System. The Sustainability Institute, Hartland, Vermont.

102. Forrester, J.W. (1969). A deeper knowledge of social systems. *Technology Review,* 71(6), 1–11.

103. Senge, P.M. (1990). *The Fifth Discipline: The Art and Practice of the Learning Organization.* New York: Doubleday/Currency.

104. Sterman, J.D. (2000). *Business Dynamics: Systems Thinking and Modeling for a Complex World.* Boston: Irwin McGraw-Hill.

105. Sterman, J. D. (1991). A skeptic's guide to computer models. In: Barney, G.O., Kreutzer, W.B., and Garrett, M.J. (Eds.). *Managing a Nation,* 2nd ed. Boulder, CO: Westview Press.

106. Sterman, J.D. (2000). *Business Dynamics: Systems Thinking and Modeling for a Complex World.* Boston: Irwin McGraw-Hill.

107. *Ibid.*

108. McArdle, W.D., Katch, F.I., and Katch, V.L. (1996). *Exercise Physiology: Energy, Nutrition, and Human Performance.* Baltimore: Williams & Wilkins.

109. Dansinger, M.L., et al. (2007). Meta-analysis: The effect of dietary counseling for weight loss. *Annals of Internal Medicine,* 147, 41–50.

110. Pi-Sunyer, F.X. (1999). Obesity. In: Shils, M.E., Olson, J.A., Shike, M., and Ross, A.C. (Eds.). *Modern Nutrition in Health and Disease.* Baltimore: Williams & Wilkins.

111. Hill, J.H. and Wing, R. (2003). The National Weight Control Registry. *The Permanente Journal,* 7(3), 34–37.

112. Peters, J.C., Wyatt, H.R., Donahoo, W.T., and Hill, J.O. (2002). From instinct to intellect: the challenge of maintaining healthy weight in the modern world. *Obesity Reviews,* 3, 69–74.

113. Koopmans, H.S. (1998). Experimental studies on the control of food intake. In: Bray, G.A., Bouchard, C., and James, W.P.T. (Eds.). *Handbook of Obesity* (pp. 273–311). New York: Marcel Dekker.

114. Flier, J.S. and Maratos-Flier, E. (2007). What fuels fat. *Scientific American*, 297(3), 72–81.

115. Whitney, E.N. and Rolfes, S.R. (1999). *Understanding Nutrition*. Belmont, CA: West/Wadsworth.

116. Brownell, K.D. and Fairburn, C.G. (Eds.). (1995). *Eating Disorders and Obesity: A Comprehensive Handbook*. New York: Guilford Press

117. Flier, J.S. and Maratos-Flier, E. (2007). What fuels fat. *Scientific American*, 297(3), 72–81.

118. Jéquier, E. and Tappy, L. (1999). Regulation of body weight in humans. *Physiological Reviews*, 79(2), 451–480.

119. Flier, J.S. and Maratos-Flier, E. (2007). What fuels fat. *Scientific American*, 297(3), 72–81.

120. *Ibid.*

121. Bell, C.G., Walley, A.J., and Froguel, P. (2005). The genetics of human obesity. *Nature Reviews Genetics*, 6, 221–234.

122. Stipanuk, M.H. (Ed.). (2000). *Biochemical and Physiological Aspects of Human Nutrition*. Philadelphia: W.B. Saunders.

123. Whitney, E.N. and Rolfes, S.R. (1999). *Understanding Nutrition*. Belmont, CA: West/Wadsworth.

124. Shell, E.R. (2002). *The Hungry Gene: The Inside Story of the Obesity Industry*. New York: Grove Press.

125. Guyton, A.C. and Hall, J.E. (1996). *Textbook of Medical Physiology*. Philadelphia: W.B. Saunders.

126. Shell, E.R. (2002). *The Hungry Gene: The Inside Story of the Obesity Industry*. New York: Grove Press.

127. Brownell, K.D. and Horgen, K.B. (2004). *Food Fight*. Chicago: Contemporary Books.

128. Pool, R. (2001). *Fat: Fighting the Obesity Epidemic*. Oxford: Oxford University Press.

129. Jéquier, E. and Tappy, L. (1999). Regulation of body weight in humans. *Physiological Reviews*, 79(2), 451–480.

130. Another is insulin.

131. Grady, D. (2002, November 26). Why We Eat (and Eat and Eat). *New York Times*, p. D1.

132. French, S. and Castiglione, K. (2002). Recent advances in the physiology of eating. *Proceedings of the Nutrition Society*, 61, 489–496.

133. Woods, S.C., Schwartz, M.W., Baskin, D.G., and Seeley, R.J. (2000). Food intake and the regulation of body weight. *Annual Review of Psychoogy*, 51, 255–277.

134. Schwartz, M.W., Baskin, D.G., Kaiyala, K.J., and Woods, S.C. (1999). Model for the regulation of energy balance and adiposity by the central nervous system. *American Journal of Clinical Nutrition*, 69, 584–596.

135. Woods, S.C., Seeley, R.J., Porte Jr., D., and Schwartz, M.W. (1998). Signals that regulate food intake and energy homeostasis. *Science*, 280(5368), 1378–1383.

136. Figlewicz, D.P. et al. (1996). Endocrine regulation of food intake and body weight. *Journal of Laboratory andClinicalMedicine*, 127, 328–332.

137. Schwartz, M.W. and Seeley, R.J. (1997). The new biology of body weight regulation. *Journal of the American Dietetic Association*, 97, 54–58.

138. Flier, J.S. (2004). Obesity wars: molecular progress confronts an expanding epidemic. *Cell*, 116, 337–350.

139. Mattes, R.D., Pierce, C.B., and Friedman, M.I. (1988). Daily caloric intake of normal-weight adults: response to changes in dietary energy density of a luncheon meal. *American Journal of Clinical Nutrition*, 48, 214–219.

140. Pool, R. (2001). *Fat: Fighting the Obesity Epidemic*. Oxford: Oxford University Press.

141. Gura, T. (1997). Obesity sheds its secrets. *Science*, 275, 751–753.

142. Pi-Sunyer, F.X. (1999). Obesity. In: Shils, M.E., Olson, J.A., Shike, M., and Ross, A.C. (Eds.). *Modern Nutrition in Health and Disease*. Baltimore: Williams & Wilkins.

143. Dullo, A.G., Jacquet, J., and Girardier, L. (1996). Autoregulation of body composition during weight recovery in human: the Minnesota Experiment revisited. *International Journal of Obesity*, 20(5), 393–405.

144. Marx, J. (2003). Cellular warriors at the battle of the bulge. *Science*, 299, 846–849.

145. Bell, C.G., Walley, A.J., and Froguel, P. (2005). The genetics of human obesity. *Nature Reviews Genetics*, 6, 221–234.

146. Shell, E.R. (2002). *The Hungry Gene: The Inside Story of the Obesity Industry*. New York: Grove Press.

147. Marx, J. (2003). Cellular warriors at the battle of the bulge. *Science*, 299, 846–849.

148. Martindale, D. (2003). Burgers on the Brain. *New Scientist*, 177(2380), 26.

149. Shell, E.R. (2002). *The Hungry Gene: The Inside Story of the Obesity Industry*. New York: Grove Press.

150. Pi-Sunyer, F.X. (1999). Obesity. In: Shils, M.E., Olson, J.A., Shike, M., and Ross, A.C. (Eds.). *Modern Nutrition in Health and Disease*. Baltimore: Williams & Wilkins.

151. Sjöström, L. (1980). Fat cells and body weight. In: Stunkard, A.J. (Ed.). *Obesity*. Philadelphia: W.B. Saunders.

152. Shils, M.E., Olson, J.A., Shike, M., and Ross, A.C. (Eds.). (1999). *Modern Nutrition in Health and Disease*. Baltimore: Williams & Wilkins.

153. A μg is a microgram, or one-millionth (10^{-6}) of a gram.

154. McArdle, W.D., Katch, F.I., and Katch, V.L. (1996). *Exercise Physiology: Energy, Nutrition, and Human Performance*. Baltimore: Williams & Wilkins.

155. Pi-Sunyer, F.X. (1999). Obesity. In: Shils, M.E., Olson, J.A., Shike, M., and Ross, A.C. (Eds.). *Modern Nutrition in Health and Disease*. Baltimore: Williams & Wilkins.

156. Whitney, E.N. and Rolfes, S.R. (1999). *Understanding Nutrition*. Belmont, CA: West/Wadsworth.

157. Spalding, K.L., et al. (2008). Dynamics of fat cell turnover in humans. *Nature*, 453(7196), 783–787.

158. Fat cell size and number can be assessed from small tissue samples obtained (usually by means of a percutaneous needle aspiration) from multiple subcutaneous sites. See: 1) Knittle, J.L., Timmers, K., and Ginsberg-Fellner, F. (1979). The growth of adipose tissue in children and adolescents. *Journal of. Clinical Investigation*, 63, 239–246; and 2) Pool, R. (2001). *Fat: Fighting the Obesity Epidemic*. Oxford: Oxford University Press.

159. McArdle, W.D., Katch, F.I., and Katch, V.L. (1996). *Exercise Physiology: Energy, Nutrition, and Human Performance*. Baltimore: Williams & Wilkins.

160. Pool, R. (2001). *Fat: Fighting the Obesity Epidemic*. Oxford: Oxford University Press.

161. Roberts, N., Andersen, D., Deal, R., Garet, M., and Shaffer, W. (1983). *Introduction to Computer Simulation: A System Dynamics Modeling Approach*. Reading, MA: Addison-Wesley.

162. Buckmaster, L. and Brownell, K.D. (1988). Behavior modification: the state of the art. In: Frankle, R.T. and Yang, M. (Eds.). Obesity and Weight Control: The Health Professional's Guide to Understanding and Treatment. Rockville, MD: Aspen.

163. Whitney, E.N. and Rolfes, S.R. (1999). *Understanding Nutrition*. Belmont, CA: West/Wadsworth.

164. Stipp, D. (2003, February 3). The quest for the antifat pill nature programmed us to overeat. Fen-Phen helped that, until it backfired. Safer drugs may be coming soon. *Fortune Magazine*, pp. 66–67.

165. Buckmaster, L. and Brownell, K.D. (1988). Behavior modification: the state of the art. In: Frankle, R.T. and Yang, M. (Eds.). Obesity and Weight Control: The Health Professional's Guide to Understanding and Treatment. Rockville, MD: Aspen.

166. Vasselli, J.R. and Maggio, C.A. (1988). Mechanisms of appetite and body-weight regulation. In: Frankle, R.T. and Yang, M. (Eds.). *Obesity and Weight Control: The Health Professional's Guide to Understanding and Treatment*. Rockville, MD: Aspen.

167. There is now evidence that the induction of *ob* mRNA is a function of fat cell size, with larger fat cells expressing more *ob* mRNA than smaller cells. See: Jebb, S.A. et al. (1996). Changes in macronutrient balance during over- and underfeeding assessed by 12-d continuous whole-body calorimetry. *American Journal of Clinical Nutrition*, 64, 259–266.

    Fat cell size may also be signaled through enzymatic mechanisms mounted on fat cell membranes. One such mechanism involves the enzyme lipoprotein lipase (LPL), which plays a key role in the process of lipid deposition in the adipose tissue. See: Whitney, E.N. and Rolfes, S.R. (1999). *Understanding Nutrition*. Belmont, CA: West/Wadsworth.

168. Jéquier, E. and Tappy, L. (1999). Regulation of body weight in humans. *Physiological Reviews*, 79(2), 451–480.

169. Buckmaster, L. and Brownell, K.D. (1988). Behavior modification: the state of the art. In: Frankle, R.T. and Yang, M. (Eds.). Obesity and Weight Control: The Health Professional's Guide to Understanding and Treatment. Rockville, MD: Aspen.

170. Pool, R. (2001). *Fat: Fighting the Obesity Epidemic*. Oxford: Oxford University Press.

171. Baumeister, R.F. and Heatherton, T.F. (1996). Self-regulation failure: an overview. *Psychological Inquiry*, 7(1), 1–15.

172. Blundell, J.E. and Tremblay, A. (1995). Appetite control and energy (fuel) balance. *Nutrition Research Reviews*, 8, 225–242.

173. Polivy, J. and Herman, P. (1985). Dieting and binging: a causal analysis. *American Psychologist*, 40(2), 193–201.

174. McArdle, W.D., Katch, F.I., and Katch, V.L. (1996). *Exercise Physiology: Energy, Nutrition, and Human Performance*. Baltimore: Williams & Wilkins.

175. Muraven, M., and Baumeister, R. F. (2000). Self-regulation and depletion of limited resources: Does self-control resemble a muscle? *Psychological Bulletin*, 126, 247–259.

176. Muraven, M., Tice, D. M., and Baumeister, R. F. (1998). Self-control as a limited resource: regulatory depletion patterns. *Journal of Personality and Social Psychology*, 74, 774–789.

177. Muraven, M., and Baumeister, R. F. (2000). Self-regulation and depletion of limited resources: Does self-control resemble a muscle? *Psychological Bulletin*, 126, 247–259.

178. *Ibid.*
179. Baumeister, R.F., Heatherton, T.F., and Tice, D.M. (1994). *Losing Control: How and Why People Fail at Self-Regulation*. San Diego: Academic Press.
180. Blundell, J.E. et al. (1996). Control of human appetite: implications for the intake of dietary fat. *Annual Review ofNutrition*, 16, 285–319.
181. Boekaerts, M., Pintrich, P.R., and Zeidner, M. (Eds.). (2000). *Handbook of Self-Regulation*. San Diego: Academic Press.
182. Muraven, M., Tice, D.M., and Baumeister, R.F. (1998). Self-control as a limited resource: regulatory depletion patterns. *Journal of Personality and Social Psychology*, 74, 774–789.
183. Boekaerts, M., Pintrich, P.R., and Zeidner, M. (Eds.). (2000). *Handbook of Self-Regulation*. San Diego: Academic Press.
184. *Ibid.*
185. Muraven, M., Tice, D.M., and Baumeister, R.F. (1998). Self-control as a limited resource: regulatory depletion patterns. *Journal of Personality and Social Psychology*, 74, 774–789.
186. Tangney, J.P., Baumeister, R.F., and Boone, A.L. (2004). High self-control predicts good adjustment, less pathology, better grades, and interpersonal success. *Journal of Personality*, 72(2), 271–322.
187. Baumeister, R.F., Heatherton, T.F., and Tice, D.M. (1994). *Losing Control: How and Why People Fail at Self-Regulation*. San Diego: Academic Press.
188. Muraven, M., Tice, D.M., and Baumeister, R.F. (1998). Self-control as a limited resource: regulatory depletion patterns. *Journal of Personality and Social Psychology*, 74, 774– 89.
189. *Ibid.*
190. Muraven, M., and Baumeister, R.F. (2000). Self-regulation and depletion of limited resources: does self-control resemble a muscle? *Psychological Bulletin*, 126, 247–259.
191. Muraven, M., and Slessareva, E. (2003). Mechanisms of self-control failure: motivation and limited resources. *Personality and Social Psychology Bulletin*, 29, 894–90.
192. Muraven, M., Tice, D.M., and Baumeister, R.F. (1998). Self-control as a limited resource: regulatory depletion patterns. *Journal of Personality and Social Psychology*, 74, 774–789.
193. *Ibid.*
194. Sterman, J.D. (2000). *Business Dynamics: Systems Thinking and Modeling for a Complex World*. Boston: Irwin McGraw-Hill.
195. Roizen, M.F. and Oz, M.C. (2006). *You on a Diet: The Owner's Manual for Waist Management*. New York: Free Press.
196. Freud, S. (1930). *Civilization and Its Discontents*. London: Hogarth.

197. Tangney, J.P., Baumeister, R.F., and Boone, A.L. (2004). High self-control predicts good adjustment, less pathology, better grades, and interpersonal success. *Journal of Personality*, 72(2), 271–322.

198. Muraven, M., and Baumeister, R.F. (2000). Self-regulation and depletion of limited resources: does self-control resemble a muscle? *Psychological Bulletin*, 126, 247–259.

199. Friedman, J.M. (2003). A war on obesity, not the obese. *Science*, 299, 856–863.

200. Muraven, M., Tice, D.M., and Baumeister, R.F. (1998). Self-control as a limited resource: regulatory depletion patterns. *Journal of Personality and Social Psychology*, 74, 774–789.

201. *Ibid.*

202. Muraven, M., and Baumeister, R.F. (2000). Self-regulation and depletion of limited resources: does self-control resemble a muscle? *Psychological Bulletin*, 126, 247–259.

203. Muraven, M., Tice, D.M., and Baumeister, R.F. (1998). Self-control as a limited resource: regulatory depletion patterns. *Journal of Personality and Social Psychology*, 74, 774–789.

204. *Ibid.*

205. Muraven, M. (2003). Blowing your diet: models of self-control. *Contemporary Psychology*, 48(6), 742–744.

206. Muraven, M., Tice, D.M., and Baumeister, R.F. (1998). Self-control as a limited resource: regulatory depletion patterns. *Journal of Personality and Social Psychology*, 74, 774–789.

207. Tangney, J.P., Baumeister, R.F., and Boone, A.L. (2004). High self-control predicts good adjustment, less pathology, better grades, and interpersonal success. *Journal of Personality*, 72(2), 271–322.

208. Muraven, M., and Baumeister, R.F. (2000). Self-regulation and depletion of limited resources: does self-control resemble a muscle? *Psychological Bulletin*, 126, 247–259.

209. Innate individual differences can now be measured. Tangney et al. developed an instrument (based on 36 dimensions) to measure self-control strength. See: Tangney, J.P., Baumeister, R.F., and Boone, A.L. (2004). High self-control predicts good adjustment, less pathology, better grades, and interpersonal success. *Journal of Personality*, 72(2), 271–322.

210. Muraven, M., Tice, D.M., and Baumeister, R.F. (1998). Self-control as a limited resource: regulatory depletion patterns. *Journal of Personality and Social Psychology*, 74, 774–789.

211. *Ibid.*

212. Muraven, M. (2003). Blowing your diet: models of self-control. *Contemporary Psychology*, 48(6), 742–744.

213. Muraven, M., Tice, D.M., and Baumeister, R.F. (1998). Self-control as a limited resource: regulatory depletion patterns. *Journal of Personality and Social Psychology*, 74, 774–789.

214. Baumeister, R.F., Heatherton, T.F., and Tice, D.M. (1994). *Losing Control: How and Why People Fail at Self-Regulation*. San Diego: Academic Press.

215. Kiley, D. (2005, September 19). My dinner with NutriSystem. *Business Week*.

216. Wing, R.R. and Hill, J.O. (2001). Successful weight loss maintenance. *Annual Review of Nutrition*, 21, 323–341.

217. Hill, J.H. and Wing, R. (2003). The National Weight Control Registry. *Permanente Journal*, 7(3), 34–37.

218. Hill, J.O. and Billington, C.J. (2002). It's time to start treating obesity. *American Journal of Cardiology*, 89, 969–970.

219. Brownell, K.D. and Rodin, J. (1994). Medical, metabolic, and psychological effects of weight cycling. *Archives of Internal Medicine*, 154, 1325–1330.

220. Foreyt, J.P. and Poston, W.S.C. (1998). Obesity: a never-ending cycle? *International Journal of Fertility*, 43(2), 111–116.

221. Wing, R.R. and Hill, J.O. (2001). Successful weight loss maintenance. *Annual Review of Nutrition*, 21, 323–41.

222. Hill, J.O., Thompson, H., and Wyatt, H. (2005). Weight maintenance: what's missing? *Supplement to the Journal of the Am Dietetic Association*, 105(5), S63–S69.

223. Polivy, J. and Herman, C.P. (2002). If at first you don't succeed: false hopes of self-change. *American Psychologist*, 57(9), 677–689.

224. Foster, G.D., Wadden, T.A., Vogt, R.A., and Brewer, G. (1997). What is a reasonable weight loss? Patients' expectations and evaluations of obesity treatment outcomes. *Journal of Consulting and Clinical Psychology*, 65, 79–85.

225. Wadden, T.A., Brownell, K.D., and Foster, G.D. (2002). Obesity: responding to the global epidemic. *Journal of Consulting and Clinical Psychology*, 70(3), 510–525.

226. McArdle, W.D., Katch, F.I., and Katch, V.L. (1996). *Exercise Physiology: Energy, Nutrition, and Human Performance*. Baltimore: Williams & Wilkins.

227. Friedman, J.M. (2003). A war on obesity, not the obese. *Science*, 299, 856–863.

228. Baumeister, R.F., Heatherton, T.F., and Tice, D.M. (1994). *Losing Control: How and Why People Fail at Self-Regulation*. San Diego: Academic Press.

229. McArdle, W.D., Katch, F.I., and Katch, V.L. (1996). *Exercise Physiology: Energy, Nutrition, and Human Performance*. Baltimore: Williams & Wilkins.
230. Walk Around Australia: A Journey for Kids. http://www.walkaroundoz.org.au
231. Pool, R. (2001). *Fat: Fighting the Obesity Epidemic*. Oxford: Oxford University Press.
232. Stipp, D. (2003, February 3). The quest for the antifat pill nature programmed us to overeat. Fen-Phen helped that, until it backfired. Safer drugs may be coming soon. *Fortune Magazine*, pp. 66–67.
233. Kolata, G. (2007, May 8). Genes take charge, and diets fall by the wayside. *New York Times*.
234. Encyclopedia Britannica Online. (1999). Nutrition, Human.
235. Heyman, M.B. et al. (1992). Underfeeding and body weight regulation in normal-weight young men. *American Journal of Physiology*, 263, R250–R257.
236. Dullo, A.G., Jacquet, J., and Girardier, L. (1997). Post-starvation hyperphagia and body fat overshooting in humans: a role of feedback signals from lean and fat tissues. *Journal ofClinical Nutrition*, 65, 717–23.
237. St-Pierre et al. (1996) have described a case study of energy balance before and after a ski expedition through Greenland in a 59-year-old man with a habitual weight maintenance of 67.2 kg. At 2–3 weeks after his return, his *ad libitum* food intake was found to be 1.5 MJ/day in excess of his habitual intake despite the fact that his body weight and body fat had already been completely restored to habitual levels. See 1) St-Pierre, S., Roy, B. and Tremblay, A. (1996). A case study on energy balance during an expedition through Greenland. *International Journal of Obesity*, 20, 493–495 ; and 2) Dullo, A.G. (1997). Human pattern of food intake and fuel-partitioning during weight recovery after starvation: a theory of autoregulation of body composition. *Proceedings of the Nutrition Society*, 56, 25–40.
238. Dullo, A.G. (1997). Human pattern of food intake and fuel-partitioning during weight recovery after starvation: a theory of autoregulation of body composition. *Proceedings of the Nutrition Society*, 56, 25–40.
239. Muraven, M., and Baumeister, R.F. (2000). Self-regulation and depletion of limited resources: does self-control resemble a muscle? *Psychological Bulletin*, 126, 247–259.
240. Friedman, J.M. (2003). A war on obesity, not the obese. *Science*, 299, 856–863.
241. Polivy, J. and Herman, C.P. (2002). If at first you don't succeed: false hopes of self-change. *American Psychologist*, 57(9), 677–689.

242. Armore, D.A. and Taylor, E.E. (1998). Situated optimism: specific outcome expectancies and self-regulation. In: Zanna, M.P. (Ed.). *Advances in Experimental Social Psychology*, Vol. 30 (pp. 309–379). New York: Academic Press.

243. Polivy, J. and Herman, C.P. (2002). If at first you don't succeed: false hopes of self-change. *American Psychologist*, 57(9), 677–689.

244. Baumeister, R.F., Heatherton, T.F., and Tice, D.M. (1994). *Losing Control: How and Why People Fail at Self-Regulation*. San Diego: Academic Press.

245. Polivy, J. and Herman, C.P. (2002). If at first you don't succeed: false hopes of self-change. *American Psychologist*, 57(9), 677–689.

246. Whitney, E.N. and Rolfes, S.R. (1999). *Understanding Nutrition*. Belmont, CA: West/Wadsworth.

247. Sterman, J.D. (2000). *Business Dynamics: Systems Thinking and Modeling for a Complex World*. Boston: Irwin McGraw-Hill.

248. Wadden, T.A. et al. (1992). Relationship of dieting history to resting metabolic rate, body composition, eating behavior, and subsequent weight loss. *American Journal of Clinical Nutrition*, 56, 203S–208S.

249. O'Neil, J. (2003, October 7). For youth, downsize to dieting. *New York Times*, p. D6.

250. Field, A.E. et al. (2003). Relation between dieting and weight change among preadolescents and adolescents. *Pediatrics*, 112(4), 900–906.

251. Polivy, J. and Herman, P. (1985). Dieting and binging: a causal analysis. *American Psychologist*, 40(2), 193–201.

252. Brownell, K.D. and Rodin, J. (1994). Medical, metabolic, and psychological effects of weight cycling. *Archives of Internal Medicine*, 154, 1325–1330.

253. Kayman, S., Bruvold, W., and Stern, J.S. (1990). Maintenance and relapse after weight loss in women: behavioral aspects. *American Journal of Clinical Nutrition*, 52, 800–807.

254. Whitney, E.N. and Rolfes, S.R. (1999). *Understanding Nutrition*. Belmont, CA: West/Wadsworth.

255. Brownell, K.D. and Rodin, J. (1994). Medical, metabolic, and psychological effects of weight cycling. *Archives of Internal Medicine*, 154, 1325–1330.

256. *Ibid.*

257. Kuhl, J. and Helle, P. (1986). Motivational and volitional determinants of depression: the degenerated-intention hypothesis. *Journal of Abnormal Psychology*, 95, 247–251.

258. Self-efficacy is not the same as self-esteem. Perceived self-efficacy is concerned with judgments of personal capability, whereas self-esteem is concerned with judgments of self-worth. Bandura (1997) highlights the distinction between the two concepts by pointing out that people can

have high self-efficacy for a task from which they derive no self-pride (e.g., being able to brush one's teeth well) or have low self-efficacy for a task but have no loss of self-worth (e.g., not being able to ride a unicycle). However, he observes that people often try to develop self-efficacy in activities that give them a sense of self-worth, so that the two concepts are frequently intertwined. See: 1) Bandura, A. (1997). *Self-Efficacy: The Exercise of Control*. New York: W.H. Freeman; and 2) Strecher, V.J., DeVellis, B.M., Becker, M.H., and Rosenstock, I.M. (1986). The role of self-efficacy in achieving health behavior change. *Health Education Quarterly*, 13(1), 73–91.

259. Glanz, K., Rimer, B.K., Lewis, F.M. (Eds.). (2002). *Health Behavior and Health Education: Theory, Research, and Practice*. San Francisco: Jossey-Bass.

260. Jairath, N. (1999). *Coronary Heart Disease and Risk Factor Management: A Nursing Perspective*. Philadelphia: W.B. Saunders.

261. Baumeister, R.F., Heatherton, T.F., and Tice, D.M. (1994). *Losing Control: How and Why People Fail at Self-Regulation*. San Diego: Academic Press.

262. Foster, G.D., Wadden, T.A., Vogt, R.A., and Brewer, G. (1997). What is a reasonable weight loss? Patients' expectations and evaluations of obesity treatment outcomes. *Journal of Consulting and Clinical Psychology*. 65, 79–85.

263. Kirschenbaum, D.S. and Fitzgibbon, M.L. (1995). Controversy about the treatment of obesity: Criticisms or challenges? *Behavior Therapy*, 26, 43–68.

264. Miller-Kovach, K., Hermann, M., and Winick, M. (1999). The psychological ramifications of weight management. *Journal of Women's Health and Gender-Based Medicine*, 8(4), 477–482.

265. Foster, G.D., Wadden, T.A., Vogt, R.A., and Brewer, G. (1997). What is a reasonable weight loss? Patients' expectations and evaluations of obesity treatment outcomes. *Journal of Consulting and Clinical Psychology*. 65, 79–85.

266. *Ibid.*

267. Hill, J.O., Thompson, H., and Wyatt, H. (2005). Weight maintenance: what's missing? *Supplement to the Journal of the Am Dietetic Association*, 105(5), S63–S69.

268. Because the National Weight Control Registry is not a randomized controlled study (people self-selected to participate in the study), and because most of the data are obtained from self-reports of participants, it is difficult to determine the degree to which this group's results are generalizable to the general population. The result, therefore, must be

interpreted with some caution. See: Hill, J.H. and Wing, R. (2003). The National Weight Control Registry. *Permanente Journal*, 7(3), 34–37.

269. Hill, J.O. et al. (2005). The National Weight Control Registry: is it useful in helping deal with our obesity epidemic? *Journal of Nutrition Education and Behavior*, 37, 206–210.

270. Klem, M.L., Wing, R.R., McGuire, M.T., Seagle, H.M., and Hill, J. (1997). A descriptive study of individuals successful at long-term maintenance of substantial weight loss. *American Journal of Clinical Nutrition*, 66, 239–46.

271. Dennis, K.E. and Goldberg, A.P. (1996). Weight control self-efficacy types and transitions affect weight-loss outcomes in obese women. *Addictive Behaviors*, 21(1), 103–116.

272. Vasselli, J.R. and Maggio, C.A. (1997). Mechanisms of appetite and body weight regulation. In: Dalton, A. (Ed.). *Overweight and Weight Management: The Health Professional's Guide to Understanding and Practice*. Gaithersburg, MD: Aspen.

273. Roberts, N., Andersen, D., Deal, R., Garet, M., and Shaffer, W. (1983). *Introduction to Computer Simulation: A System Dynamics Modeling Approach*. Reading, MA: Addison-Wesley.

274. Richardson, G.P. and Pugh, G.L. (1981). *Introduction to System Dynamics Modeling and Dynamo*. Cambridge, MA: MIT Press.

275. Forrester, J.W. (1993). System dynamics as an organizing framework for pre-college education. *System Dynamics Review*, 9(20), 183–194.

276. McArdle, W.D., Katch, F.I., and Katch, V.L. (1996). *Exercise Physiology: Energy, Nutrition, and Human Performance*. Baltimore: Williams & Wilkins.

277. Sterman, J.D. and Booth Sweeney, L. (2002). Cloudy skies: assessing public understanding of global warming. *System Dynamics Review*, 18, 207–240.

278. Wilson, E.O. (1998). *Consilience: The Unity of Knowledge*. New York: Alfred A. Knopf.

279. Sterman, J.D. (1991). A Skeptic's Guide to Computer Models. In: Barney, G.O., Kreutzer, W.B., and Garrett, M.J. (Eds.). *Managing a Nation*, 2nd ed. Boulder, CO: Westview Press.

We Can't Manage What We *Mis*-Predict

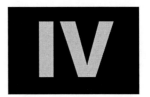

Learning by Doing

14

Life must be understood backward. But . . . it must be lived forward.
—Soren Kierkegaard

Part III focused on understanding system structure: how system variables, such as energy consumed and expended in the human system of energy and weight regulation, are related; how they influence one another; and how they are influenced by our external environment. Along the way, this discussion helped us clear up some of the public's muddled thinking about human energy and weight regulation, such as the limitations of the energy balance equation. However, as I noted at the close of Chapter 13, understanding system structure is not enough. Effective control of any complex dynamic system, such as the human body, requires a second essential skill: the ability to predict the system's behavior. The ability to infer system behavior is essential if we are to know how actions taken would influence the system, and thus is essential in devising appropriate interventions for change. So, in Part IV we shift our attention from understanding to predicting.

Psychology theorists have long recognized that predictive judgment plays a crucial role in human behavior. For example, "Kelly's first postulate states, 'A person's processes are psychologically channelized by ways in which he anticipates events.'"[1] Translation: Many of the judgment calls that people make in their daily lives, whether professionally or privately, are predictive judgments about behavior and its effects, that is, about the relation between contemplated actions and outcomes.[2] The *expectancy-valence theory* in behavioral decision making adds a sort of a psychological fine-tuning to this, further postulating that human behavior is jointly influenced by "the expectancy that behaving in a particular way will lead to a given outcome *and* the desirability of that outcome" [emphasis added].[3]

The crucial role of predictive judgment is not limited to humans. Organisms of all kinds rely on their predictive skills to survive. Whether big or small, organisms rely on their abilities to interpret warning signals of

T.K.A. Hamid, *Thinking in Circles About Obesity*,
DOI 10.1007/978-0-387-09469-4_14, © Springer Science+Business Media, LLC 2009

threatening conditions, to predict what is likely to happen (as a rabbit can predict that he is likely to be attacked when he smells a fox), and then to take preventive measures. But, perhaps out of sheer necessity—because we can neither fight nor run well enough to survive attack from major predators—humans have come to rely, more than most other species, on their predictive skills.[4]

In managing personal health, predictive judgment clearly is a crucial skill, especially when it comes to managing chronic conditions such as obesity. Without accurate predictions about the relationship between interventions and outcomes, one cannot know with certainty what resources to commit to a treatment effort or, in retrospect, how well these resources were used. Perhaps even more important is that, in matters of health, an inaccurate prediction can be extremely costly (even deadly), such as when exaggerated expectations in weigh-loss treatment sap motivation, undermine beliefs in self-efficacy, and drive patients to give up.[5,6]

How Hard Can It Be?

Because success in predicting the future depends, to a considerable degree, on making sense of the past, there is a common misperception that once a system's structure is understood, predicting system behavior should follow naturally and easily. While this may be true in the case of simple systems, it is a serious misconception about complex systems.[7,8]

As was noted earlier, research with human subjects has shown that, while people may learn to understand the detailed relationships in complex environments, they are usually unable to figure out the dynamic behavior that these relationships imply. That is, even when we have an accurate model of the system—the system's key variables, how they are related, how they influence one another, and how they are influenced by the system's external environment—being able to mentally "run" the model to predict the system's dynamic behavior over time is a much more difficult task.[9]

In his classic book, *The Sciences of the Artificial*,[10] Herbert Simon, winner of the 1978 Nobel Memorial Prize in Economic Science, argued that when it comes to complex systems, "even when we have the correct premises, it may be very difficult to discover what they imply," which, Simon suggested, is a direct consequence of *bounded rationality,* the term he coined to encompass "the many limitations of attention, memory, recall, information processing capability, and time that constrain human decision making."[11]

In Chapter 13, we got a taste of our own bounded rationality when we tried to discern the dynamic behavior of a mere three-feedback system, only to discover it was not all that obvious (even though the behavior of each of the individual loops, in isolation, was obvious). Our goal in this chapter is to go a step farther. Beyond merely discussing the difficulties of correctly inferring how a complex system will behave, this chapter gives you an opportunity to "experience" that first hand.

Trying Your Hand at Predicting Dynamics

> I forget what I hear; I remember what I see; I know what I do.
>
> —Chinese proverb

As this Chinese proverb suggests, personal experience provides for both a deeper appreciation of a challenge and a more memorable one.

The purpose of this hands-on exercise is to give you the opportunity to assess for yourself the ease or difficulty of figuring out how a system's functioning changes over time. We will use a familiar system, namely, the plumbing analogy we used in earlier chapters: the bathtub with an inflow from a faucet and an outflow through a drain. While this will have you thinking about things like water flow, bathtubs, faucets, and drains, remember that these parts reflect similar structures and processes that determine how food intake (the inflow rate) and energy expenditure (the outflow rate) regulate changes in human body weight (the stock). Indeed, the stock-and-flow structure of this exercise—basically a stock of "stuff" with an inflow that replenishes it and an outflow that drains it—extends well beyond weight and energy regulation to many types of real-life systems and everyday tasks, such as managing a checking account or a company's inventory.

The system and its simple stock-and-flow structure are redrawn below for your convenience (Figure 14.1). Your task, specified in more detail below, is

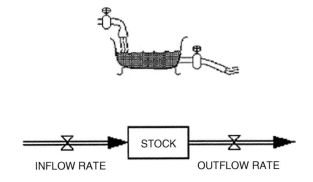

Figure 14.1 Stock-and-flow structure

to determine how changes in the inflow and outflow rates cause the quantity in the stock (the bathtub) to vary over time.

The Bathtub Exercise

The exercise is a slightly adapted version of one devised by professors John Sterman and Linda Booth Sweeney of MIT and Harvard University, respectively, to assess the innate skill of their incoming graduate students to think dynamically.[12] Originally conceived as a one-time experiment, the exercise proved so popular and insightful, and even fun, that it quickly caught on, becoming a requisite class exercise in many introductory systems-thinking courses around the world, including my own course at the Naval Postgraduate School.

The exercise form you will need to use is provided in Figure 14.2. At the top of the figure is a depiction of the plumbing system, consisting of the bathtub with water flowing in and water draining out. Below the bathtub, graph A depicts how the inflow and outflow rates change over time.

As indicated by the initial conditions on the figure, the system starts at time zero, with the bathtub holding 100 liters (L) and in a state of equilibrium, that is, with the inflow from the faucet exactly equaling the outflow at the drain (both at 50 L/min). As long as the amount of water flowing in equals what is draining out, the water level in the bathtub remains unchanged. This steady-state situation, however, holds for only the first 2 minutes, after which things start to change. Specifically, the inflow into the bathtub changes into the sawtooth pattern shown in graph A: at 2 minutes, it starts to progressively rise in a straight-line fashion, peaking at 100 L/min at 4 minutes; it then declines in a straight-line fashion for 4 minutes, dropping to zero at 8 minutes; the inflow rate then turns around and starts rising again, and so on. All the while, the outflow at the drain remains constant, at the 50-L/min level.

Given this scenario for the inflow and outflow rates, your task now is to infer how the quantity of water in the bathtub changes over time. (That would be analogous, in the case of human weight and energy regulation, to inferring how body weight would change in response to changes in food intake when the level of daily physical activity remains constant.) Your task is to sketch on the blank graph B how the quantity of water in the bathtub changes over the 16-minute duration. Note that I have already plotted the first 2 minutes, when the water level starts and remains at the 100-L level.

Now, stop reading and spend a few minutes thinking about and then sketching your answer on graph B.

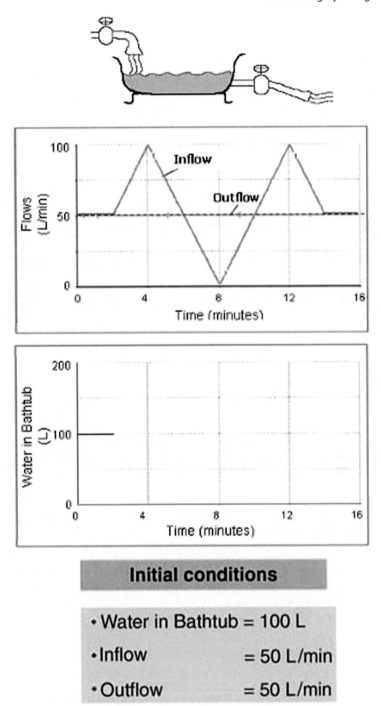

Figure 14.2 Graph A shows how the inflow and outflow rates change over time. From that information, sketch on graph B how the quantity of water in the bathtub changes over time. L, liter

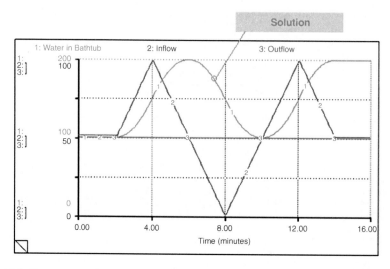

Figure 14.3 The correct solution to the problem. Notes: The left vertical axis garnishes two sets of scales. The top set of numbers (0, 100, 200) apply to the "Water in Bathtub," and the lower set (0, 50, 100) apply to the flows.

The Answer

The correct solution to the problem is provided in Figure 14.3.

A correct solution must exhibit the following two features[13]:

1. Whenever the inflow exceeds the (steady) outflow, the water level rises.
2. Whenever the inflow drops below the outflow (i.e., below 50 L/min), the water level declines.

Obeying these two rules of conservation and accumulation is enough to obtain a very good approximation of the correct answer (and would earn you close to a full mark in my class).

But you must obey the rules, which is what would allow you to correctly determine, for example, that the water level must continue to increase after 4 minutes, even as the inflow rate starts declining—a result that many participants find counterintuitive, as discussed below—because, while the inflow starts falling at 4 minutes, its magnitude at that point (and for a couple of minutes longer) is still *greater* than that of the outflow.

If you are more ambitious, you can trace the shape of the water level's trajectory more precisely by following one additional rule:

3. The peaks and troughs of the water level occur when the inflow crosses the outflow, that is, when the *net* inflow is equal to zero. That happens at 6, 10, and 14 minutes.

Notice that the above three rules describe qualitative features of the behavior and do not require any arithmetic whatsoever.

Finally, to earn a gold star, you can bound the qualitative pattern of the water level by quantitatively assessing the precise level at which the water level peaks. For that, however, you would need to apply some modest arithmetic:

4. To figure out at what level the water quantity first peaks, one would need to calculate the quantity added to the bathtub during the interval of time between the second and sixth minutes (that's the 4-minute interval where the magnitude of the inflow exceeds the outflow). That would be the area enclosed by the graph of the *net* rate, that is, a triangle with area (½ * 50 L/ min * 4 minutes = 100 L). Since the bathtub initially contains 100 L of water, the water level must peak at 100 + 100 = 200 L.

Note that to attain a gold-star performance on the exercise (which was beyond what Sterman and Booth Sweeney expected from their students) requires little calculation (the formula for calculating the area of triangles), but nothing beyond high school arithmetic.

So how did Sterman's and Booth Sweeney's high-powered MIT and Harvard graduate students do? The students' performance was surprisingly poor. Fewer than half the students (48 percent) got the qualitative behavior right, that is, correctly sketching a rising water level when the inflow exceeded the outflow, and vice versa. Only 40 percent placed the peaks and troughs of the stock at the right times (at 6, 10, and 14 minutes). Only a third figured out the correct numeric value (200 L) at which the water level peaks.[14]

These disappointingly poor results were no fluke. Since Sterman's and Booth Sweeney's first experiment at MIT and Harvard, the results have been replicated many times and over a diverse set populations, from Austrian university students,[15,16] to MBAs at the University of Chicago,[17] to sophomores at the California Institute of Technology,[18] to my students at the Naval Postgraduate School.

What Do These Results Tell Us?

An examination of the poor performance by the many students who participated in the exercise over the past few years, with a wide range of backgrounds and training, suggests that the errors were systematic errors, not merely calculation errors. Participants, for example, frequently violated fundamental relationships between stocks and flows such as those relating to conservation of matter (that is, that the quantity in a stock must increase whenever the inflow rate exceeds the outflow, and vice versa).[19] Also, in attempting to figure out how the interrelated quantities in the system change over time, many of the participants relied consistently on heuristics that seem intuitive, but that are (dynamically) erroneous. This invariably led them to commit gross errors.

To illustrate, let me provide two examples. The first relates to a common tendency among participants to match the shape of the bathtub water level to that of the inflow. Did you? Such a response is shown in Figure 14.4, which clearly illustrates that the subject matched the quantity of water in the bathtub (the stock) with the sawtooth trajectory of the inflow.[20] This so-called pattern-matching heuristic may seem intuitively correct but is utterly wrong.

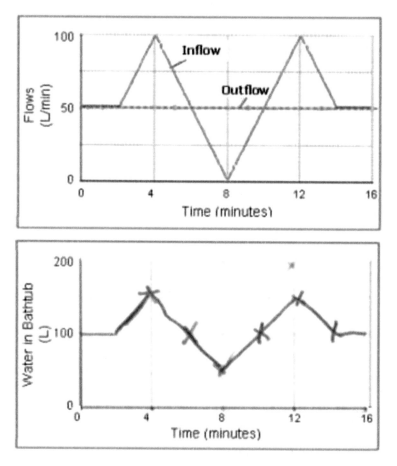

Figure 14.4 A typical erroneous response

Notice, by contrast, that in the solution graph in Figure 14.3, at 4 minutes, the inflow rate starts declining, and yet the water level in the bathtub continues to increase. It must, of course! The water level should rise as long as the inflow, though falling, remains greater than the outflow, which is indeed the case until 6 minutes. The key to whether the stock level increases or decreases is not whether the inflow rate is rising or falling, but rather whether its *magnitude* is greater than or less than that of the outflow rate. If it is greater, then that would mean more water is being added to the bathtub than is being drained out. The correct implication of a declining inflow at between 4 and 6 minutes is that the water level in the bathtub would rise at a *decreasing* rate (see Figure 14.5).

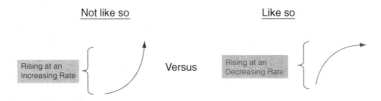

Figure 14.5   Rising at a *decreasing* rate

The widespread tendency to match the trajectories of the bathtub's water level to the faucet's inflow pattern illustrates a basic misunderstanding of the difference between causing *a flow* to move in a certain direction and causing the associated *stock* to move in that *same* direction. Just because one reduces a rate of inflow does not mean that the stock fed by that inflow has likewise been reduced. Beyond bathtubs or human weight and energy regulation, this insight is handy because it applies to so many aspects of our lives. Consider global warming. If you read in tomorrow's newspaper that a new worldwide agreement has miraculously been reached to immediately decrease greenhouse gas emissions by 10 percent per decade, would that reverse the global warming trend? No, it would not, because decreasing the emissions by 10 percent from current levels would not decrease the *stock* of greenhouse gases in the atmosphere. For that to happen, emissions must decrease to a level below the rate at which greenhouse gas particles are naturally removed from the atmosphere, that is, below the system's outflow rate. And that, experts estimate, would require a much steeper reduction—close to 50 percent—from current levels.[21]

The same pattern-matching thought process causes people to dramatically underestimate the degree to which the process of stock accumulation provides systems with *inertia* and *memory*. Notice that, in the last 2 minutes in Figure 14.3, even as the inflow falls back to its start-up level, the water level in the bathtub does not return to its original level. Instead, the water remains at its maximum level, because, at any point in time, the amount of water in the tank reflects the *cumulative* effect of the net inflows over outflows, not merely what is going on at that very moment. Thus, at 14 minutes, the amount of water in the tank reflects the cumulative effect of the net inflows over outflows over the first 14 minutes, a net addition of some 100 L. When, at 14 minutes, the inflow drops to its original 50 L/min and stays there, the inflow into the tank from that point onward will be exactly equal to the outflow, causing the level in the tank to remain steady *at its peak value.*

Stocks are, therefore, said to provide systems with inertia because they provide a "memory" of all past events in the system—in this case, a memory of the fact that in the preceding 14 minutes the inflow has exceeded the outflow most of the time.

It is serendipitous that I happen to be writing this chapter in late November, just before the holiday season—a time of year when many of us subject our bodies to a tsunami of caloric intake. I have to remind myself at this festive time of year that any body weight I gain will not go away once I revert back to my pre-holiday food intake levels (just as the bathtub level did not revert back to its initial value even as the inflow rate did). Perhaps this seems obvious to you, but most people tend to misperceive or choose to ignore this fact.[22] This was aptly demonstrated in a recent two-phase study in which scientists at the National Institutes of Health tracked the amount of weight gained by 195 adults between Thanksgiving and New Year's Day, and then, in phase two, checked on them a year later. Not surprisingly, the research team found that most of their experimental subjects did gain weight over the holidays. What was of greater concern, however, was the striking lack of after-holidays compensation by most of the participants.[23] As a result, for most subjects (165 out of the 195 [85 percent]) the amount of weight gained during the holidays never came off.[24,25]

Most of us, it appears, either do not realize or do not *want* to realize that our bodies (like all stocks) do have memory!

Beyond Bathtubs

The difficulties people have with this exercise often surprise them, because the system is rather simple: there is only one stock, the outflow is constant, and the inflow follows a simple pattern. The key underlying process in the task—a process of replenishment/depletion regulating the quantity in a stock—is a familiar one, and the task requires only a little calculation and no knowledge of higher mathematics; it does not require any of the analytic tools of calculus, such as derivatives and integrals.

Surprise notwithstanding, the results do provide some very useful insights. They suggest that inferring the dynamic behavior of even a simple system (a single stock with two flows) is perhaps not as intuitive as we think. They also suggest that our collective poor performance arises not from a faulty understanding of system structure (in this case, we had perfect knowledge about the system's pieces and their relationships), but from the apparently innate inability to use our knowledge to properly infer system behavior. That is, even when we have an accurate mental picture or model of a system's structure, with human intuition alone we cannot reliably deduce its dynamics.[26]

According to Sterman, part of the problem is simply that we have not been trained to distinguish between what is a stock and what is a rate and how they relate to each other.[27] The other part is more fundamental:

> [The exercise] exposes us to one of the most fundamental bounds on human cognition: our inability to simulate mentally the dynamics of ... systems. Indeed, our experimental studies show that people are unable to accurately infer the behavior of even the simplest systems.[28]

Experiments in which people perform in dynamic environments have consistently shown that, while the human mind is an excellent recorder of decisions, reasons, motivations, and structural relationships, it is not that good (or reliable) at inferring the behavioral implications of interactions over time.[29] That is, being able to mentally "run" our mental model of some system or situation to figure out how it behaves over time is a much more difficult task for us. This holds true even for systems that are far simpler than those we encounter in our daily lives, as we saw here.[30,31]

Is there anything we can do to overcome that difficulty? Yes. The next few chapters demonstrate how—even if we are not innately wired for the task— with the proper tools we can infer the dynamics of not just our bathtubs, but even of highly complex systems, such as the multiloop nonlinear feedback system of human weight and energy regulation.

"Give Us the Tools, and We Will Finish the Job"   **15**

> Give us the tools, and we will finish the job
> —Winston Churchill

Sources of Complexity in Systems

Invariably at the conclusion of these bathtub exercises, after the group's collective performance is analyzed and discussed, most of the participants tend to have the mixed feeling of having taken one step forward and another step backward. On the positive side, participants realize that they have gained a deeper appreciation of their strengths and weaknesses in reasoning about systems. They realize they have done reasonably well in comprehending system structure, although not as well in inferring system behavior. On the negative side, there is an almost palpable disappointment from having struggled (and failed) with a task that is actually quite simple.

Their worry is understandable. After all, the bathtub system is as simple a stock-and-flow structure as you can find. In contrast to real-life systems that we manage in our private or professional lives, "there are no feedback processes, no time delays, no nonlinearities. There is only one stock. The outflow is constant, and the inflow follows a simple pattern."[32] Real-life systems, such as human weight and energy regulation, are not quite that simplistic or that transparent.

Complexity in systems is driven by two primary factors: (1) the number of elements or parts in the system, and (2) the degree and nature of the interactions between them (such as feedback and nonlinearities). The significance of the number of elements is obvious. Having to grapple with a large number of variables obliges us to attend to a great many features imultaneously. The larger the number of parts, the more involved the process of investigating or controlling the behavior of a system becomes.[33] Complexity also increases

T.K.A. Hamid, *Thinking in Circles About Obesity*,
DOI 10.1007/978-0-387-09469-4_15, © Springer Science+Business Media, LLC 2009

when there is a dense network of interactions among system elements. With many interdependent or correlated variables, actions that affect or are meant to affect one part of the system tend to have side effects on other parts of the system.[34] So much will be going on, and some of the things that are going on will cause still other things to go on, so making sense of it all quickly becomes a daunting task.[35]

Both factors of complexity characterize the human bioenergetics system. Using the bathtub system as a sort of a benchmark, let's extrapolate a little and contemplate how much more unwieldy such a real system would be. Unlike the bathtub system (with its single stock, one constant outflow, and an inflow that follows a simple predetermined pattern), the human bioenergetics system would have several stocks and flows; the outflows would not be constant, and the inflows would assume many complex patterns. Let's think about each of these complications in turn.

First, rather than a single stock (the bathtub), we would have several. In the human bioenergetics system, the intake—food energy—is used to accomplish two primary tasks: fueling the body's metabolic and physical activities, and providing the major building blocks for the synthesis of body tissue (with the excess energy stored in the body's energy depots). This suggests a system not only with multiple stocks, but also with multiple *types* of stocks. For example, we would have at least two aggregate stocks for the body's mass compartments: fat mass and fat free mass. Similarly, we would need at least two stocks to accumulate the body's energy reserves: a fat stock and a glucose stock.

On the output side, in contrast to the single bathtub drain, we would need an outflow for each of the three forms of energy expenditure: resting energy expenditure (REE); the thermic effect of activity (TEA); and the thermic effect of food (TEF). Similarly, on the input side, multiple inflows (spigots) are required to properly capture human food intake. Humans do not eat pure energy; we eat nutrients—the predominant nutrients being protein, carbohydrate, and fat—that are oxidized by the body to provide the energy we need. The three macronutrient inputs need to be captured separately (not as a single spigot) because of the significant metabolic differences among them (as will be explained in Chapter 16).

Next, consider the degree and nature of interrelationships among the system's parts. In contrast to the bathtub's open-loop structure, in human energy regulation, the system's stocks and flows are not independent components, each marching to its own tune. They are *interdependent*. For example, there are feedback effects among the stocks and flows—body weight affects energy expenditure, and energy expenditure affects body weight; appetite shapes body weight, and body weight influences appetite. Unlike the bathtub system, where the inflow was an external variable with a simple, predetermined (and recurring) pattern, the inflows in the case of human appetite are much more nuanced—driven not only by internal biological and psychological states of need, but also by external cultural and social factors. Finally, unlike the bathtub, with its constant outflow rate, body weight is not lost at a constant (linear) rate throughout a period of caloric deprivation (because of the concomitant drop in the body's maintenance energy requirements that accompanies weight loss).

In the simplistic bathtub exercise, because the inflow and outflow variables were both external—each doing its own thing, independent of the other components in the system—the arithmetic was straightforward. By contrast, the dense interactions among the many more stocks and flows in the human energy regulation system complicate the bookkeeping required to "run" the model.

But why? Why can we fairly easily extend a static mental picture of some system by incorporating additional elements and interrelationships, as we just did, but we struggle to accurately determine the dynamic behavior of the simpler bathtub system?

The KISS Acronym: "Keep It Simple, Stupid"

The finding that human information processing, as marvelous as it is, falters when it comes to dynamic behavior is by no means unique to the bathtub exercise—far from it. As mentioned earlier, it has been a robust finding in experimental studies of behavioral decision making in a wide variety of problem-solving settings.[36]

As already noted, among the most notable experts to draw attention to human cognitive limitations was Nobel laureate Herbert Simon, in his groundbreaking work on the "bounded rationality" of human judgment.[37] Subsequently, the work of Jay Forrester and others in the field of system dynamics further demonstrated that deficiencies in dynamic reasoning are particularly acute in the case of *complex nonlinear feedback systems*. This ongoing research effort is clearly showing that human intuition is neither efficient nor reliable in inferring the behavior of systems of interconnected feedback structures, especially where multiple loops interact in complex nonlinear fashions (as in our system of weight and energy regulation).[38]

Behavior-decision scientists and cognitive psychologists have long sought to explain why this is so. Why have we not evolved an innate simulation capacity to run the complex mental models we hold of our world? And how do we manage without it? Now, they think they know why.

When tackling dynamic decision tasks, such as those in which the task or situation changes over time, autonomously, or in reaction to our decisions or actions, we can use one of two primary strategies: feedforward and feedback. For our purposes, the important difference is that feedforward involves basing our actions on predictions of the state of the system, whereas feedback involves basing our actions on current information we receive about the system (so-called outcome feedback). The two strategies differ quite significantly with respect to the kind of model needed and the cognitive skills required. Specifically, the feedback-based strategy requires a much simpler model than feedforward does, and this, in turn, translates into a significantly simpler cognitive task. Not surprisingly, feedback is, more often than not, the strategy we deploy.[39]

Consider, for example, a common task such as passing another car while driving on the highway. To do that, we do not make an a priori judgment as to the best path—a (predictive) task that would require some heavy-duty computation. Instead, we rely on a series of incremental judgment–action–outcome steps to accomplish the task. That is, rather than computing an optimal one-step response, a series of action-and-adjustment responses, all of which may be relatively inaccurate, takes us progressively to the target. Notice that such corrective feedback "allows [it] to appear as though complex sequences of behavior had been planned in detail when, in fact, only relatively simple actions need to be coordinated across time."[40]

Sterman and Booth Sweeney[41] provide a very plausible evolutionary explanation for the apparently innate limitation to reason dynamically, and they use the bathtub exercise as the context for their point:

> [As in many real life situations,] it is not necessary to understand the relationship between flows and stocks to fill a bathtub—nature accumulates the water "automatically." It is far more efficient to simply monitor the level of water in a tub and shut off the tap when the water reaches the desired level—a simple, effectively [goal-seeking] negative feedback process, which, experiments ... show, people can do well. Thus for a wide range of everyday tasks, decision makers have no need to infer how the flows relate to the stocks—it is better to simply wait and see how the state of the system changes, and then take corrective action. In such settings [dynamic reasoning about] stocks and flows offers no survival value and is unlikely to evolve.[42]

Unfortunately, the wait-and-see strategy can fail spectacularly in systems with long time delays and where effects are irreversible, as in the case of human health and disease.[43] When it comes to our bodies, many processes can be hard, if not impossible, to reverse, and even when self-repair is possible, the often long delays mean that there is little opportunity for corrective action through outcome feedback.

Argument for a Calculus

Engineers have long appreciated that the structures of complex technological systems often lead to unanticipated, and even puzzling, behavior, and that intuitive judgment alone is unreliable in estimating how these systems behave dynamically, even with good knowledge of the system's individual parts. Engineers, thus, long ago turned to computer models and laboratory experiments to manage complex technological systems.

Biological systems (such as the human body) are far more complex and harder to predict than many of our technological systems. So why do we not use the same approach of modeling and experimentation to anticipate our bodies' behavior before trying new interventions and treatments?

The typical answer is that the average person's ability to properly use models of a system as complex as the human body is grossly insufficient. But what justification can there be for the apparent assumption that ordinary people do not know enough to use models of their health, but believe that they do know enough to directly intervene in managing their weight and energy regulation?[44]

I contend (and substantial supporting evidence is beginning to accumulate) that people do know enough to use such tools. People have already learned to rely on computer-based tools to handle the complexities of managing their financial portfolios, preparing their taxes, and getting a good deal on eBay. By contrast, in managing personal health and well-being, we continue to rely on intuition and raw judgment. Yet, more than engineering or personal finance, personal health is precisely the setting in which the complexities may be the most problematic and the stakes are the highest.

As noted earlier, it is perhaps paradoxical that the recent advances in medicine have made the task of personal health management more, not less, complex. This is partly because the elimination of infectious diseases has increased life expectancy, so that minor dysfunctions have more time to develop into chronic diseases.

Computer modeling tools can help. Using today's affordable desktop computers, we can now construct silicon surrogates of human physiology that faithfully mimic our bodies' functions. With increasingly user-friendly software, ordinary people, for the first time in history, have access to and can learn to make effective use of models of systems as complex as their own bodies. Using these tools, dieters or patients, like engineers, can have a laboratory in which to conduct thought experiments to test myriad sorts of what-if scenarios and learn quickly and cost-effectively answers that would seldom be obtainable through raw intuition.

Leveraging Computer Technology

A key message is this book is that we cannot and should not rely on intuition alone in managing our bodies. To effectively manage a system as complex as our bodies, we need a reliable and efficient system of dynamic "book-keeping." The digital computer, a complementary innovation to systems thinking, provides that function.

> [C]omputer [models] represent a kind of "telescope for the mind"—[they multiply] our powers of analysis and insight just as a telescope does our powers of vision.[45]

The type of computer model I am talking about here is referred to as a simulation or microworld. This kind of computer program is built to simulate or mimic the real-life system that is modeled. (A simulation or microworld for human physiology is analogous to the "flight simulators" that many people are familiar with. Instead of piloting an aircraft, it is a tool for "flying" our bodies.) In essence, it is a silicon replica of a real-life system. Unlike a mental model, a computer simulator can reliably and efficiently trace through time the implications of a messy maze of interactions. "It is just in this area of deducing the behavior implied by a set of [interactions] that the human mind is the weakest, but computer simulation is beyond question."[46] Computer simulation, thus, fills the gap where human judgment is suspect, keeping track of how the known interrelated components of a system interact to produce system behavior. It provides a tool of "bookkeeping" that is more reliable, and far more efficient, than human intuition.

In the next chapters, we will see an example of just such a model in action and demonstrate the many virtues of simulation-type models. Perhaps the most important is that they make perfectly controlled experimentation possible, because in the microworld, unlike in real life, the effect of changing one treatment intervention or environmental factor can be observed while all other factors are held unchanged. In real life, by contrast, many variables change simultaneously, confounding the interpretation of treatment results. Such controlled experimentation can not only yield useful insights into the efficacy of different treatment options, but also predict treatment outcomes.

Computer models do not have to be passive sorts of things, simply, "telling us about some slice of reality but not really giving us any special insight into how to perhaps shape that reality to our own ends."[47] These models are at their best when they allow us to create what-if scenarios to see how that reality might be bent to our will (e.g., by intervening in different ways to modify the reality or situation that the model represents).[48]

A Microworld for Weight and Energy Regulation

Telescopes for the Mind

Prior to the development of modern computers, formal modeling of real-life systems was limited to pencil-and-paper mathematical formulations. This imposed certain limitations. For example, it was often necessary to make simplifying—even heroic—assumptions when dealing with complex phenomena (such as to assume that relations between system variables are well-behaving *linear*, straight-line relations). To render our models mathematically tractable, we often needed to break large systems into manageable "analytical bites" and analyze the simplified fragments in isolation, "with the hope that we [could] then re-assemble these chunks of partial knowledge into an understanding of the overall system."[49]

The advent of computers in the middle of the 20th century, and the subsequent explosive proliferation of microcomputers, was a signal development in the analysis of complex systems. It has given rise to the development of new computational (rather than algebraic) tools for tackling complex systems. This chapter introduces what is perhaps the largest cannon in this arsenal: simulations (or microworlds) constructed inside the digital computer.[50]

Though only a few decades old, computer modeling of complex systems has had a profound impact on the so-called new sciences of complexity. "Dubbed the 'third branch' of science (after theory and experiment), [computer] simulation is now an essential tool in research on problems from galaxy formation to protein folding to epidemiology."[51]

Simulation's particular advantage is its greater fidelity in modeling processes, making possible both more complex models and models of more complex systems, because, in contrast to traditional mathematical analysis, computer modeling removes much of the pressure to strip problems of their complicating features before solving them. Today, thanks to the availability of affordable, high-quality computing capabilities, we can construct silicon models that are faithful surrogates of our most complex real-world processes.[52]

T.K.A. Hamid, *Thinking in Circles About Obesity*,
DOI 10.1007/978-0-387-09469-4_16, © Springer Science+Business Media, LLC 2009

While computer simulation is becoming increasingly commonplace in the military, pilot training, power plant operations, economic development, financial engineering, and many other engineering and economic tasks, it is still underused in health management. Yet, as argued earlier, this is precisely the setting in which dynamic complexity is most problematic and where the stakes are the highest.

My objective in this part of the book is to demonstrate both the feasibility and utility of such tools for personal health care management. A major part of my research leading up to this book was in the development of integrative computer models that serve as a laboratory in which to learn about obesity and weight management as well as serve as tools to support decision making about treatment options. This chapter provides a brief overview of such a tool. The discussion is somewhat brief and largely nontechnical. The interested reader can find more details on the model's technical formulation in a number of publications in the academic literature.[53] The rest of the chapters in Part IV demonstrate the model's utility in gaining insight into and ultimately managing human weight and energy regulation. Before discussing the model, however, it will be useful to clarify some important distinctions between simulation models, or microworlds, and the more common computer models that you may already have used or are familiar with.

Simulation Models Are *Operational* Models

The type of computer model I am talking about is different from the models you are apt to read about in the newspaper or hear about on television. Many of those models, typically used for business and economic applications, are statistical models that aim to capture the associations among two or more variables (e.g., the relation between price and demand of a product or service), and are typically derived from the number crunching of historical time-series data.

Simulations (or microworlds) are different. The aim with such models is not to capture correlations between variables, but to emulate a system's operation, that is, to look at the activity, process, or system in terms of how it really works and to replicate that in silicon.[54] Let me use a simple example to demonstrate this correlational versus operational distinction.

Let's say that we are interested in forecasting aggregate milk production in the United States. What would such a model look like? An example of an actual econometric-type model that appeared in a leading economics journal looks something like this[55]:

$$\text{Milk Production} = \alpha_1 * GNP + \alpha_2 * \text{Interest Rates} + \ldots + \beta$$

The structure of the model follows a commonly used statistical form. The equation states that milk production is a function of a set of macroeconomic variables (e.g., the gross national product [GNP], interest rates, etc.), each with its own weighting factor (α_1 and α_2). According to the journal article, the model was, by all statistical measures, quite sound, which is to say, the values of milk production it generated closely tracked historically observed values,[56] and that's a good thing.

However, the model's equation clearly does not purport to represent how milk actually is produced. For nowhere in the expression do we see any *cows*—the primary "engine" for the production of milk!

By contrast, from an operational point of view, cows would be the first variable we would include in a model for milk production, for example, formulating milk production as a function of cows and their milk-producing productivity. That would be step one. Next, because production of milk replenishes the nation's milk inventory, while milk consumption depletes it, the operational thinker would then seek to specify the consumption process. For example, milk consumption could similarly be modeled as a product of consumers and their consumption rate. This is operational thinking! The resulting operational picture would look something like what you see pictured in Figure 16.1.[57]

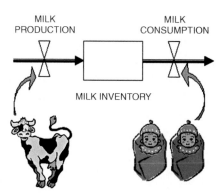

Figure 16.1 What an *operational* model looks like

What does operational thinking buy us? The real benefit from thinking operationally is that it enhances our understanding of how the real system actually works. Knowing how a system works is the first step toward being able to change how it functions.

Rather than trying to predict the behavior of a system through a series of high-level, abstract, correlational relationships, operational thinking has you getting right down to the utter facts of what's really going on. And, when you do, you gain a much deeper insight into how one might go about *changing* the way the system is working! Operational thinking helps you to identify the levers for change that actually are available to a change agent. For example, in the [milk] illustration, if we want to increase milk production, we have two options: (1) increase the number of cows producing milk, and (2) increase average productivity per cow (e.g., by increasing dairy farmers' knowledge of productivity-enhancing techniques, providing incentives for investing in state-of-the-art automated milking technology, and so on)....

By thinking in terms of how a process or system really works (i.e., its "physics"), we have a much better chance of understanding how to make it work better! This is what operational thinking does for you.[58]

Another attractive, though often underappreciated, feature of operational-type models is that they tend to be easier for nontechnical users to understand and relate to, because, as the above picture demonstrates, the variables in these types of models correspond to real variables in the real system. In our example above, each variable had a corresponding meaning or counterpart in the real system (cows, cows' productivity in producing milk, milk inventory, consumers and their consumption rate). This contrasts with statistical and econometric-type models, which often incorporate artificial variables (technically referred to as arbitrary scaling factors) that are routinely added to improve their fit to the historical time series data.[59]

Once the model's building blocks have been assembled, and their relationships have been established (such as specifying that Total Milk Production equals Number of Cows times Average Productivity per Cow) and fed into the computer, the computer then performs the critical bookkeeping function of keeping track of how the system variables interact to produce system behavior. A simulation model, thus, is not a static representation of the underlying system, but a model of the system as an operating (running) system. To accomplish that, simulation models rely on a set of rules for computing how the values of variables change over time.[60] The basic computation scheme is quite simple.

For example, the rule for tracking changes in a stock-type variable (such as the milk inventory above or the bathtub water level discussed earlier) goes like so: the value of the stock, say, a minute from now is equal to the value of the stock now plus the inflow into the stock over the next minute minus the outflow. Once the status of the system a minute from now is computed, the computer can then repeat the process to calculate the value of the stock for the minute after that (i.e., 2 minutes from now). To increase our computational accuracy, rather than perform these computations once a minute, we would instead perform them every second or even every millisecond. This would increase the number crunching that would be necessary, but computers are perfectly suited to the task.

With this understanding of what computer simulation models are, we can now move on to discuss the structure of our microworld of human weight and energy regulation. Again, the intent of this discussion is not to delve into the model's mathematical formulations, but, rather, to use the model to give you a sort of tutorial in how the processes of energy and weight regulation operate.

Overview of Model Structure

Figure 16.2 provides an overview of the model's four major subsystems: body composition, energy intake (EI), energy expenditure (EE), and energy metabolism and regulation. These subsystems are not independent, stand-alone systems, but, as the interconnections in the figure suggest, they interact with one another.

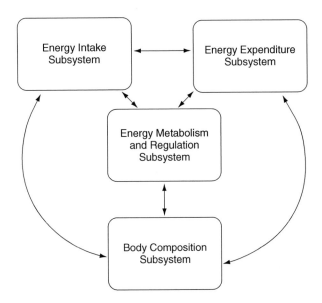

Figure 16.2 Overview of the model's four subsystems

By incorporating these multiple interrelated subsystems, the model provides an integrated holistic perspective of the key functions and processes comprising human weight and energy regulation (including metabolism, hormonal regulation, body composition, nutrition, and physical activity). As such, it allows us to capture the various interdependencies and interactions, for example, how changes in one subsystem can be compensated for by other subsystems and where interventions in one domain will influence or be influenced by the state of variables elsewhere.[61] Such an integrative perspective provides a striking contrast with much of the discourse—both academic and popular—about the obesity problem, where the tendency is to emphasize one aspect or problem area in isolation, such as nutrition, physical activity, hormonal regulation, metabolism, or body composition.

The model, furthermore, is not merely a static snapshot of the system's constituent parts and their interdependencies. As a dynamic simulation model, it allows us to view the system as it is in real life—as an operating system. For example, it captures how energy input derived from food consumption processes in the energy input subsystem is channeled to yield the energy used to fuel energy expenditure in the energy expenditure subsystem and provide the major building blocks for the synthesis of body tissue in the body composition subsystem. In the model, as in reality, the body uses the nutrients to fuel its metabolic and physical activities and rearranges any excess into storage compounds (also in the body composition subsystem). In orchestrating all of this, the body relies on an elaborate system of hormonal mechanisms in the energy metabolism and regulation subsystem.

Figure 16.2 provides only a high-level overview of the model's four major subsystems and hints of their interrelationships. The complete model is much more detailed and contains more than six hundred causal links and hundreds of variables. (For example, envision within the energy input subsystem multiple stock-and-flow type variables plumbed together to capture the intake of the proteins, carbohydrates, and fats, while in the body composition subsystem, multiple types of stocks capture the body's fat and fat-free mass compartments and accumulate the body's energy fat and glucose reserves.)

The rest of this chapter expands upon this high-level view and delineates in more detail the inner workings of the four interrelated subsystems. It will not be a balanced discussion, though. The energy metabolism and energy regulation subsystem (at the center of the model) is discussed in somewhat greater detail than the other three. This investment will come in handy in later chapters in helping us better interpret the results of the simulation experiments we will run.

After completing the discussion of the model's structure in this chapter, we will proceed in subsequent chapters to investigate the model's behavior. Specifically, we will conduct a number of experiments designed to provide a better understanding of how this type of model can fulfill its twofold purpose: to serve as a personal laboratory for learning about how our physiology and metabolism work, and to serve as a personal decision support tool to assess treatment options and predict treatment outcomes.

Energy Intake (EI) Subsystem

The body derives all the energy and structural materials it needs from the foods we eat. The principal substances from which the body's cells extract energy are oxygen together with one or more of the foodstuffs that react with the oxygen, namely, fats, carbohydrates (CHO), and proteins. (Alcohol consumption can also be a source of energy.) When completely broken down in the body, a gram of carbohydrate yields about 4 kilocalories (kcal) of energy; a gram of protein also yields 4 kcal; and a gram of fat yields 9 kcal.[62,63]

The three macronutrients—fat, carbohydrate, and protein—however, do not constitute an interchangeable energy currency within the body, as is often assumed.[64] Recent research has clearly shown that isocaloric quantities of these macronutrients are not equivalent as calorie sources in the human body,[65] primarily because the efficiency with which the body extracts and stores excess energy varies substantially among the three nutrients. Furthermore, the body appears to have metabolic priorities that dictate how much of a given nutrient is deployed for its different activities and the form in which the excess energy is stored (e.g., fat versus glycogen)—all factors that can significantly influence body weight and composition over time. Such differences among the three macronutrients highlight the need for distinguishing their respective inflows when studying (and modeling) energy intake.[66]

Therefore, in the model, energy input is modeled not as a single inflow but as three separate (though interrelated) flows: fat, CHO, and protein. The stock-and-flow structure looks something like the simplified picture in Figure 16.3.

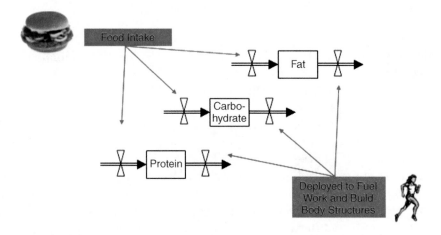

Figure 16.3 Inside the energy intake subsystem

The digestive system is the body's ingenious way of breaking down foods into nutrients ready for absorption into the bloodstream. In the model (as in our bodies), essentially all carbohydrates are converted into glucose by the digestive tract and liver before they reach the cells. Similarly, the proteins are converted into amino acids and the fats into fatty acids. Once a nutrient has entered the bloodstream, it may be transported to any of the cells in the body where it is deployed (e.g., allowed to react chemically with oxygen under the influence of various enzymes) to do the body's work (biological and/or mechanical).[67]

The body uses the nutrients to fuel its metabolic and physical activities and rearranges any excess into storage compounds to be used between meals and overnight, when fresh energy supplies run low. When more energy is consumed than expended, the body's energy reserves are replenished. Conversely, if less energy is consumed than expended, the result is depletion of energy reserves and weight loss.[68]

Energy Expenditure (EE) Subsystem

In the model, the body's total energy expenditure is divided conceptually into three components: resting energy (also referred to as maintenance), physical activity, and food processing. All three were discussed in Chapter 10, but for completeness and because they constitute an important part of model structure, we review them here briefly.

The largest of the three components is the resting energy expenditure (REE), defined as the energy expended to sustain the basic metabolic functions of an awake individual at rest. It is the amount of energy required to maintain the basic internal housekeeping functions of the body—to keep our heart beating, our nerves transmitting, and our lungs breathing.[69] In most sedentary adults, the REE makes up about 60 to 70 percent of total energy expenditure.

Two factors establish the value of REE: body composition and energy balance. A person's body composition establishes his or her body's nominal resting energy expenditure level—a baseline level—that is then adjusted upward or downward as a function of the person's energy balance (i.e., as a function of what the person does with his or her body).

As we shall see in the body composition subsystem, human body composition can be viewed as being composed of two main compartments: fat-free mass (FFM) and fat mass (FM). The two tissue types have very different qualitative and quantitative fuel requirements. Fat tissue, which is primarily composed of inert triglyceride, is less metabolically active than FFM, and thus has a lower rate of fuel consumption per unit mass.[70] This explains, for example, why men have higher metabolic rates than women (women have relatively more fat and less muscle than men) and why metabolic rates decrease with age (because we often lose muscle mass as we get older).[71,72]

The second factor affecting REE is the body's energy balance. As we have already discussed, during caloric deprivation the body adapts physiologically to the negative energy balance by decreasing the metabolic activity of the tissue mass at the cellular level in order to conserve energy and restrain the rate of weight loss. In the event of overconsumption and weight gain, there is, conversely, an increase in REE per unit mass; that is, there is an exaggerated increase in daily REE beyond that effectuated by the increase in tissue mass.[73] The REE per unit of metabolic mass, in other words, increases with positive energy balance and decreases with negative energy balance. These up/down adjustments in REE, experimental research findings have demonstrated, can increase/decrease a person's daily REE by as much as 20 percent.[74-76]

The second largest component of daily energy expenditure is the energy expended for muscular work, known as the thermic effect of activity (TEA). The TEA of an individual not engaged in heavy labor accounts for 15 to 20 percent of daily energy expenditure, but with heavy and regular exercise, TEA can be easily doubled or even tripled.[77]

The third component of energy expenditure is the thermic effect of food (TEF), which constitutes the various metabolic costs associated with processing a meal, including the costs of digestion, absorption, transport, and storage of nutrients within the body. (It is referred to as the *thermic* effect of food because the acceleration of activity that occurs when we eat—as the gastrointestinal (GI) tract muscles speed up their rhythmic contractions, and the cells that manufacture and secrete digestive juices begin their tasks—produces heat.) The TEF accounts for approximately 10 percent of total daily energy expenditure in moderately active people, but obviously can increase or decrease depending on the amount and the composition of a person's diet.[78]

Energy Metabolism and Regulation Subsystem

In the human body, the chemical energy trapped within the bonds of food nutrients is initially stored in its chemical form within the body's tissues, ready to be transformed into mechanical energy (and, ultimately, heat) by the action of the musculoskeletal system or to be used to build body structures. In essence, living cells are energy transducers with the capacity to extract and utilize the potential energy stored in the chemical bonds of carbohydrates, fats, and proteins.[79] *Metabolism* is defined as the sum total of all the chemical reactions that go on in living cells by which nutrients are broken down to yield energy or rearranged into body structures.

The cells of the body—heart cells, muscle cells, lung cells, and so on—require an uninterrupted supply of metabolic fuel whether they are at rest or carrying out their unique specialized functions. To accomplish this, the body relies on an elaborate system of hormonal mechanisms to maintain the right amounts of blood nutrients that meet the varied demands of the body's specialized tissues. The body's subsystem of energy metabolism and regulation also provides the capacity to store energy-rich substrates in times of plenty and to draw on these stores in times of want, thus liberating us from the necessity of constant food intake.[80]

Glucose and Free Fatty Acid Metabolism

As was mentioned earlier, essentially all carbohydrates are converted into glucose by the digestive tract and liver before they reach the cells. Similarly, the proteins are converted into amino acids and the fats into fatty acids.

In a normal individual, the blood's glucose concentration is maintained within the narrow range of 70 to 100 mg/deciliter (dL).[81] It is important to maintain the blood glucose concentration at a sufficiently high level because glucose is the only nutrient that can normally be used by the cells of the brain. Even though the mass of the brain is only 2 percent of the total body, under resting conditions, the metabolism of the brain accounts for about 15 percent of the total metabolism in the body. At the same time, it is also important that the blood's glucose concentration does not rise too high because excessive levels of glucose concentration can cause considerable cellular dehydration.[82]

Because maintaining glucose balance is critical, the body uses glucose frugally when the diet provides only small amounts (relying more on fat as a source of energy) and freely when stores are abundant (displacing fat in the fuel mix).[83] This homeostatic regulation is achieved primarily by two hormones: *insulin*, which moves glucose from the blood into the cells for use as an energy source, and *glucagon*, which brings glucose out of storage (primarily in the liver) when necessary.

The principal way that insulin controls glucose use in the body is by facilitating the diffusion of glucose across cell membranes. This process works as follows: After a meal, as blood glucose rises, special cells of the pancreas (called beta cells) respond by secreting insulin into the blood. → In the presence of insulin, glucose combines with glucose receptors located on the cells' plasma membranes. → The receptors respond by ushering glucose from the blood into the cells. In the absence of insulin, on the other hand, the amounts of glucose that can diffuse to the insides of most cells of the body to serve as fuel for their work is minimal. In effect, then, the rate of carbohydrate utilization by most cells is controlled by the rate of insulin secretion from the pancreas.[84]

The process of glucose regulation in the human body provides a good example for us to peek inside the energy metabolism and regulation subsystem and get a deeper understanding of the model's (and the body's) inner workings. It is an interesting system, yet simple enough for demonstrating how, like most systems, it can be naturally modeled as accumulations and rates of flow threaded together by feedback loops.

Not unlike water in a tank, the glucose in the bloodstream is essentially a stock that increases with the release of glucose into the bloodstream and decreases by the cells' glucose uptake. Similarly, insulin is a stock that increases as insulin is secreted by the pancreas beta cells and decreases when insulin breaks down and is cleared. Insulin has a so-called plasma half-life of about 6 minutes, which means it degrades 10 to 15 minutes after being released into the bloodstream, losing its ability to influence glucose uptake and release. This relatively rapid clearing rate provides the body with the ability to rapidly turn insulin off when needed.[85]

The glucose and insulin stock-and-flow processes interact with one another, forming a classic negative feedback mechanism. It is this homeostatic feedback process that effectively regulates the body's glucose concentration to within desired levels. Figure 16.4 shows how the loop is formed as each stock influences the flow to the other.

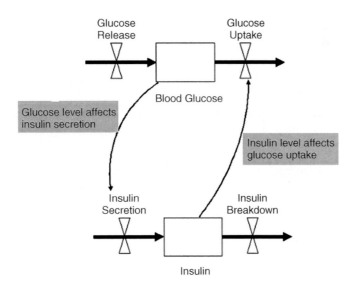

Figure 16.4 Inside the energy metabolism subsystem

Specifically, the insulin stock (that is, the amount of insulin in the plasma) affects the uptake of glucose (that is the outflow of the glucose stock), while the amount of glucose in the bloodstream (the glucose stock) regulates the rate at which insulin is secreted. The glucose stock acts as a catalyst for the inflow rate to the insulin stock, and, likewise, insulin acts as a catalyst for the outflow from the glucose stock.

To see the negative feedback loop in action, we can take a walk around the loop with a pencil in hand. After a meal is consumed, glucose from the ingested food is absorbed in the intestine, causing the level of glucose in the blood to rise. We would indicate this increase in the glucose level with an up arrow (↑) to the left of the *blood glucose* stock in Figure 16.4. The elevated level of glucose stimulates beta cells in the pancreas to release insulin, inducing an increase in the *insulin secretion* rate (↑) and, in turn, the *insulin* stock (↑). Because insulin facilitates the uptake of glucose by many cells of the body, the elevated insulin levels increases the rate of *glucose uptake* (↑), and that causes the *blood glucose* level to decrease (↓). Adding this last down arrow (↓) to the right of the *blood glucose* stock in Figure 16.4 closes the loop. It also demonstrates the feedback effect, that is, how the loop acts to counter-act (reverse) the initial rise of the glucose level in the blood (lowering it back down).[86] Working to counteract change (or disturbance) is what negative loops do.

Figure 16.5 (produced by the model) shows how the above process is repeated following the three regular meals over a 24-hour period. Before a person's first meal, the blood glucose is normally in the range of 80 to 90 mg/dL, a level high enough to keep insulin secretion at its minimal rate. After a meal, blood glucose concentration quickly increases to a level that is two to three times above normal (typically peaking 30 to 60 minutes after the start of the meal).[87] This, in turn, induces insulin secretion to increase markedly (and rapidly), as much as tenfold, facilitating the uptake of glucose by many cells of the body.[88]

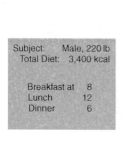

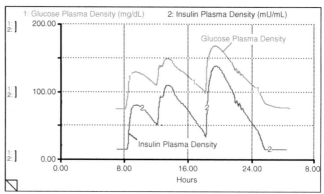

Figure 16.5 The "synchronized" cycles of glucose and insulin levels over a 24-hour period

Most of the cells take only the glucose they can use for energy right away, but the liver and muscle cells can assemble the small glucose units into long, branching chains of glycogen for storage, a process called *glycogenesis*. After the liver and muscle cells have stored as much glycogen as they can—an amount sufficient to supply the energy needs of the body for only 12 to 24 hours—any additional glucose is converted by the liver into fat and is stored in the fat cells. Thus, high blood glucose returns to normal as excess glucose is stored as glycogen (which can be converted back to glucose) and fat (which cannot be).[89]

Fat synthesis from carbohydrates (referred to as *de novo lipogenesis*) is especially important for two reasons. First, as mentioned above, the ability of the liver and muscles to store carbohydrates in the form of glycogen is generally slight; a maximum of only a few hundred grams of glycogen can be stored in the liver and the skeletal muscles.[90] Therefore, fat synthesis provides a means by which excess ingested carbohydrates can be stored for later use. Second, each gram of fat contains almost two-and-one-half times as many calories of energy as each gram of glycogen. Therefore, for a given weight gain, a person can store several times as much energy in the form of fat as in the form of carbohydrate, which is exceedingly important when an animal must be highly motile to survive.[91] The cost the body pays is that some energy is lost in the transformation. On average, storing excess energy from dietary carbohydrate in body fat requires an expenditure of 25 percent of ingested energy.[92]

As mentioned above, the body uses glucose freely (displacing fat in the fuel mix) when its carbohydrate stores are abundant.[93] On the other hand, when carbohydrates are in short supply, all the fat-sparing effects of carbohydrates are lost and actually reversed. This is achieved through several hormonal changes that take place to promote rapid fatty acid mobilization from adipose tissue and its utilization for energy in place of the absent carbohydrates. Among the most important of these is a marked decrease in pancreatic secretion of insulin caused by the absence of carbohydrates. In the absence of insulin, the enzyme *hormone-sensitive lipase* in the fat cells becomes strongly activated. This causes hydrolysis[94] of the stored triglycerides, releasing large quantities of fatty acids and glycerol into the circulating blood. (The fat in foods and in fat tissue is called neutral fat or *triglycerides*.) Consequently, the plasma concentration of free fatty acids begins to rise within minutes. Free fatty acids then become the main energy substrate used by essentially all tissues of the body besides the brain.[95]

In the meantime, when the hormonal system senses a drop in the blood glucose concentration level (as may occur between meals), the alpha cells of the pancreas respond by secreting the hormone glucagon into the blood.

Glucagon raises blood glucose by signaling the liver to dismantle its glycogen stores and release glucose into the blood, a process called *glycogenolysis*.[96] If a person does not eat carbohydrates to replenish the liver's limited glycogen stores, he or she will be quickly depleted. If this happens (e.g., due to dietary restriction or prolonged exercise), body proteins are dismantled to make glucose to fuel the brain's special cells. The conversion of protein to glucose, a process called *gluconeogenesis*, is the body's metabolic pathway to augment glucose availability and maintain plasma glucose levels in the face of depleted glycogen stores.[97] The price paid, however, is a temporary reduction in the body's protein stores, particularly muscle protein. In extreme conditions, this causes a significant reduction in the lean tissue mass and an accompanying solute load on the kidneys, which must increase their workload to excrete the nitrogen-containing byproducts of protein breakdown.[98]

Protein/Amino Acid Metabolism

Unlike glucose and free fatty acids (FFAs), whose primary task is to fuel biological work, amino acids provide the major building blocks for the synthesis of body tissue.[99] The importance of dietary protein to sustaining life was demonstrated in the early 1800s by the nutritional experiments of François Magendie, who found that adult dogs fed diets containing only flour (carbohydrate) or oil (fat) died, whereas dogs lived indefinitely on diets of eggs or cheese—that is, on diets containing protein.[100]

Twenty to 30 grams of the body's proteins are degraded daily and used to produce other body chemicals, a process referred to as the daily *obligatory loss of proteins*. Therefore, all cells must continue to form new proteins to take the place of those that are being destroyed. To prevent a net loss of protein from the body, a daily supply of protein is needed in the diet. Once the cells replenish their protein stores, any additional amino acids in the blood are used for energy (displacing fat in the fuel mix) or stored as fat.[101]

Even though amino acids are needed to do the work that only they can perform—building vital proteins—they will be sacrificed to provide energy and glucose if need be. When this occurs, the protein is not extracted from specialized storage depots; rather, protein in the body is available only as the working and structural components of the tissues. Thus, to supply the needed energy when supplies of glucose or FFAs are inadequate, the body, in effect, dismantles its own tissues and uses them for energy. While this may sound like a heavy price to pay, it is a lifesaving adaptation, for without energy, cells die, and without glucose, the brain and nervous system falter.

Exercise Metabolism

During physical activity, the muscles' requirements for fuel are met by mobilization of reserves within muscle cells and from extramuscular fuel depots. How much of which fuels they use depends on an interplay among the fuels available from the diet, the intensity and duration of the activity, and the degree to which the body is conditioned to perform that activity.[102]

During low- to moderate-intensity physical activity, the lungs and circulatory system have no trouble keeping up with the muscles' need for oxygen. The individual breathes easily, and the heart beats steadily—the activity is aerobic. With the availability of oxygen, the muscles can derive their energy from both glucose and fatty acids since both can be oxidized to provide energy.[103,104]

Early in a session of moderate exercise, approximately half the energy expended is derived from glucose and half from FFAs. To maintain the supply of glucose in circulation, liver glycogen is converted into glucose and released into the bloodstream. The muscles use both this glucose and their own private glycogen stores to fuel their work. But as exercise continues for an hour or more, two things happen. First, the liver's limited store of glycogen is depleted. As this happens, glucose output by the liver fails to keep pace with muscle use, and so blood glucose concentration drops.[105]

Second, the hormone *epinephrine* (more commonly known as adrenaline) is released by the adrenal medullae (a gland) as a result of sympathetic stimulation. In response, the fat cells begin to rapidly break down their stored triglycerides, liberating fatty acids into the blood. The FFA concentration in the blood can rise as much as eightfold, and the use of these fatty acids by the muscles for energy is correspondingly increased.[106] This causes a steady decline in the combustion of glucose for energy, with a concomitant increase in FFA utilization. Toward the end of prolonged exercise, FFA may supply as much as 80 percent of the total energy required.

Intense activity presents a different metabolic situation. Whenever a person exercises at a rate that exceeds the capacity of the heart and lungs to supply oxygen to the muscles, aerobic metabolism cannot meet energy needs. Instead, the muscles must draw more heavily on glucose, which is the only fuel that can be used anaerobically, that is, that can be metabolized to produce energy without the simultaneous use of oxygen.[107] A selective dependence on glucose metabolism during intense physical activity has an additional advantage: its rapidity of energy transfer compared to fats (about twice as fast).[108]

At the start of an intense exercise session, glucose energy is supplied from the glycogen stored in the active muscles. As exercise continues and the muscles' glycogen stores decline, blood glucose becomes the major source of glucose energy.[109] Muscle glycogen depletion causes muscle fatigue, which, in turn, greatly diminishes exercise capacity, making continued exertion more and more difficult. With the depletion of liver and muscle glycogen and a continued large use of blood glucose by active muscle, blood glucose can fall to hypoglycemic levels (less than 45 mg glucose per 100 mL blood). The symptoms of a reduction in blood glucose (hypoglycemia) include feelings of weakness, hunger, and dizziness. Endurance athletes commonly refer to this sensation of fatigue as "bonking" or "hitting the wall."[110]

Body Composition Subsystem

Clinically, body composition is viewed in terms of two compartments: fat-free mass (FFM) and fat mass (FM). Fat-free mass constitutes the skeleton, muscle, connective tissue, organ tissues, skin, bone, and water. Fat mass is composed of two types: (1) *essential fat*, which is the fat associated with bone marrow, the central nervous system, viscera (internal organs), and cell membranes; and (2) *storage fat*, which is fat stored in adipose tissue.[111] The percent distribution of the FFM and FM compartments can vary quite significantly among people as a result of physical and behavioral differences, but a major determinant is a person's gender. "A normal-weight man, for example, has from 12 to 20 percent body fat; a woman, because of her greater quantity of essential fat (in mammary glands and the pelvic region) 20 to 30 percent."[112]

"Overweight" and "over-fat" are not necessarily synonymous. This point is clearly illustrated in athletes, many of whom are muscular and exceed some average weight for their sex and height, but are otherwise quite lean in body composition.[113] Thus, one person may be very muscular and lean, with a substantial percentage of the weight coming from metabolically active muscle tissue, whereas another person of the same weight may be very sedentary and pudgy, with a large percentage of the weight accounted for by inert fat tissue. No problem for the first person, but perhaps a big problem for the second. For either individual, body composition would not be a static attribute to be measured once and then forgotten. It is very dynamic. For most people, changes in body composition do occur over time with changes in nutrition, physical activity, and aging.[114,115]

To capture body composition as a variable in a model to be used as a personal health support tool, one needs to be able to assess it. In practice, this is not difficult to do. Today, modern techniques make it possible to carry out a "bloodless dissection" to assess human body composition (see

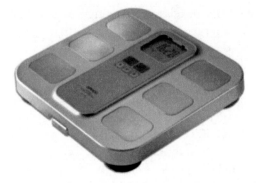

Figure 16.6 "Fat-analysis scales- intorduced more than fifteen year ago- are so main stream today, they can be found in most home, hardware, and department stores alongside traditional mechanical and digital scales.

They look like traditional bathroom scales, and, in one respect, act like them too: they weigh the body when they are stepped on. But placing your feet on a fat-analysis scale also puts them in contact with electrodes that send a small (and undetectable) electrical current through the body. The scale compares the current entering the body with the current leaving it and calculates body fat composition using bioelectric impedance analysis, or B.I.A., which is based on the difference in the ways that an electrical current is affected by muscle and fat. Because muscle and fat have differenct electrical properties, the current passing through the body will be affected more or less depending on the proportions of muscle and fat. By combining this information with data like height, weight, and age, and comparing it with data from the general population, a body-fat percentage can be determined." (*Source*: Karen Bannan, No Calipers of Cringing: A Discreet Gauge of Body Fat, *New York Times*, November 28, 2002)

Figure 16.6). Accurate but expensive laboratory methods include densitometry (also known as underwater weighing), magnetic resonance imaging (MRI), and radiography. Less accurate and less expensive field test methods include ultrasound, anthropometry, skinfold measurement, and electrical impedance.[116]

Fat Mass (FM)

Body fat generally has negative implications because so many people have more of it than they wish. But a certain level of fat is necessary for normal function. The important functions of fat in the body include (1) providing the body's largest store of potential energy, (2) serving as a cushion for the protection of vital organs, and (3) providing insulation from the thermal stress of a cold environment.[117]

After digestion and absorption, nutrient fat is used mainly to fill the triglyceride stores in adipose tissue.[118] The fat stored in these cells represents the body's main storehouse of energy-giving nutrient that can later be dissoluted and used for energy wherever in the body it is needed. Triglycerides are particularly suited for energy storage because they are, by far, the most concentrated storage form of high-energy fuel (9 kcal/g). This allows us to carry substantial amounts of "fuel" reserves without being too bulky to walk or run. For example, the potential energy stored in the fat molecules of an average 160-lb (lb) collage-aged male with the average 15 percent body fat (amounting to about 94,500 kcal) is enough to fuel a run from New York City to Madison, Wisconsin.[119] (By contrast, our relatively limited reserves of glucose—around 2,500 calories—is enough energy for only a 20-mile run!)

When stored fat is to be used elsewhere in the body, usually to provide energy, it must first be transported to the other tissues in the form of FFAs. This is achieved by hydrolysis of the triglycerides into fatty acids and glycerol. Both the fatty acids and the glycerol then enter the bloodstream and are transported to the active tissues where they can be oxidized to give energy.[120]

The most dramatic increase that occurs in fat utilization occurs during heavy exercise. As a result of sympathetic stimulation that occurs during exercise, the adrenal medullae releases epinephrine. This directly activates an enzyme called hormone-sensitive lipase that is present in abundance in the fat cells, which, in turn, causes the rapid breakdown of triglycerides and the mobilization of fatty acids.[121]

Conversely, when glucose is abundant in the blood (for example, after a high-carbohydrate meal), the body's reliance on FFA fuel decreases. The FFAs, thus, are removed from blood circulation, made into triglycerides, and stored back into the adipose tissue. (This process of making triglycerides from FFAs is called *esterification* because it involves attachment of a fatty acid to glycerol by means of an oxygen atom.)

At any point in time, the total amount of fat in a person's body reflects both the number and size of the fat cells. Although fat-cell size is generally tightly regulated between 0.3 and 0.9 µg, their number is more expandable. For comparison, an average person has between 20 billion and 30 billion fat cells, whereas a severely obese person may have as many as 160 billion.[122] Nutritional excess causes fat cells to expand in size as they fill with fat droplets until they reach their biological upper limit (about 1.0 µg of fat).[123] When the cells reach their maximum size, they divide, increasing the numbers of cells. Thus, obesity develops when a person's fat cells increase in number, in size, or, quite often, both.

Once fat cells are formed, however, the number seems to remain fixed even if weight is lost. That is, with fat loss, the size of fat cells dwindles but not their number.[124,125]

Fat-Free Mass (FFM)

Whenever significant amounts of body weight are lost, both FFM and FM participate in the weight loss process. Similarly, a significant weight gain almost always consists of a mixture of FFM and FM. "In a sense, these two body components are companions in that significant changes in body weight involve both, albeit in variable proportions."[126] The relative contribution of these two body components to weight gain/loss depends, in part, on a person's initial body composition.

Two decades ago, Forbes[127] in a series of body-composition studies of individuals of varying body-fat content, was able to derive an empirical relationship that is remarkably accurate in predicting the relative changes in body composition when body weight (W) is gained or lost. (His mathematical formulation is incorporated in the model; see endnote.[128]) A key finding that came out of Forbes's experiments was the revelation that the composition of the tissue lost (or gained) during weight reduction (increase) depends, all other things being equal, on the initial body fat content of the subject.

Specifically, during weight loss, obese people lose more weight as fat than do lean people, and the fatter a person is, the more will be the relative contribution of FM to total weight loss. Conversely, during weight gain, obese people add more weight as fat than do lean people, who add more lean tissue. (There are, of course, situations in which this is not the case. For example, exercising makes it possible to lose some weight without sacrificing FFM.[129])

A person's initial body composition, thus, affects the composition of tissue lost during energy deprivation, and this, in turn, will affect the trajectory and the magnitude of the weight ultimately lost. The relationship, in other words, is circular.

Taking Off

Ultimately, the purpose of computer modeling is to facilitate understanding of and make predictions about system behavior. For this, system modelers rely on running computer simulations.

In this respect, our microworld of human physiology and metabolism is very much analogous to the "flight simulators" that pilots use to learn about the complexities of flying an aircraft; instead of learning to pilot an aircraft, here the aim is to learn to "fly" our bodies. Using such a tool, the dieter, like the pilot, can have a laboratory in which to conduct thought experiments and test what-if scenarios before implementing a new intervention or treatment, and without any risk of ill effects. "In the virtual world you can find the maximum dive angle—'crashing' hurts no one, and you walk away every time, better prepared for a real emergency."[130]

To demonstrate the model's utility for learning and problem solving, in the next four chapters, we use the model to play out some familiar scenarios and, in the process, help debunk a number of misconceptions about human weight and energy regulation.

Experiment 1: Assessing Weight Loss—Reality Versus Fiction

17

Assessing weight loss of dieters is a good place to start to demonstrate both the utility of and need for personal computing tools in managing personal health.

The calculus that dieters most often use (and that we see in the popular press) for estimating weight loss goes something like this: 1 lb of body tissue contains, say, 2,800 kcal. (The specific value used varies to reflect assumptions about the composition of tissue loss. The most naive—and extreme—value used is 3,500 kcal, which assumes that tissue loss is composed *entirely* of fat tissue.) Thus, a negative energy balance of 400 kcal per day would shed 1 lb in a week and 52 lb in a year.

Such a simplistic model implies (and it is widely believed) that adherence to some diet regimen would cause body weight to drop in a straight-line (linear) fashion in direct proportion to the size of the caloric deficit, and that body weight would continue to drop as long as one adheres to the particular diet. The underlying assumptions of this model are that the energy cost of lost tissue is fixed (e.g., at 2,800 or 3,500 kcal/lb) and that the body's energy requirements remain steady, even as body size decreases.[131]

By now you know that this simplistic model is grossly inaccurate because both of these assumptions are wrong. Let's briefly recap. Whenever significant amounts of body weight are lost (or gained), both fat-free mass (FFM) and fat mass (FM) participate in the weight loss/gain process, albeit in variable proportions. At the start of a diet, the relative contributions of these two body components to weight loss depends, in part, on the person's initial body composition. As body composition changes with weight loss, the FM/FFM ratio also changes. For example, a dieter may start off losing 70 percent FM and 30 percent FFM for each pound of weight lost, but then progressively loses less fat as a percentage of the total as the diet progresses and his overall body fat content decreases. Because fat and lean tissue are not energetically equivalent, how many pounds of body weight a person sheds as

T.K.A. Hamid, *Thinking in Circles About Obesity*,
DOI 10.1007/978-0-387-09469-4_17, © Springer Science+Business Media, LLC 2009

a result of a particular caloric deficit will vary as the mix of lost tissue (FM and FFM) changes over the course of the diet.[132]

Also, losing weight as a result of caloric restriction affects *involuntary* energy expenditure—all three forms of it. The most obvious is the drop in the thermic effect of feeding (TEF), since eating less on a diet naturally lowers the metabolic cost of processing the smaller meals. But, because TEF accounts for only 10 percent of total daily energy expenditure, the drop is typically not very significant in absolute terms. If dieting persists long enough and the dieter loses an appreciable amount of weight, the thermic effect of activity (TEA), which is the energy expended for muscular work, can be expected to decline slightly, as well, because, as body weight drops, the energy cost of weight-bearing physical activity decreases.

The biggest impact on involuntary energy expenditure occurs as a result of the decline in resting energy expenditure (REE), which for most sedentary people constitutes the largest component of total energy expenditure. The REE drops for two reasons. The first is the loss of body mass (especially lean body tissue, which is the more metabolically active component). The second is the diet's induced negative energy balance. The body interprets caloric deficits as a deprivation "crisis" that needs to be contained. To compensate, the body decreases metabolic activity at the cellular level in order to conserve energy and restrain the rate of weight loss. Because resting energy expenditure accounts for a whopping 60 to 70 percent of total energy expenditure, the decline in REE is often significant enough to alter the body's energy balance and, in turn, the rate of weight loss.[133]

In reality, then, decreases in body weight are accompanied by continuous changes in the body's composition and in its total energy requirements. As a result, the rate of weight loss does not remain constant, but, instead, tends to decline with time, even if the prescribed diet is maintained. As a diet progresses, the changes in the body's composition and in its maintenance energy requirements constantly modify the subsequent pattern of weight loss until a new equilibrium body weight is reached, often at a level substantially higher than expected. "Weight [loss] can therefore be viewed not only as the consequence of an initial [negative] energy balance, but also as the mechanism by which energy balance is eventually restored."[134] Energy balance affects weight loss and, simultaneously, is itself controlled by it—the causation (as is depicted in Figure 17.1) is circular.

Understanding that weight loss in dieting can be significantly less than those off-the-shelf calculators suggest—and why—is certainly an important step forward, but it is not quite enough. It would be even more useful to quantify *by how much less*.

Unfortunately, that answer is not as clear. Incorporating the various homeostatic mechanisms of human weight and energy regulation into our

Simplistic View

Reality

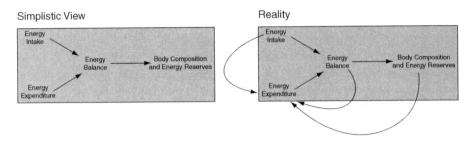

Figure 17.1 Our body work in circles not straight lines

model (as depicted in the *reality* panel of Figure 17.1), though it provides us with a more realistic picture of what goes on in our bodies, also seriously complicates the arithmetic. Not only do we need to contend with the continuously changing composition of the weight loss (FM versus FFM), we must also account for *dynamics*—the fact that as weight is (continuously) lost, the associated depression in energy expenditure effectively (and continuously) shrinks the size of the diet's energy deficit. Figuring out the net effect of these continuously interacting and changing variables is undoubtedly a messier computational task than the constant weight-for-energy conversion-type calculation. It is, however, the type of dynamic bookkeeping task that computers can easily (and reliably) perform.

The Experiment

Our objective in this first experiment is to ascertain the magnitude of the gap (the error) between the commonly used simplistic linear calculations of weight loss and the true curvilinear pattern we experience in reality.

For this and all our subsequent experiments, we will use as our experimental subject a hypothetical overweight sedentary man with an initial total weight of 220 lb (100 kg) and 25 percent body fat. Our subject maintains a relatively steady weight, albeit with occasional modest up/down fluctuations, on an average daily dietary input of 3,400 kcal. At 6 feet (1.83 meters) tall, his body mass index (BMI) is 30.[135]

In these types of experiments, the International System of Units is increasingly becoming the preferred standard for measuring energy and weight. In that system, food energy would be expressed in megajoules (MJ) rather than kilocalories (1 MJ is equivalent to 238 kcal) and body weight in kilograms (kg) rather than pounds (1 kg is equivalent to 2.2 lb). For our series of four experiments, I have chosen to adhere to these international units to align us with the rest of the literature. Thus, it will be easier to compare and cross-reference our results with those obtained elsewhere. An added bonus is that the numbers will be smaller, saving us some real estate on the many plots we will use. For ease of understanding, though, I will always provide the equivalent values in kilocalories and pounds.

Experiment 1 is conducted in two phases, as is customary in human underfeeding studies. During an initial maintenance phase (1 month in duration), our experimental subject is fed a balanced diet to maintain his weight and energy balance at normal levels. After the maintenance month, the subject's diet is then reduced during the underfeeding phase—in this case, a 5-month (22-week) period.

Specifically, during the experiment's underfeeding phase, the subject's daily caloric intake is cut to 12.25 MJ/day (2,926 kcal/day), which translates into a 2-MJ (478-kcal) daily caloric deficit for him. In terms of composition, the reduced diet is balanced, with 50 percent carbohydrate, 35 percent fat, and 15 percent protein. The size of the caloric deficit at 2 MJ/day is consistent with common treatment practice for overweight patients with BMIs in the typical range of 27 to 35. It provides a moderate caloric deficit that induces a manageable weight loss of about 1 to 2 kg/month (2 to 4 lb/month) for most patients.[136]

Experimental Results

Figure 17.2 depicts the drop in body weight during the 22-week underfeeding period. After 5 months of dieting, our experimental subject's weight has dropped from 100 to 92.35 kg (from 220 to 204 lb), a 7.65 percent decline.

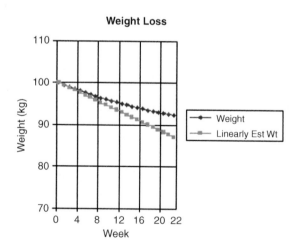

Figure 17.2 Drop in body weight—reality versus fiction

In the figure, this is compared to the decline in weight that would have been expected if we had used a typical linear type calculation, that is, with a constant weight-for-energy–type conversion. For that calculation, we assume our 100-kg man with 25 percent body fat loses approximately 70 percent FM and 30 percent FFM.[137] This means that 1 kg of lost body tissue would have an energy content of 24 MJ, equivalent to 2,606 kcal/lb.[138] Given the diet's 2 MJ/day caloric deficit, we would estimate a constant rate of weight loss of 0.083 kg/day, equivalent to 0.183 lb/day, and a total of 12.83 kg (28.3 lb) for the 22-week period. This estimate is depicted in Figure 17.2 as the linearly estimated weight (Est Wt) curve.

The simplistic linear estimate overestimates weight loss by 4.8 kg (or 10.6 lb)—that is 63 percent more than the subject's actual 7.75-kg loss over the 22-week period. Failure to account for the decline in maintenance energy expenditure that accompanies weight loss is largely responsible for this error.[139]

The shapes of the two curves are also different. While the rate of weight loss in the linear calculation is constant, dropping in a straight-line fashion, the actual rate with which weight is lost is not—it is curvilinear. Figure 17.3 highlights this phenomenon even more. It shows how the amount of weight lost every 1-month interval decreases overtime (shown here at the end of 4th, 12th, and 20th weeks).

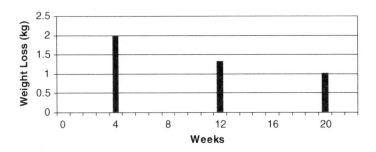

Figure 17.3 Weight lost in 1-month period

In this experiment's 5-month underfeeding intervention, weight continues to drop until the end, although at an ever-decreasing rate. If we were to extend the experiment long enough, body weight would eventually decrease to the point where this diet's energy intake level (12.25 MJ/day) would represent a new maintenance level for our experimental subject, and, at that point, weight loss would cease (with an asymptote at this new level).[140]

Looking Inside a White Box

> In order to understand the relations between . . . actions and outcomes, one needs a causal model of the process.
>
> —Einhorn and Hogarth[141]

Operational-type models (in which a system is modeled in terms of how it actually works, and system variables capture the cause-and-effect relationships among real system components) are useful not only in making predictions— *what* will happen—but also for making diagnostic inferences—*why* it happened. These models, thus, are like white boxes—devices, programs, or systems whose internal workings are well understood—in that we can trace the mechanisms underlying system behavior by appealing to the causal relations among the model's variables.[142] This is particularly valuable in the health domain because even after a correct prediction is made, it would be very useful (e.g., for prevention purposes) to be able to explain why the system (the body) behaves as it does. In contrast, models like the energy balance equation have very limited explanatory power. This point was, perhaps, best articulated by the famous physiologist Claude Bernard almost two centuries ago when he characterized the limitation of the balance technique as "trying to tell what happens inside a house by watching what goes in by the door and what comes out of the chimney."[143]

In the case of our dieting scenario, by allowing us to see clearly (and quantitatively) the multiple mechanisms by which the body accommodates energy imbalance, the model can help us understand *why* we tend to lose less weight than we expected to. Specifically, in the case of our 100-kg subject, the model allows us to quantify the role of adaptations in energy expenditure in curtailing weight loss.

Figure 17.4 shows how total energy expenditure declines for our experimental subject over the 5-month underfeeding period. Note that this decline is totally involuntary. In other words, it is not due to any changes in lifestyle, such as deciding to exercise more. As the figure shows, total energy expenditure drops by 1.28 MJ (a 9 percent drop) during the 22-week period. Interestingly, the decrease in the energy expenditure level was proportionately greater than the decrease in body weight: 9 percent versus 7.65 percent. As total energy expenditure drops, the size of the energy deficit effectively shrinks, which, in turn, slows down the rate at which weight is lost.

What accounts for this 9 percent drop in total energy expenditure? Figure 17.5 provides the answer. A small part of the total drop was due to a decline in the thermic effect of food (the metabolic cost of processing the smaller diet). The TEF drops by 0.2 MJ (equivalent to a 48-kcal drop).

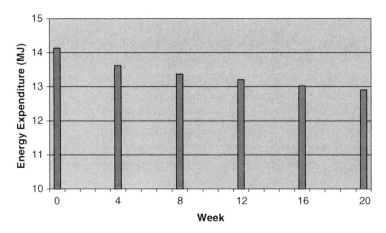

Figure 17.4 Total daily energy expenditure

A bigger part, but not much bigger, is the drop in energy expended in moving around (the TEA); it drops by 0.28 MJ (67 kcal). The bulk of the drop in energy expenditure, as clearly seen from Figure 17.5, is due to the diet-induced depression in REE. The REE drops from a pre-diet level of 9.1 MJ (2,174 kcal) to 8.3 MJ (1,983 kcal) at the conclusion of the 5-month underfeeding period. That accounts for 63 percent of the total drop in energy expenditure.

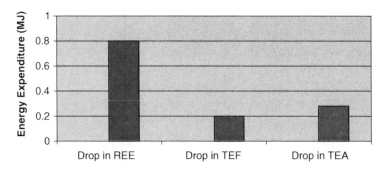

Figure 17.5 Drops in the three components of energy expenditure

These results underscore the fact that energy balance is not entirely under voluntary control. By quantifying the effects of these involuntary adaptations, our results clearly demonstrate that involuntary adaptations in energy expenditure have a significant impact on energy balance and are a big part of the reason why people tend to lose less weight than they expect to—much less. Ignoring these physiological adaptations may sell more diet books, but will inevitably lead to inaccurate predictions of treatment outcomes.

It Is Not Academic

Effective prediction of treatment outcomes is critically important in managing personal health. Treatment targets provide benchmarks that allow people to appraise how well the treatment is working. Without accurate predictions, the patient cannot know, in retrospect, how good the treatment was. Effective prediction is obviously key in setting attainable treatment goals. If one's goals are unrealistic, then failure is inevitable regardless of how hard one tries. In weight management, this matters a great deal because patients' expectations and the degree to which they are met (or not met) can affect their self-efficacy and long-term commitment.

Experiment 2: Going Ballistic—On a Diet

18

Chasing a Moving Target

In Chapter 17, the diet intervention mirrors the way most dieters try to lose weight—in a *ballistic* sort of way. They determine a caloric deficit to achieve a desired weight loss and then maintain it for the duration of the diet. More often than not, the result of such a ballistic approach is disappointment.

To understand what I mean by *ballistic behavior,* think of a cannonball (Figure 18.1).

> Once we have fired [the cannonball], we have no further influence over it. The course it takes is determined entirely by the laws of physics. This is not true of a rocket, which does not behave ballistically but is subject to the control of a pilot or the remote control of an operator who can alter its flight path if it appears that it is deviating from the designated path.[144]

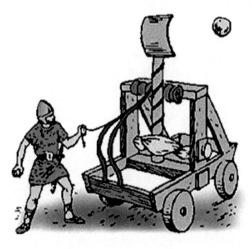

Figure 18.1 The catapult—precursor to the modern cannon—is also ballistic

T.K.A. Hamid, *Thinking in Circles About Obesity,*
DOI 10.1007/978-0-387-09469-4_18, © Springer Science+Business Media, LLC 2009

While a ballistic approach to planning or decision making may work well for some tasks (e.g., deciding on what graduate school to attend), when managing *adaptive* biological or social systems, it is often an inappropriate strategy. This certainly applies to managing human weight and energy regulation, as we saw in Chapter 17. The body's metabolism not only responds almost immediately to caloric deprivation, but the energy-sparing adaptations are substantial enough to cause the loss in body weight—over the few months of the typical diet—to diverge by a significant margin from the initial (ballistic) expectations.

Because our bodies are continuously changing and adapting over time, both autonomously as well as in reaction to our lifestyle choices, managing our bodies can be likened to pursuing a target that not only moves, but also reacts to the actions of the pursuer. This compounds the planning task for the dieter since "we have to know not only what [the] current status [of the system] is [and] what its status will be ... in the future, [but, in addition,] we have to know how certain actions we take will influence the situation."[145] This is why weight loss is rarely as straightforward an affair as dieters bargain for.

Clearly, then, in managing an adaptive system (such as our body), our plans for change should account for the fact that our very actions in a particular period can change outcomes in subsequent periods, which means that if our strategy is to be effective, we will need to continuously adjust our actions after launching them.

In this second experiment, we explore what it takes to do just that. Specifically, our goal is to devise an *adaptive* diet plan. Such a plan properly accounts for the body's energy-sparing adaptations in order to achieve a constant and steady weight loss throughout the diet and, ultimately, to reach the weight-loss target. Engineering such a steady (linear) decrease in body weight is, after all, the implicit goal for most dieters.

Obviously, as the body adapts downward in involuntary energy expenditure as weight is lost, in order to maintain a steady rate of weight loss the daily caloric deficit must progressively increase over time. But by how much?

The Experiment

Our aim in this experiment is to demonstrate how our simulation model can be used to create a diet plan that accounts for the body's energy-sparing adaptations and achieves a steady weight loss. Specifically, we aim to devise a plan to achieve a weight-loss rate of 0.5 kg (1.1 lb) per week over a 12-week period, achieving a total weight loss of 6 kg (13.2 lb) for our 100-kg experimental subject. I selected both the desired weekly weight loss and the experiment's 12-week duration to match the targets and durations of typical diet programs.[146]

Assessing how big the initial caloric deficit needs to be is not too hard. As was argued in Chapter 17, our experimental subject—100 kg, 25 percent fat, and on a 14.25 MJ/day maintenance diet—can be expected to lose body weight with a tissue composition that is approximately 70 percent FM and 30 percent FFM and with an energy content of 24 MJ per kilogram. Thus, to lose 0.5 kg per week, the subject initially needs to induce a weekly caloric deficit of 12 MJ, which translates into 1.71 MJ (410 kcal) per day. His daily caloric intake, therefore, must be reduced from 14.25 to 12.54 MJ (2,996 kcal).

This one calculation, however, serves only as an initial step in the diet plan. To properly account for the reciprocal and continuous diet–body interactions that will ensue (as the initial caloric deficit leads to weight loss, which leads to an involuntary drop in energy expenditure, which leads to shrinking the daily caloric deficit, and so on) requires an iterative process of calculation and recalculation to make a series of adjustments to caloric intake.

"No scientist or mathematician [let alone layman] can solve such a system mentally."[147] However, a dynamic type of bookkeeping task such as this is ideally suited for computers. Once relationships among the many system variables are established, codified, and fed into the computer, the computer can reliably and efficiently trace their implications over time.

The results for our experimental subject are shown in Figure 18.2, which depicts the dieting scheme needed to achieve the desired constant rate of weight loss, and in Figure 18.3, which plots the subject's resultant steady drop

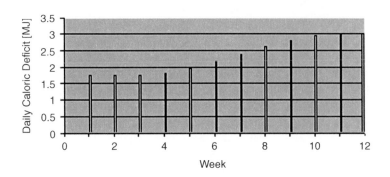

Figure 18.2 Daily caloric deficit to maintain steady loss in weight

in body weight for the 12-week period.

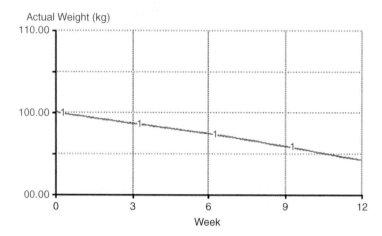

Figure 18.3 A plot of the subject's steady drop in body weight for the 12-week period

The results clearly demonstrate that in order to sustain a constant rate of weight loss, which is most people's expectation when starting a diet, the caloric deficit must progressively increase over time, not by a little, but by a significant amount. By the 12th week, the daily caloric deficit almost doubles from the original 1.71 MJ (410 kcal) to 3 MJ (717 kcal). That, it is safe to say, is substantially more than what most dieters bargain for.

A ballistic mindset, therefore, seriously underestimates the increasing hardship that dieters must endure to achieve the steady (linear) weight loss that they expected their diet plan to accomplish. It is no wonder, then, that most dieters never reach their goal.

It Is No Passive Tool

In many cases of self-regulation, failure often occurs not because of a lack of trying but because of *misregulation*.

> The essence of misregulation is that the person tries to engage in self-regulation and knows what effect is wanted, but the regulatory methods produce the wrong effect. ... [T]he majority of misregulation patterns involve some kind of deficiency in knowledge, especially self-knowledge.[148]

In experiment 1 (Chapter 17), not unlike many a dieting effort, failure to meet expectations occurs not because of a lack of effort, but because of an inaccurate prediction. The deficiency is not in self-control, but in self-knowledge concerning the body's involuntary adaptations to energy deficits and the inability to properly account for their impact.[149]

It may seem paradoxical, but persistence in such cases of misregulation *increases the costs* (e.g., time, effort, and money) that accompany the failure, rather than increasing one's chances of success.[150,151] One reason the duration in experiment 1 was extended to 5 months—somewhat longer than the average diet—was to demonstrate quantitatively how persistence only widens the gap between the initial ballistic target and the actual weight loss.

Like any other complex endeavor, effective self-regulation of body weight cannot be achieved solely through an act of will; it requires certain skills[152] and the proper tools. People need, first, to understand the multiloop nonlinear feedback system of human weight and energy regulation, and, second, to have cognitive tools to support their diagnostic and predictive abilities.

As we saw in experiments 1 and 2, because the problem is quantitative and dynamic, computer-based simulation tools are well suited for providing such support. In experiment 1, we used the computer microworld in a passive way, to show us the reality of the human weight and energy regulation system. In experiment 2, we used it in a proactive, prescrritive mode to gain insight into how to shape that reality.[153]

Experiment 3: Understanding Why 250 Pounds Does Not Equal 250 Pounds

19

Individual Differences: More than Meets the Eye

It is a common observation that people differ widely in responding to life's health challenges. Obesity is no exception. We know, for example, that some individuals are more susceptible than others to gaining weight, and that the ease of losing weight (and maintaining weight loss) can vary greatly between people, so that one person may succeed while another fails on the same diet.[154,155]

Invariably, when we think and talk about such individual differences, we tend to think and talk in terms of *static* attributes, such as differences in body composition and metabolism. And that is perfectly appropriate. But it is important to realize that differences among individuals have *dynamic* dimensions as well. For example, it turns out (as we will see in this chapter) that the ease of losing weight and keeping it off depends not only on how overweight a person is to begin with (a static attribute),[156] but also on the history or time course of weight gain (a dynamic one). Dynamic aspects, such as the time history of weight gain, are particularly interesting (and potentially problematic) in health management because they imply that, *for the same individual*, response to treatment can change over time.

One good way to distinguish between the static and the dynamic for any type of system is to perform this simple thought experiment: Imagine that you can instantly "freeze" all activity within the system, as though taking a snapshot. Static features are what you can count or measure in the frozen system. To return to an earlier example, if the system of interest is the bathtub, we would be able to measure the amount of water in the frozen bathtub (the value of the stock), but would not be able to tell whether the water level is rising or falling (the values of the rates of flow). If, on the other hand, our object of analysis is a person, at any (frozen) point in time, we would be able to measure the person's weight or fat content, but not whether the person has been gaining or losing weight of late.

T.K.A. Hamid, *Thinking in Circles About Obesity*,
DOI 10.1007/978-0-387-09469-4_19, © Springer Science+Business Media, LLC 2009

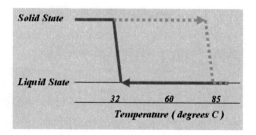

Figure 19.1 Hysteresis (agar). The notion that the condition of a person or a system at a particular point in time depends not only on contemporary conditions, but also on how that current state was reached is not unique to the human condition, it applies to many types of systems and phenomena (BK82, p. 38). In physical science, the phenomenon is known as *hysteresis*. A manifestation of hysteresis is that is easy to visualize is the transition in the state of substances for which melting temperature and freezing temperature are not identical. An example is *agar*. Agar melts at 85°C and solidifies from 35 to 40°C. This is to say that once agar is melted at 85 degrees, it retains a liquid state until cooled to 40 degrees Celsius. Therefore the temperatures of 40 to 85 degrees Celsius, agar can be either solid or liquid, depending on which state it was before. *Source*: wikipedia.org

Our objective in experiment 3 is to explore the role that individual differences—both static and dynamic—play in human weight and energy regulation and the implications for weight-loss treatment. To accomplish this, we play out a scenario of two friends with similar weights who decide to buddy-diet. At the start of the diet, they both weigh 250 lb (114 kg). Their body-weight histories, however, are quite different. One of the two has been chronically overweight at the 250-lb level, while the other just recently put on some extra weight (gaining as much as 15 percent). The question we seek to answer is this: What will the outcome be when the two friends go on the same diet? That is, how will two subjects with similar weights (but different histories of weight gain) respond to an identical dieting intervention?

The Experiment

This experiment is also conducted in two phases: phase 1, overfeeding, followed by phase 2, underfeeding (dieting). (Phase 1 is a slightly modified version of an experiment I conducted a few years ago[157] to demonstrate how well the simulation model replicates observed results of an overfeeding experiment conducted on human subjects.)

Phase 1: Overfeeding
For our experimental subject in phase 1, we re-enlist the 100-kg man from experiments 1 and 2. Let's call him subject A. Recall that he has a body

composition that is 25 percent fat, and he maintains his normal body weight of 100 kg on an average daily dietary input of 14.25 MJ.

For the experiment's initial overfeeding phase, subject A is fed a daily diet that is 50 percent above his maintenance level, that is, a diet providing a daily caloric intake of 21 MJ (5,016 kcal). The diet's composition, however, remains balanced, with 50 percent carbohydrate, 35 percent fat, and 15 percent protein. The overfeeding phase lasts for 3 months.

Figure 19.2 plots the trajectory of subject A's weight gain (the lower curve, designated as curve 1). After 3 months on the 21-MJ diet, subject A has gained 14 kg and now weighs 114 kg (250 lb).

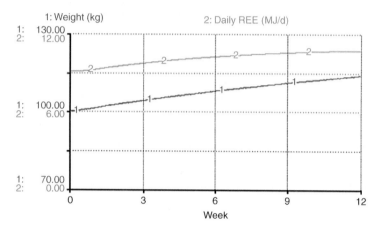

Figure 19.2 Changes in A's weight and REE over a 12-week period

As subject A gains weight, both fat-free mass (FFM) and fat mass (FM) participate in the weight gain. As I explained earlier, the relative contributions of these two body components to weight gain depend, in part, on a person's initial body composition. For subject A, whose initial body composition was 25 percent FM, approximately three quarters of the added weight will be FM.[158–160] As subject A accumulates relatively more FM with each extra kilogram of weight, his body's fat percent increases above the initial 25 percent. At the end of the 3-month period, at his new weight of 114 kg, his body's fat composition has grown to 31 percent.

Notice, in Figure 19.2, that I also show the changes in subject A's resting energy expenditure (REE) level (shown as curve 2). This is to underscore the important fact that change in body weight is not the only mechanism by which the body accommodates a positive energy balance. As body weight increases during overfeeding, the body's maintenance energy requirements also increase.[161] This is driven by two mechanisms. The primary one is the increase in lean body tissue (FFM). In addition, metabolic adaptations during food energy overconsumption also induce increases in REE.[162,163] With positive energy, in other words, REE per unit of metabolic mass also increases. (This is the converse of what happens during caloric deprivation, when metabolic activity decreases in order to conserve energy.) These energy-conserving or energy-dissipating mechanisms in REE protect against the full extent of overeating or undereating and serve to minimize the effects of short-term fluctuations in energy balance.

During the 3-month overfeeding phase, subject A's REE increases by as much as 18 percent, from a level of 9.1 MJ/day to 10.73 MJ/day. This significant elevation, as we shall soon see, has consequences.

Phase 2: Dieting

By the conclusion of phase 1, subject A's static specifications are identical to those of our second subject, B. The objective of phase 2 of the experiment is to assess the differences, if any, in how the two subjects, who now have identical weight (114 kg) and body composition (31 percent FM), respond to the same diet. Specifically, for the underfeeding phase of the experiment, both men are put on a balanced diet of 14 MJ (3,345 kcal). That level of caloric intake would be slightly below subject A's old maintenance level of 14.25 MJ/day (a value that no longer holds for him at his new higher weight) and substantially below subject B's maintenance daily diet of 15.35 MJ (3,667 kcal).[164]

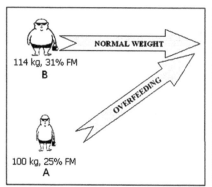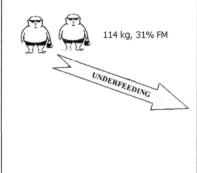

Figure 19.3 Left: phase 1. Right: phase 2

Note that the *static* similarities between our two subjects fail to capture an important difference between the two. For subject A, the extra 14 kg is a recent weight increase, while for the chronically overweight subject B, the 114-kg overweight condition constitutes his normal (steady-state) weight. This distinct difference in their weight timelines is enough to differentiate them metabolically, even though both have the same weight and body composition. Specifically, subject A's elevated REE level (as a result of his recent overfeeding behavior) pushes his REE rate (at 10.73 MJ/day) 10 percent higher than subject B's (at 9.71 MJ/day).[165]

The difference is significant because it appreciably alters the effective values of the caloric imbalance experienced by the two men. An elevation in the body's total energy expenditure (as in subject A's case) effectively expands the size of the diet's energy deficit and, in turn, accelerates the loss of body weight. After 3 months, subject A loses 5.68 kg (12.5 lb), dropping to a weight of 108.23 kg (238.6 lb). In comparison, subject B drops to 110.87 kg (244.4 lb), a loss of only 3.04 kg (8.9 lb). Not only is there a difference in the amount of weight lost on the same diet, but the difference is quite substantial, with one losing half as much as the other.

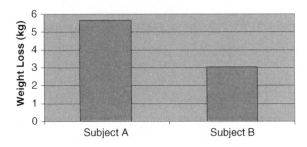

Figure 19.4 Weight loss after 3 months on a 14-MJ diet: two subjects

114 kg ≠ 114 kg ≠ 114 kg!

The above results underscore the important (albeit subtle) role that dynamic factors play in influencing the magnitude and time course of weight loss and, hence, the outcome of diets. But this is not to say that they are the only important factors. *Static* individual differences (i.e., those that we can measure if we take a snapshot) can also have a significant impact on treatment outcome. Body composition is one such factor.

Body composition is a particularly interesting attribute to investigate because there is so much variation among people. Indeed, one of the remarkable features of human adipose tissue is the extraordinary range of its capacity to store fat. At the low end, for example, a well-trained marathon runner may have a fat content as low as 8 percent, whereas the fat content of a morbidly obese person may be around 50 percent.[166] The fattest human on record, Jon Minnoch of Bainbridge Island, Washington, weighed an estimated 1400 lb at his death in 1983 and was about 80 percent fat.[167] The average middle-aged American lies somewhere between Minnoch and the marathon runner. "A normal-weight man [has] 12 to 20 percent body fat; a woman, because of her greater quantity of essential fat [in mammary glands and the pelvic region], 20 to 30 percent."[168]

To assess the impact of body composition, I reenacted phase 2 of experiment 3 with a third man, subject C. Like subject B, our new subject has been chronically overweight at 114 kg. But, unlike both subjects A and B, who have similar body composition, subject C's percent FM is substantially higher, at 40 percent.

When all three men are put on the same 14 MJ/day balanced diet for 3 months, the results are even more dramatic: subject C does not lose even a pound!

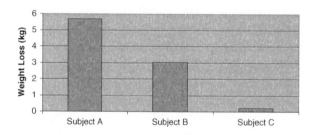

Figure 19.5 Weight loss after 3 months on a 14-MJ diet: two subjects

The reason is body composition. Subject C does not lose much weight because the 14-MJ diet is very close to his maintenance energy level, that is, the level of caloric intake that would maintain his weight at its current 114-kg level. Recall that a person's nominal resting energy expenditure (REE) is a function of metabolic mass rather than absolute body mass. Because lean body tissue is the principal metabolically active component of total body mass, the contribution of the FFM to the REE is much greater per kilogram than that of body fat. Subject C's relatively low maintenance energy level, compared to subject A's and subject B's, is a direct result of his body's composition, specifically, his lower percent of FFM.

One Size Does Not Fit All

Overall, the results of experiment 3 underscore the fact that obese patients are not a single homogeneous group, and that different people, however similar they may look superficially (e.g., weigh the same), need different goals and different regimens for weight loss.[169] Static individual differences such as body composition must be considered, as should an individual's weight and dieting histories.

The results, thus, highlight the need for adopting more personalized models in weight management. The traditional search for the one-size-fits-all model (such as the energy balance equation) that is applied en masse is a bankrupt strategy that we need to abandon.

Mass customization, as this concept is known, is not unique to health and in fact is taking root in a wide range of industries. Rather than continuing to mass produce for the increasingly elusive average customer, many businesses are already using state-of-the-art information technology to build and deliver products and services designed to fit the precise specifications of each individual customer. As consumers, we expect that in everything else we do, and now it needs to happen in health.

Experiment 4: Trading Treatment Options—Diet Versus Exercise

20

Energy Is Not a Single Currency

More than a century ago, William James articulated, most romantically, how human behavior is purposeful, and (indefinitely) adaptive:

> Romeo wants Juliet as filings want a magnet, and if no obstacles intervene he moves toward her by as straight a line as [the filings move to the magnet]. But Romeo and Juliet, if a wall be built between them, do not remain idiotically pressing their faces against its opposite sides like the magnet and the filings with the (obstructing) card. Romeo soon finds a circuitous way, by scaling the wall or otherwise, of touching Juliet's lips directly. With the filings the path is fixed; whether it reaches the end depends on accidents. With the lover it is the end which is fixed, the path may be modified indefinitely.[170]

In personal health regulation, as in romance and most other endeavors, people have a spectrum of options they can choose from to achieve their goals, which is a good thing, for it allows us to both choose interventions that best suit our needs and change treatment paths when our needs or life's circumstances change. However, as the previous chapters have explained, selecting the option that works better for us requires knowledge and skill, as well as appropriate decision-support tools.

"Appropriate" is a key qualifier here. A serious limitation of the energy balance equation is that it does not provide the patient—the decision-maker—with enough discriminatory power to compare weight-loss treatment options. The energy balance equation suggests (and it is widely held) that a decline in body weight is determined solely by the size of the energy deficit, regardless of how that deficit is induced. Energy, in other words, is treated as though it were a single currency. In reality, how an energy deficit is created does matter. A daily energy deficit of 500 kcal can be induced, for example, by eliminating soft drinks (two cans) and dessert (cheese cake, for example) from the daily diet or by jogging 4 miles in an hour. Statically, both

T.K.A. Hamid, *Thinking in Circles About Obesity*, DOI 10.1007/978-0-387-09469-4_20, © Springer Science+Business Media, LLC 2009 strategies would create the same caloric deficit. Over time, however, the patterns of weight change that result from these two isocaloric strategies could be quite different.

Specifically, the two strategies have different impacts on the *composition* of weight loss—fat mass versus fat-free mass—which, in turn, affects the body's involuntary adaptations to its maintenance energy requirements and, ultimately, energy balance. When exercise is used to create a desired energy deficit, it tends to protect against the loss in fat-free mass (FFM).[171,172] (This favorable impact on body composition occurs partly because of increases in muscle size through increased protein synthesis during exercise.) By conserving and even increasing fat-free body mass (the principal metabolically active component of total body mass), exercise partially blunts the diet-induced depression in metabolic energy expenditure that typically accompanies diet-based weight loss.[173,174]

The bottom-line question, however, is: What impact do such differences have on weight loss? Are the differences only in the quality (i.e., composition) of weight loss or in quantity as well?

Our objective in this fourth experiment is to explore these highly pertinent questions. Specifically, I use the model as a vehicle to compare (and quantify) the impacts of food restriction and exercise on the amount and composition of weight loss under a number of different scenarios. In terms of William James's characterization above, we will use the simulation to support Romeo's decision-making process—not necessarily to reach Juliet, but to compare and evaluate the possible routes to her.

To address the above issues, this experiment contains three steps. In all three, the experimental subject is, as before, our overweight sedentary man with an initial weight of 100 kg and 25 percent body fat living on a maintenance daily diet of 14.25 MJ.

Diet Versus Exercise: Do 500 kcal = 500 kcal?

In step one, we tackle the basic apples-versus-oranges question, comparing the amount of weight loss on comparable diet and exercise regimens. Specifically, we compare changes to our subject's body weight and composition after undertaking two separate calorically equivalent treatments. In the first treatment, the subject consumes a 12.25-MJ/day diet for 12 weeks, inducing a daily caloric deficit of 2 MJ (478 kcal). The result of that diet is then compared to his weight loss if, instead, he participates in an exercise program that induces an identical daily caloric deficit of 2 MJ.

To accommodate the fact that overweight sedentary individuals are usually physically unfit, a limitation that undoubtedly hampers their capacity to exercise, the daily 2-MJ (478-kcal) exercise regimen is stretched over a 2-hour period. This allows for a modest intensity level of 1 MJ/hour (which, for example, could be achieved by leisurely walking). (Note that while the daily 2-hour session admittedly exceeds the U.S. government's recommended minimum guidelines for physical activity—60 minutes of moderate to vigorous exercise—it is right in line with levels recommended by the American College of Sports Medicine, as well as exercise levels reported by successful weight "losers" in practice.[175])

A comparison of the changes in body weight over the 12-week period for both the dieting and exercising interventions is shown in Figure 20.1. The first thing to notice is that at the end of the 3-month period, the difference in weight loss from dieting versus exercising is quite small—almost negligible, in fact. After 12 weeks of dieting, body weight drops by 4.9 kg (10.8 lb) to 95.1 kg, while a calorically equivalent daily exercise regimen causes weight to drop a comparable 4.7 kg (10.3 lb).

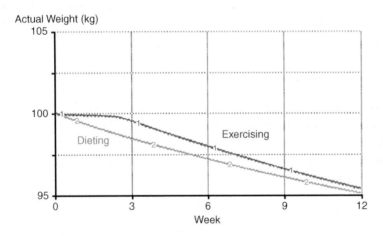

Figure 20.1 Comparing weight loss from diet- and exercise-interventions

The weight-loss trajectories of the two interventions are quite different, however. With dieting, the subject starts losing weight almost immediately, while in the exercise scenario, body weight drops very little in the early phases. This flat start in the exercise treatment can be attributed to the increase in muscle size that our sedentary overweight subject enjoys as he embarks on the 2-MJ/day exercise regimen. The initial buildup of the subject's muscle mass (an addition to his FFM compartment) counterbalances what his body loses in fat mass (FM), causing a minimal net change in total body weight. This exercise effect, however, is transitory, because the gains in muscle mass a person makes when embarking on a new exercise regimen depend on the relative intensity of the exercise overload—relative, that is, to the subject's fitness level. Thus, as exercise continues at the same intensity level, the subject's fitness invariably improves, which causes this adaptive physiological response (the gain in muscle mass) to eventually level off.

During the first few weeks of the exercise regimen, the body relies on its fat fuel reserves to compensate for both the daily caloric deficit and the initial buildup of muscle mass. While this obviously induces larger losses in FM (in comparison to dieting), it also (perhaps less obviously) precipitates less of a net loss in *total* body mass. Since FM has a much larger energy density than FFM, smaller losses in FM tissue are used to fuel larger gains in FFM. Eventually, though, as the buildup of muscle mass levels off, total weight starts to decline under the cumulative burden of the sustained 2-MJ daily energy deficit.

The distinctively different trajectories of weight loss from dieting versus exercising have important implications on how people interpret (or misinterpret) treatment outcomes. Consider this: If the duration of the weight-loss treatment were shorter, say 4 weeks instead of 12, our subject may conclude, as many probably do, that exercise is an ineffective weight-loss strategy. But that would be both premature and wrong.

In the case of exercise, not only does size (of the caloric deficit) matter, but so does duration. Indeed, failure to properly account for this "delay effect" may help explain why published research results on the efficacy of exercise as a treatment option have been rather mixed. On the one hand, numerous studies have found that increased levels of physical activity are as effective as dieting (with some studies showing exercise to be more effective than dieting for long-term weight control). On the other hand, there is an equally abundant set of studies reporting just the opposite—that exercise has less (or significantly less) effect on weight loss than food restriction does.[176,177] Such mixed findings, not surprisingly, have caused confusion in the public and have led some investigators to discount the importance of exercise in the treatment of obesity.[178]

A few years ago, an American College of Sports Medicine scientific panel was assembled to review the issue. The panel concluded that the inconsistent results can be attributed, in part, to the complexity and expense of performing longer-term studies, thus limiting many experiments to relatively short durations.[179] Because significant weight changes from exercise occur after a delay, as the above results suggest, short-duration studies do not allow for the full estimation of the potential effects of exercise on weight loss.[180]

Difference in the time course of weight loss is not the only difference between the exercise and diet options. The two treatment strategies also have different impacts on the composition of lost tissue. Figure 20.2 shows a comparison between the changes in body weight and composition (FFM, FM, and percent body fat) in dieting versus exercising. The key finding here is that, while the difference in *total* weight loss is not significant, the difference in the composition of the weight that was lost is. As the figure shows, in the exercise treatment (the dashed bars), FM drops by 4.2 kg, accounting for almost 90 percent of the total loss in weight, while FFM drops by only 0.5 kg. This contrasts with the diet treatment, in which 70 percent of the weight loss was FM and 30 percent was FFM (FM drops by 3.4 kg, while the FFM loss was 1.5 kg).[181]

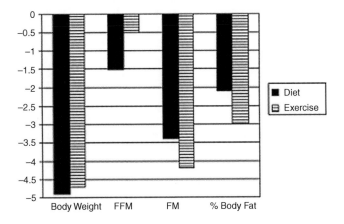

Figure 20.2 Diet versus exercise

Overall, then, we can draw two conclusions from these results. First, given enough time, exercise—even at a moderate level—induces a comparable loss in body weight to food restriction. This should provide a more palatable option to people who would prefer exercise as a strategy to help maintain weight loss while allowing the consumption of enough calories to supply the body with adequate nutrients and energy.

Second, and perhaps more important, the experiment quantifies the significant degree to which exercise protects against the loss of FFM, as well as the favorable impact it has on changes in the percent of body fat. This is potentially quite significant since maximizing fat loss yields the greatest reduction in coronary heart disease risk.[182] In addition, the conservation of muscle mass during exercise-induced weight loss maintains a person's ability to perform daily tasks requiring strength or muscular staying power.

Trading Exercise Intensity for Exercising Time

Because, for many people, the most costly aspect of exercise is the time spent doing it, there is an understandable inclination to aim at exercising at the highest possible level of intensity in order to induce the largest possible energy deficit per exercise session. The objective of part 2 of the experiment is to assess the viability of such a strategy, that is, trading exercise intensity for exercise time.

We will assume that the subject's time constraints allow him to exercise only 3 days a week, say, Mondays, Wednesdays, and Fridays. The subject's decision task, then, is to replace the current regimen—exercising daily for 2 hours at the light rate of 1 MJ/hour—with a new exercise schedule that allows him to achieve the same weekly energy deficit of 14 MJ (3,345 kcal) in just three weekly sessions. A reasonable strategy to accomplish that would be to double the exercise intensity level from 1 MJ/hour to 2 MJ/hour and to extend the duration to from 2 hours to 2 hours and 20 minutes on each of the three exercise days. (Cycling would be an exercise option that would fit that bill.)

The loss in body weight and change in percent of body fat attained after exercising for 12 weeks at this new high-intensity level are compared in Figure 20.3 to the results obtained earlier. The outcome is somewhat surprising. While exercising at the lower intensity level caused total body weight to drop by 4.7 kg, as a combination of a

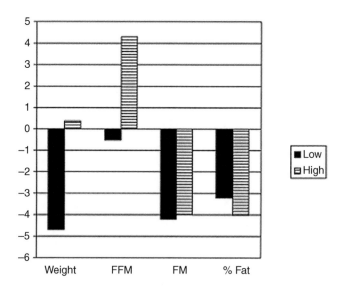

Figure 20.3 Low versus high exercise intensity

modest 0.5-kg drop in FFM and a more substantial 4.2-kg drop in FM, we now see that no weight is lost when exercise intensity doubles to 2 MJ/hour (in fact, total body weight increases slightly from 100 to 100.37 kg).

Two factors contribute to this counterintuitive result. First, the increased level of exercise intensity induces a rather significant 4.3-kg (9.5-lb) increase in FFM (mainly muscle mass), a value that exceeds the simultaneous 4-kg (8.8-lb) loss in FM. The differential induces a net increase in total body weight (albeit only a minimal 0.37 kg), but also produces a very favorable 4 percent drop in our subject's body-fat percentage, lowering it from 25 percent to 21 percent.

The second factor behind the unexpected change in body weight at the higher intensity level is somewhat more subtle. When put on the high-intensity exercise regimen, our sedentary obese subject ends up expending less cumulative exercise energy per exercise session (and for the entire treatment period). The cause of this unintended outcome lies in the body's selective dependence on different energy sources to fuel differing levels of exercise activity and a person's capacity to meet the body's specific energy needs.

As explained in Chapter 10, during intense exercise, the muscles draw more heavily on glucose, primarily in the form of muscle glycogen, for energy.[183] How much exercise can be sustained by any particular person's glycogen reserves would depend on the intensity and duration of effort, as well as on the fitness and nutritional status of the exerciser. An overweight sedentary person, such as our 100-kg subject, embarking on a new exercise regimen not only starts with more limited glycogen stores but also tends to use his reserves at a faster rate than does a trained athlete. (In athletes, muscle cells that repeatedly deplete their glycogen through exercise adapt to store greater amounts of glycogen to support that work. Conditioned muscles also rely less on glycogen and more on fat for energy, so glycogen utilization occurs more slowly in trained than in untrained individuals at a given work intensity.[184]) Generally, glycogen depletion occurs within 1 to 2 hours from the onset of intense activity. As glycogen is depleted, the muscles become fatigued. This, in turn, greatly diminishes the capacity to continue exercising at a high intensity level. This dynamic is what causes our subject's energy expenditure level to drop at the higher intensity level in the experiment; the high-intensity exercise regimen collides head on with his biological limitations, and biology wins the battle.[185]

The weekly energy expenditure totals for the two intensity levels are plotted in Figure 20.4. At the low-intensity level, the subject's actual energy expenditure matches the weekly target level of 14 MJ. In the high-intensity scenario, by contrast, he expends only 11 MJ, or 78 percent of the weekly target. This suggests that, for an overweight sedentary subject, a high -intensity level exercise regimen can prove counterproductive as a weight-reducing strategy.

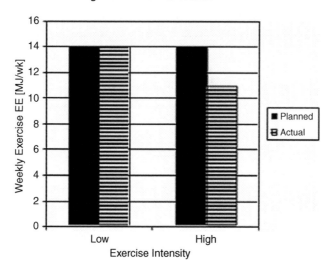

Figure 20.4 Actual versus planned weekly exercise energy expenditures at low and high intensity levels

For our sedentary subject, failure in the high-intensity exercise scenario occurs not because of a lack of effort, but because of pursuing what is for him a futile endeavor. This echoes a lesson we learned earlier: the importance of setting realistic goals. Trying harder, no matter how much harder, to attain unrealistic goals, whether for exercising or dieting, is often a recipe for failure and disappointment.

Manipulating Diet Composition

Because the body's glycogen stores are relatively limited, the composition of one's diet can have a great effect on the recovery time from glycogen depletion.[186] For example, people on a high-fat/high-protein diet or on no food at all show extremely little recovery, even after as long as 5 days.[187] However, with a high-carbohydrate diet, full recovery typically occurs in about 2 days. This suggests that manipulating the carbohydrate content of the daily diet may help enhance a person's capacity to sustain a high-intensity exercise regimen. Professional athletes have long known this and have learned to load up on carbohydrates to fill up their muscle and liver carbohydrate stores before a taxing event.[188]

The third, and last, part of the experiment assesses the degree to which this approach applies to an overweight nonathlete. To do this part, I changed the composition of the subject's daily diet from the (relatively) balanced 50 percent carbohydrate, 35 percent fat, and 15 percent protein, to a high-carbohydrate diet composed of 75 percent carbohydrate, 10 percent fat, and 15 percent protein, and reenacted the high-intensity exercise scenario.

The adjusted diet does indeed prove effective for our sedentary subject. As with professional athletes, the higher dose of carbohydrates in the diet replenishes our subject's glycogen stores sufficiently to sustain his capacity to complete the 2-hour high-intensity exercise session and to recover fast enough to do it three times a week. This boosts his exercise energy expenditure totals over the entirety of the 12 weeks to the planned weekly level of 14 MJ, and, in turn, it induces the hoped-for drop in total body weight. (Comparable results were reported by Brown,[189] where a switch to a high-carbohydrate diet allowed runners to extend their exercise duration from 1½ hours to up to 4 hours.) Total body weight drops by 5.54 kg, compared to the minimal gain in total body weight (of 0.37 kg) in the balanced-diet case (Figure 20.5).[190]

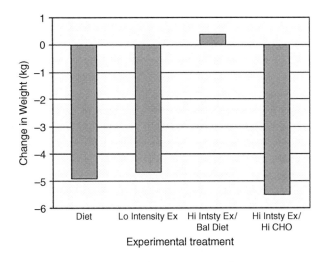

Figure 20.5 Change in body weight in the four experimental treatments

These results underscore the significant interaction effects between diet composition and physical activity and emphasize the critical role that diet composition can have in exercise-based treatment interventions. On the flip side, the results allude to the potential risks in the many quick-loss diets that promote low—sometimes seriously low—carbohydrate intake levels. A diet deficient in carbohydrates results in dehydration as muscle and liver glycogen stores are depleted, thus diminishing exercise capacity and putting serious limits on physical activity as a way to expend calories.

More generally, the results of experiment 4 underscore the value of an integrative perspective on obesity treatment. The tendency for most people (and many health care professionals) is still to emphasize one aspect or treatment strategy, such as focusing too narrowly on the effects of diet versus exercise, or on one type of diet or one type of physical activity.[191] As we know, the human body is truly a marvel of system integration, a conglomerate of interrelated and interdependent control processes and subsystems, and where changes in one subsystem affect and are affected by others. The significant interaction we observed here between diet composition and physical activity is a good example of that. It clearly demonstrates the need to devise interventions that capitalize on, rather than ignore, the interactions between the body's multiple subsystems.

Don't Trade . . . Integrate

Perhaps the most convincing data on the value of integrating physical activity and dieting, instead of choosing one over the other, to achieve and maintain weight loss come from the "successful losers" of the National Weight Control Registry:

> Almost 100 percent of them use a combination of diet and exercise to lose weight, and about 95 percent use a combination of diet and exercise to maintain their loss. . . . How much exercise? Far more than the recommended minimum. On average they expend 2,800 kcal (12 MJ) a week through physical activity, the equivalent of walking four miles a day every day, although most use a mixture of different activities, including walking, aerobic dancing, tennis, cycling, running and lifting weights.[192]

Granted, thermodynamic principles make it difficult for humans to lose weight quickly by exercise alone; an hour-long jog may burn 300 calories, the same 300 calories that are in a single candy bar.[193,194] This surprises and discourages many people, but it should not.

Although in comparison with weight loss from dieting, weight loss from exercise takes longer, "regular exercise appears to be one of the major factors determining the long-term success of weight loss programs."[195] That may be due to its effect in conserving and even increasing fat-free body mass.

Apart from its effects on body weight and composition, regular exercise has many other potential benefits for overweight people. Indeed, a remarkable and consistent finding "is that heavy people who are fit have lower risk [for major killers like heart disease] than thin people who are unfit."[196]

PhDs for the Masses?
(That's *Personal Health Decision support*)

My objective in Part IV is twofold: first, to make the case that we cannot and should not rely either on intuition or on simplistic models to manage a system as complex and important as our bodies; and second, to demonstrate the feasibility and potential utility of a new generation of dynamic computer-based tools for personal weight and energy regulation.

Already, the explosive proliferation of microcomputers is empowering people in all sorts of ways. As computers continue to become faster, cheaper, and more widely available, even more of our decisions and everyday choices will involve the results of computer models. Many, myself included, expect that in the next few years, computer-based tools will prove to be a critical technology for personal health care.[197]

The potential value of such tools is twofold. First, they serve as tools for learning and understanding. Recall our flight simulator example: Pilots use simulations to understand and learn how to handle their complex flying machines. A "flight simulator" of human physiology can be just as useful for understanding and learning to "fly" our bodies (without crashing!). As a metaphor for learning and problem solving, the flight simulator has several virtues. For example, it makes perfectly controlled experimentation possible. As we saw in the experiments described in the previous chapters, in the simulated system, as opposed to real systems, the effect of changing one factor can be observed while all other factors are held unchanged. In real life, by contrast, many variables change simultaneously, confounding the inter-pretation of treatment results.[198] As we will see in Part V, using such tools to help people better understand what works for them and what does not—and why—can be very useful in prevention efforts.

In addition to being laboratories for learning, computer-based tools also can serve as personal health decision support systems, allowing people to assess treatment options and predict treatment outcome. As already argued, with a complex dynamic system such as human physiology, having perfect understanding of system structure is not enough. The ability to infer system

T.K.A. Hamid, *Thinking in Circles About Obesity*,
DOI 10.1007/978-0-387-09469-4_21, © Springer Science+Business Media, LLC 2009

behavior is essential if decision makers are to know the consequences of their actions and devise appropriate weight-control strategies, such as dieting versus exercising versus a combination of both. As we saw in Chapter 14 (the bathtub exercise), accurately determining the dynamic behavior of a complex system is tough, even with perfect knowledge of the system's structure. The beauty of computer models is that they can reliably and efficiently trace, over time, the implications of a messy maze of interactions.

In performing its twin roles—learning and decision support—computer technology offers an added attraction: facilitating mass customization. As we saw in the experimentation chapters, the quantity and quality of weight loss, whether by dieting or exercising, depends on a host of personal factors that can vary significantly among individuals (e.g., initial body weight and composition, past history of weight gain, stamina, and fitness). Because computer-based tools can be highly personalized, by tailoring model parameters to account for such individual differences, they can provide specific, tailored solutions to patients' individual problems.[199] This is particularly important in obesity treatment. Given the sheer number of obese individuals who need help, there simply are not enough health professionals available to provide personalized long-term treatment.[200]

To me, this suggests a pressing need for a bold new public policy initiative to "confer" PhDs on the masses—*personal health decision support* tools that ordinary people can use to manage their health and well-being.

Thanks to the great advances in systems sciences, medicine, and computer technology over the last few decades, we are in a position to do this and to do it right away. The model presented in the previous few chapters is one concrete example of such technology in action. As an academic and a researcher, my goal was not to demonstrate an off-the-shelf product with all the bells and whistles, but rather to demonstrate both the feasibility and value of such tools. My hope is that the concept proves enticing enough for consumers to demand these tools and for businesses to build them.

Using today's affordable desktop computers, we can now construct and run computer models of complex systems and do it at an affordable price. With increasingly user-friendly software, ordinary people, for the first time in history, can access and make effective use of such models. Using these tools, dieters or patients, like engineers and pilots, can have a laboratory in which to conduct thought experiments to test myriad sorts of what-if scenarios before attempting a weight-loss strategy. They can learn quickly and at low cost the answers that would seldom be obtainable by raw intuition.

To paraphrase Dr. David Eddy, developer of an up-and-running PHDS tool called Archimedes, "Our mission is that in 10 years, no one will make an important decision in health care without first asking: 'What does [my PHDs] say?'"[201]

Notes

1. Hogarth, R.M. (1981). Beyond discrete biases: functional and dysfunctional aspects of judgmental heuristics. *Psychological Bulletin,* 90, 197–217.
2. Plous, S. (1993). *The Psychology of Judgment and Decision Making.* New York: McGraw-Hill.
3. Bandura, A. (1997). *Self-Efficacy: The Exercise of Control.* New York: W.H. Freeman.
4. Laszlo, E. (1996). *The Systems View of the World: A Holistic Vision for Our Time (Advances in Systems Theory, Complexity, and the Human Sciences).* Cresskill, NJ: Hampton Press.
5. Brownell, K.D. (1991). Personal responsibility and control over our bodies: when expectation exceeds reality. *Health Psychology,* 10, 303–310.
6. Foster, G.D., Wadden, T.A., Vogt, R.A., and Brewer, G. (1997). What is a reasonable weight loss? Patients' expectations and evaluations of obesity treatment outcomes. *Journal of Consulting and Clinical Psychology.* 65, 79–85.
7. Forrester, J.W. (1996). System Dynamics and K-12 Teachers: A lecture at the University of Virginia School of Education. System Dynamics Group report number D-4665–4, Sloan School of Management, MIT. Also System Dynamics Group report number D-4224–1, Sloan School of Management, MIT.
8. Sterman, J.D. (2000). *Business Dynamics: Systems Thinking and Modeling for a Complex World.* Boston: Irwin McGraw-Hill.
9. Richardson, G.P. and Pugh, G.L. (1981). *Introduction to System Dynamics Modeling and Dynamo.* Cambridge, MA: MIT Press.
10. Simon, H.A. (1970). *Sciences of the Artificial.* Cambridge, MA: MIT Press.
11. Sterman, J.D. (2000). *Business Dynamics: Systems Thinking and Modeling for a Complex World.* Boston: Irwin McGraw-Hill.

12. Booth Sweeney, L. and Sterman, J. D. (2000). Bathtub dynamics: initial results of a systems thinking inventory. *System Dynamics Review,* 16, 249–294.

13. *Ibid.*

14. *Ibid.*

15. Kainz, D. and Ossimitz, G. (2002). Can students learn stock–flow thinking? An empirical investigation. In: *Proceedings of the 2002 International System Dynamics Conference.* Albany, NY: System Dynamics Society.

16. Ossimitz, G. (2002). Stock-flow-thinking and reading stock-flow-related graphs: an empirical investigation in dynamic thinking abilities. Proceedings of the 2002 International System Dynamics Conference. Albany, NY: System Dynamics Society.

17. Sterman, J.D. and Booth Sweeney, L. (2002). Cloudy skies: assessing public understanding of global warming. *System Dynamics Review,* 18, 207–240.

18. Sterman, J. D. (2002) All models are wrong: reflections on becoming a systems scientist. *System Dynamics Review,* 18, 501–531.

19. Sterman, J.D. (2006). Learning from evidence in a complex world. *American Journal of Public Health,* 96(3), 505–514.

20. Sterman, J.D. and Booth Sweeney, L. (2002). Cloudy skies: assessing public understanding of global warming. *System Dynamics Review,* 18, 207–240.

21. *Ibid.*

22. Sterman, J. D. (2002) All models are wrong: reflections on becoming a systems scientist. *System Dynamics Review,* 18, 501–531.

23. Brownell, K.D. and Horgen, K.B. (2004). *Food Fight.* Chicago: Contemporary Books.

24. Yanovski, J.A. et al. (2000). A prospective study of holiday weight gain. *New England Journal of Medicine,* 342(12), 861–867.

25. Parker-Pope, T. (2005, December 13). The skinny on holiday weight gain: it's not as bad as you think, but it sticks. *Wall Street Journal,* p. D1.

26. Forrester, J.W. (1996). System Dynamics and K-12 Teachers: A lecture at the University of Virginia School of Education. System Dynamics Group report number D-4665–4, Sloan School of Management, MIT. Also System Dynamics Group report number D-4224–1, Sloan School of Management, MIT.

27. Sterman, J. D. (2002) All models are wrong: reflections on becoming a systems scientist. *System Dynamics Review,* 18, 501–531.

28. *Ibid.*

29. Forrester, J.W. (1979). System Dynamics: Future Opportunities. Paper D-3108–1, The System Dynamics Group, Sloan School of Management, Massachusetts Institute of Technology.

30. Sterman, J. D. (2002) All models are wrong: reflections on becoming a systems scientist. *System Dynamics Review,* 18, 501–531.
31. Booth Sweeney, L. and Sterman, J. D. (2000). Bathtub dynamics: initial results of a systems thinking inventory. *System Dynamics Review,* 16, 249–294.
32. Sterman, J. D. (2002) All models are wrong: reflections on becoming a systems scientist. *System Dynamics Review,* 18, 501–531.
33. Mackinnon, A. J. and Wearing, A. J. (1980) Complexity and decision making. *Behavioral Science,* 25, 285–296.
34. Dörner, D. (1989). *The Logic of Failure.* New York: Metropolitan Books.
35. Wegner, D.M. (2002). *The Illusions of Conscious Will.* Cambridge, MA: Bradford Books.
36. Sterman, J. D. (2002) All models are wrong: reflections on becoming a systems scientist. *System Dynamics Review,* 18, 501–531.
37. Simon, H.A. (1970). *Sciences of the Artificial.* Cambridge, MA: MIT Press.
38. Sterman, J.D. (2000). *Business Dynamics: Systems Thinking and Modeling for a Complex World.* Boston: Irwin McGraw-Hill.
39. Brehmer, B. (1990). Strategies in real-time, dynamic decision making. In: Hogarth, R. (Ed.). *Insights in Decision making: A Tribute to Hillel J. Einhorn.* Chicago: University of Chicago Press.
40. Hogarth, R.M. (1981). Beyond discrete biases: functional and dysfunctional aspects of judgmental heuristics. *Psychological Bulletin,* 90(2), 197–217.
41. Sterman, J.D. and Booth Sweeney, L. (2002). Cloudy skies: assessing public understanding of global warming. *System Dynamics Review,* 18, 207–240.
42. *Ibid.*
43. *Ibid.*
44. Forrester, J.W. (1971). Counterintuitive behavior of social systems. *Technology Review,* 73(3), 52–68.
45. Buchanan, M. (2005). Supermodels to the rescue. *Strategy+Business,* Spring, 2005.
46. Forrester, J.W. (1979). System Dynamics: Future Opportunities. Paper D-3108-1, The System Dynamics Group, Sloan School of Management, Massachusetts Institute of Technology.
47. Casti, J.L. (1997). *Would-Be Worlds: How Simulation Is Changing the Frontiers of Science.* New York: John Wiley .
48. *Ibid.*
49. *Ibid.*
50. *Ibid.*
51. Sterman, J.D. (2006). Learning from evidence in a complex world. *American Journal of Public Health,* 96(3), 505–514.

52. Casti, J.L. (1997). *Would-Be Worlds: How Simulation Is Changing the Frontiers of Science*. New York: John Wiley.

53. Abdel-Hamid, T. (2002). Modeling the dynamics of human energy regulation and its implications for obesity treatment. *System Dynamics Review*, 18(4), 431–471.
    Abdel-Hamid, T.K. (2003). Exercise and diet in obesity treatment: an integrative system dynamics perspective. *Medicine and Science in Sports and Exercise*, 35(3), 400–413.

54. High Performance Systems. (2001). *An Introduction to Systems Thinking*. Hanover, NH: High Performance Systems.

55. *Ibid.*

56. *Ibid.*

57. *Ibid.*

58. *Ibid.*

59. Sterman, J.D. (2000). *Business Dynamics: Systems Thinking and Modeling for a Complex World*. Boston: Irwin McGraw-Hill.

60. In a system dynamics model, this is accomplished through the use of simultaneous difference equations.

61. Blundell, J.E. et al. (1996). Control of Human Appetite: Implications for the Intake of Dietary fat. *Annual Review of Nutrition* , 16, 285–319.

62. Food energy was formerly measured in kilocalories, which is commonly abbreviated as kcal. One kcal is the amount of heat necessary to raise the temperature of 1 kg of water 1°C. When, in popular books and magazines, they write that an apple provides "100 calories," it really means 100 kcal.

63. Whitney, E.N. and Rolfes, S.R. (1999). *Understanding Nutrition*. Belmont, CA: West/Wadsworth.

64. Stubbs, J., Murgatroyd, P.R., Goldberg, G.R., and Prentice, A.M. (1993). Carbohydrate balance and the regulation of day-to-day food intake in humans. *American Journal of Clinical Nutrition*, 57, 897–903.

65. Stipanuk, M.H. (Ed.). (2000). *Biochemical and Physiological Aspects of Human Nutrition*. Philadelphia: W.B. Saunders.

66. Stubbs, J., Murgatroyd, P.R., Goldberg, G.R., and Prentice, A.M. (1993). Carbohydrate balance and the regulation of day-to-day food intake in humans. *American Journal of Clinical Nutrition*, 57, 897–903.

67. Guyton, A.C. and Hall, J.E. (1996). *Textbook of Medical Physiology*. Philadelphia: W.B. Saunders.

68. Whitney, E.N. and Rolfes, S.R. (1999). *Understanding Nutrition*. Belmont, CA: West/Wadsworth.

69. Kaufman, F.R. (2005). *Diabesity: The Obesity-Diabetes Epidemic that Threatens America—And What We Must Do to Stop It*. New York: Bantam.

70. Wadden, T.A. and Stunkard, A.J. (Eds.). (2002). *Handbook of Obesity Treatment*. New York: Guilford Press.

71. The following empirically derived formulation is used in the model by Westerterp et al.: Nominal REE = 0.024 * FM + 0.102 * FFM + 0.85 (MJ/day). See: Westerterp, K.R., Donkers, J., Fredrix, E., and Boekhoudt, P. (1995). Energy Intake, physical activity and body weight: a simulation model. *British Journal of Nutrition, 73,* 337–347.

72. Pi-Sunyer, F.X. (1999). Obesity. In: Shils, M.E., Olson, J.A., Shike, M., and Ross, A.C. (Eds.). *Modern Nutrition in Health and Disease*. Baltimore: Williams & Wilkins.

73. Leibel, R.L., Rosenbaum, M., and Hirsch, J. (1995). Changes in energy expenditure resulting from altered body weight. *New England Journal of Medicine, 332,* 621–628.

74. Dullo, A.G. and Jacquet, J. (1998). Adaptive reduction in basal metabolic rate in response to food deprivation in humans: a role for feedback signals from fat stores. *American Journal of Clinical Nutrition, 68,* 599–606.

75. Heshka, S. Yang, M., Wang, J., Burt, P. and Pi-Sunyer, F.X. (1990). Weight loss and change in resting metabolic rate. *American Journal of Clinical Nutrition, 52,* 981–986.

76. Saltzman, E. and Roberts, S.B. (1995). The role of energy expenditure in energy regulation: findings from a decade of research. *Nutrition Reviews 53,* 209–220.

77. Whitney, E.N. and Rolfes, S.R. (1999). *Understanding Nutrition*. Belmont, CA: West/Wadsworth.

78. *Ibid.*

79. McArdle, W.D., Katch, F.I., and Katch, V.L. (1996). *Exercise Physiology: Energy, Nutrition, and Human Performance*. Baltimore: Williams & Wilkins.

80. Johnson, L.R. (1998). *Essential Medical Physiology*. Philadelphia: Lippincott-Raven.

81. *Ibid.*

82. Guyton, A.C. and Hall, J.E. (1996). *Textbook of Medical Physiology*. Philadelphia: W.B. Saunders.

83. Whitney, E.N. and Rolfes, S.R. (1999). *Understanding Nutrition*. Belmont, CA: West/Wadsworth.

84. Guyton, A.C. and Hall, J.E. (1996). *Textbook of Medical Physiology*. Philadelphia: W.B. Saunders.

85. *Ibid.*

86. Sterman, J.D. (2000). *Business Dynamics: Systems Thinking and Modeling for a Complex World*. Boston: Irwin McGraw-Hill.

87. Flatt, J.P., Ravussin, E., Acheson, K.J., and Jéquier, E. (1985). Effects of dietary fat on postprandial substrate oxidation and on carbohydrate and fat balances. *Journal of Clinical Investigation*, 76, 1019–1024.
88. Guyton, A.C. and Hall, J.E. (1996). *Textbook of Medical Physiology*. Philadelphia: W.B. Saunders.
89. *Ibid.*
90. Johnson, L.R. (1998). *Essential Medical Physiology*. Philadelphia: Lippincott-Raven.
91. Guyton, A.C. and Hall, J.E. (1996). *Textbook of Medical Physiology*. Philadelphia: W.B. Saunders.
92. Whitney, E.N. and Rolfes, S.R. (1999). *Understanding Nutrition*. Belmont, CA: West/Wadsworth.
93. *Ibid.*
94. Hydrolysis is a chemical process in which a molecule is cleaved into two parts by the addition of a molecule of water. See: Wikipedia. Hydrolysis. <wikipedia.org/wiki/Hydrolysis>.
95. Guyton, A.C. and Hall, J.E. (1996). *Textbook of Medical Physiology*. Philadelphia: W.B. Saunders.
96. Whitney, E.N. and Rolfes, S.R. (1999). *Understanding Nutrition*. Belmont, CA: West/Wadsworth.
97. *Ibid.*
98. McArdle, W.D., Katch, F.I., and Katch, V.L. (1996). *Exercise Physiology: Energy, Nutrition, and Human Performance*. Baltimore: Williams & Wilkins.
99. *Ibid.*
100. Stipanuk, M.H. (Ed.). (2000). *Biochemical and Physiological Aspects of Human Nutrition*. Philadelphia: W.B. Saunders.
101. Guyton, A.C. and Hall, J.E. (1996). *Textbook of Medical Physiology*. Philadelphia: W.B. Saunders.
102. Whitney, E.N. and Rolfes, S.R. (1999). *Understanding Nutrition*. Belmont, CA: West/Wadsworth.
103. During exercise, glucose can be metabolized by muscle tissue without requiring large amounts of insulin because the contraction process itself makes exercising muscle fibers permeable to glucose even in the absence of insulin.
104. Whitney, E.N. and Rolfes, S.R. (1999). *Understanding Nutrition*. Belmont, CA: West/Wadsworth.
105. McArdle, W.D., Katch, F.I., and Katch, V.L. (1996). *Exercise Physiology: Energy, Nutrition, and Human Performance*. Baltimore: Williams & Wilkins.
106. Guyton, A.C. and Hall, J.E. (1996). *Textbook of Medical Physiology*. Philadelphia: W.B. Saunders.

107. Whitney, E.N. and Rolfes, S.R. (1999). *Understanding Nutrition.* Belmont, CA: West/Wadsworth.

108. McArdle, W.D., Katch, F.I., and Katch, V.L. (1996). *Exercise Physiology: Energy, Nutrition, and Human Performance.* Baltimore: Williams & Wilkins.

109. Glycogen depletion usually occurs within 1 to 2 hours from the onset of intense activity. See: McArdle, W.D., Katch, F.I., and Katch, V.L. (1996). *Exercise Physiology: Energy, Nutrition, and Human Performance.* Baltimore: Williams & Wilkins.

110. McArdle, W.D., Katch, F.I., and Katch, V.L. (1996). *Exercise Physiology: Energy, Nutrition, and Human Performance.* Baltimore: Williams & Wilkins.

111. Spirduso, W.W. (1995). *Physical Dimensions of Aging.* Champaign, IL: Human Kinetics.

112. Whitney, E.N. and Rolfes, S.R. (1999). *Understanding Nutrition.* Belmont, CA: West/Wadsworth.

113. McArdle, W.D., Katch, F.I., and Katch, V.L. (1996). *Exercise Physiology: Energy, Nutrition, and Human Performance.* Baltimore: Williams & Wilkins.

114. Spirduso, W.W. (1995). *Physical Dimensions of Aging.* Champaign, IL: Human Kinetics.

115. Whitney, E.N. and Rolfes, S.R. (1999). *Understanding Nutrition.* Belmont, CA: West/Wadsworth.

116. Brooks, G.A., Fahey, T.D., White, T.P., and Baldwin K.M. (2000). *Exercise Physiology: Human Bioenergetics and its Applications.* Mountain View, CA: Mayfield.

117. McArdle, W.D., Katch, F.I., and Katch, V.L. (1996). *Exercise Physiology: Energy, Nutrition, and Human Performance.* Baltimore: Williams & Wilkins.

118. Jungermann. K. and Barth, C.A. (1996). Energy Metabolism and Nutrition. In: Greger, R. and Windhorst, U. (Eds.). *Comprehensive Human Physiology*, Vol. 2 (pp. 1425–1457). Berlin, Heidelberg: Springer-Verlag.

119. Assuming an energy expenditure of about 100 calories per mile.

120. Guyton, A.C. and Hall, J.E. (1996). *Textbook of Medical Physiology.* Philadelphia: W.B. Saunders.

121. *Ibid.*

122. Pi-Sunyer, F.X. (1999). Obesity. In: Shils, M.E., Olson, J.A., Shike, M., and Ross, A.C. (Eds.). *Modern Nutrition in Health and Disease.* Baltimore: Williams & Wilkins.

123. McArdle, W.D., Katch, F.I., and Katch, V.L. (1996). *Exercise Physiology: Energy, Nutrition, and Human Performance.* Baltimore: Williams & Wilkins.

124. Pi-Sunyer, F.X. (1999). Obesity. In: Shils, M.E., Olson, J.A., Shike, M., and Ross, A.C. (Eds.). *Modern Nutrition in Health and Disease*. Baltimore: Williams & Wilkins.

125. Whitney, E.N. and Rolfes, S.R. (1999). *Understanding Nutrition*. Belmont, CA: West/Wadsworth.

126. Forbes, G.B. (1987). *Human Body Composition: Growth, Aging, Nutrition and Activity*. New York: Springer-Verlag.

127. *Ibid*.

128. Forbes derived empirical relationship is: $\partial(\text{FFM})/\partial(\text{FM}) = 10.4/\text{FM}$, which can be rewritten as $\partial(\text{FFM})/\partial(\text{W}) = 10.4/(\text{FM} + 10.4)$. See: Forbes, G.B. (1987). *Human Body Composition: Growth, Aging, Nutrition, and Activity*. Berlin, Heidelberg: Springer-Verlag.

129. Ballor, D.L. and Poehlman, E.T. (1994). Exercise-training enhances fat-free mass preservation during diet-induced weight loss: a meta-analytical finding. *International Journal of Obesity*, 18, 35–40.

130. Sterman, J.D. (2006). Learning from evidence in a complex world. *American Journal of Public Health*, 96(3), 505–514.

131. Weinsier, R.L., Bracco, D., and Schultz, Y. (1993). Predicted Effects of small decreases in energy expenditure on weight gain in adult women. *International Journal of Obesity*, 17, 693–699.

132. Stipanuk, M.H. (Ed.). (2000). *Biochemical and Physiological Aspects of Human Nutrition*. Philadelphia: W.B. Saunders.

133. Novotny, J.A. and Rumpler, W.V. (1998). Modeling of energy expenditure and resting metabolic rate during weight loss in humans. In: Clifford, A.J. and Muller, H.G. (Eds.). *Mathematical Modeling in Experimental Nutrition*. New York: Plenum Press.

134. Wadden, T.A. and Stunkard, A.J. (Eds.). (2002). *Handbook of Obesity Treatment*. New York: Guilford Press.

135. According to World Health Organization's (WHO) reference standards, the energy cost of routine physical activity is determined as the product of the REE and an appropriate activity factor referred to as the *physical activity ratio (PAR)*. Total 24-hour energy expenditure (EE), thus, would be equal to the REE multiplied by the physical activity factor (PAR) and added to the energy cost of processing food intake. For free-living conditions, an average PAR value of 1.4 would be typical. This is the value used for our experimental subject. See: 1) Weinsier, R.L., Bracco, D., and Schultz, Y. (1993). Predicted effects of small decreases in energy expenditure on weight gain in adult women. *International Journal of Obesity*, 17, 693–699; and 2) McArdle, W.D., Katch, F.I., and Katch, V.L. (1996). *Exercise Physiology: Energy, Nutrition, and Human Performance*. Baltimore: Williams & Wilkins.

136. National Institutes of Health (1998). *Clinical Guidelines on the Identification, Evaluation, and Treatment of Overweight and Obesity in Adults.* U.S. Department of Health and Human Services, NIH Publication No. 98-4083.

137. Forbes, G.B. (1987). *Human Body Composition: Growth, Aging, Nutrition, and Activity.* Berlin, Heidelberg: Springer-Verlag.

138. The energy content of fat is 0.032 MJ/g, and that of pure protein is 0.017 MJ/g. Using the most commonly used hydration constant for FFM of 0.73 (i.e., assuming FFM to being 73 percent water and 27 percent protein) one arrives at the energy densities of FFM and FM to be 4.6 MJ/kg and 32 MJ/kg, respectively. Thus, 1 kg of body tissue (70 percent FM, 30 percent FFM) has an energy content of 24 MJ. (This is equivalent to 2,606 kcal/pound.) These estimates are comparable to those used in Brownell, K.D. and Fairburn, C.G. (Eds.). (1995). *Eating Disorders and Obesity: A Comprehensive Handbook.* New York: Guilford Press. Also see Whitney, E.N. and Rolfes, S.R. (1999). *Understanding Nutrition.* Belmont, CA: West/Wadsworth.

139. Ravussin, E., Schutz, Y., Acheson, K.J., Dusmet, M., Bourquin, L. and Jequier, E. (1985). Short-term, mixed-diet overfeeding in man: no evidence for "luxuskonsumption." *American Journal of Physiological and Endocrinological Metabolism,* 249, E470–E477.

140. Forbes estimates that this new equilibrium would be approached with a half-time of approximately 9 months. See: Forbes, G.B. (1987). *Human Body Composition: Growth, Aging, Nutrition and Activity.* New York: Springer-Verlag.

141. Einhorn, H. J. and Hogarth, R. M. (1982). Prediction diagnosis and causal thinking in forecasting. *Journal of Forecasting,* 1, 23–36.

142. Einhorn, H. J. and Hogarth, R. M. (1987). Decision making: going forward in reverse. *Harvard Business Review,* 65(1): 66–70.

143. Young, V.R., Yu, Y.M., and Fukagawa, N.K. (1992). Whole body energy and nitrogen (protein) relationships. In: Kinney, J.M. and Tucker, H.N. (Eds.). *Energy Metabolism: Tissue Determinants and Cellular Corollaries* (pp. 139–161). New York: Raven Press.

144. Wegner, D.M. (2002). *The Illusions of Conscious Will.* Cambridge, MA: Bradford Books.

145. Brehmer, B. (1990). Strategies in real-time, dynamic decision making. In: Hogarth, R. (Ed.). *Insights in Decision Making: A Tribute to Hillel J. Einhorn.* Chicago: University of Chicago Press.

146. Williamson, D.F. ,et al. (1992). Weight loss attempts in adults: goals, duration, and rate of weight loss. *American Journal of Public Health,* 82(9), 1251–1257.

147. Forrester, J.W. (1991). System Dynamics and the Lessons of 35 years. Working paper No. D-4224-4, System Dynamics Group, Sloan School of Management, Massachusetts Institute of Technology Cambridge, MA 02139

148. Baumeister, R.F., Heatherton, T.F., and Tice, D.M. (1994). *Losing Control: How and Why People Fail at Self-Regulation*. San Diego, CA: Academic Press.

149. *Ibid.*

150. *Ibid.*

151. Baumeister, R.F. and Heatherton, T.F. (1996). Self-regulation failure: an overview. *Psychological Inquiry*, 7(1), 1–15.

152. Bandura, A. (1997). *Self-Efficacy: The Exercise of Control*. New York: W. H. Freeman.

153. Casti, J.L. (1997). *Would-Be Worlds: How Simulation Is Changing the Frontiers of Science*. New York: John Wiley.

154. Bouchard, C. and Pérusse, L. (1993). Genetics of Obesity. *Annual Review of Nutrition*, 13, 337–354.

155. Baumeister, R.F., Heatherton, T.F., and Tice, D.M. (1994). *Losing Control: How and Why People Fail at Self-Regulation*. San Diego: Academic Press.

156. *Ibid.*

157. Abdel-Hamid, T. (2002). Modeling the dynamics of human energy regulation and its implications for obesity treatment. *System Dynamics Review*, 18(4), 431–471.

158. Brownell, K.D. and Fairburn, C.G. (Eds.). (1995). *Eating Disorders and Obesity: A Comprehensive Handbook*. New York: Guilford Press

159. Sjöström, L. (1980). Fat cells and body weight. In: Stunkard, A.J. (Ed.). *Obesity*. Philadelphia: W.B. Saunders.

160. Forbes, G.B. (1987). *Human Body Composition: Growth, Aging, Nutrition and Activity*. New York: Springer-Verlag.

161. *Ibid.*

162. Keesey, R.E. (1993). Physiological regulation of body energy: implications for obesity. In: Stunkard, A.J. and Wadden, T.A. (Eds). *Obesity: Theory and Therapy*. New York: Raven Press.

163. Saltzman, E. and Roberts, S.B. (1995). The role of energy expenditure in energy regulation: findings from a decade of research. *Nutrition Reviews* 53, 209–220.

164. This is roughly calculated as follows: Total daily energy expenditure (EE) is equal to the REE multiplied by an appropriate physical activity factor (e.g., a value of 1.4 would be typical) and added to the energy cost of diet-induced thermogenesis. REE can be estimated using an empirically derived formulation proposed by Westerterp et al (1995), shown below.

165. Westerterp et al. empirically derived formulation is used to calculate nominal REE as follows: Nominal REE = 0.024*FM + 0.102*FFM + 0.85 (MJ/day). See: Westerterp, K.R., Donkers, J., Fredrix, E., and Boekhoudt, P. (1995). Energy intake, physical activity and body weight: a simulation model. *British Journal of Nutrition, 73,* 337–347.

166. Van Itallie, T.B. and Kissileff, H.R. (1990). Human obesity: a problem in body energy economics. In: Stricker, E.M. (Ed.), *Handbook of Behavioral Neurolobiology Volume 10 Neurobiology of Food and Fluid Intake* (pp. 207–240). New York: Plenum Press.

167. Shell, E.R. (2002). *The Hungry Gene: The Inside Story of the Obesity Industry.* New York: Grove Press.

168. Whitney, E.N. and Rolfes, S.R. (1999). *Understanding Nutrition.* Belmont, CA: West/Wadsworth.

169. Uma, G. and Siva Perraju, T. (2000). Services on the Net: an agent based approach. Database and Expert Systems Applications, Proceedings of the 11th International Workshop (pp. 770–774). London, UK.

170. Vancouver, J.B. (1996). Living systems theory as a paradigm for organizational behavior: understanding humans, organizations, and social processes. *Behavioral Science,* 41(3), 165–204.

171. Ballor, D.L. and Poehlman, E.T. (1994). Exercise-training enhances fat-free mass preservation during diet-induced weight loss: a meta-analytical finding. *International Journal of Obesity,* 18, 35–40.

172. McArdle, W.D., Katch, F.I., and Katch, V.L. (1996). *Exercise Physiology: Energy, Nutrition, and Human Performance.* Baltimore: Williams & Wilkins.

173. Also, the thermic effect of food (TEF) will be higher in an exercise scenario since more food energy will be consumed.

174. McArdle, W.D., Katch, F.I., and Katch, V.L. (1996). *Exercise Physiology: Energy, Nutrition, and Human Performance.* Baltimore: Williams & Wilkins.

175. Brody, J.E. (2000, October 17). One-two punch for losing pounds: exercise and careful diet. *New York Times.*

176. McArdle, W.D., Katch, F.I., and Katch, V.L. (1996). *Exercise Physiology: Energy, Nutrition, and Human Performance.* Baltimore: Williams & Wilkins.

177. Andrews, J. F. (1991). Exercise for slimming. *Proceedings of the Nutrition Society.* 50, 459–471.

178. Melby, C.L., Commerford, S.R., and Hill, J.O. (1998). Exercise, macronutrient balance, and weight control. In: Lamb, D.R. and Murray, R. (Eds.) *Perspectives in Exercise Science and Sports Medicine (Volume II): Exercise, Nutrition, and Weight Control.* Carme, IN: Cooper Publishing Group.

179. Grundy, S.M., Blackburn, G., Higgins, M., Lauer, R., Perri, M.G.,and Ryan, D. (1999). Physical activity in the prevention and treatment of obesity and its comorbidities: evidence report of independent panel to assess the role of physical activity in the treatment of obesity and its comorbidities. *Medicine and Science in Sports and Exercise*, 31, 1493–1500.
180. Kirk, E.P., Jacobsen, D.J., Gibson, C., Hill, J.O., and Donnelly, J.E. (2003). Time course for changes in aerobic capacity and body composition in overweight men and women in response to long-term exercise: the Midwest Exercise Trial (MET). *International Journal of Obesity*, 27, 912–919.
181. The composition of weight loss is clearly a function of the type of exercise. Resistance training, for example, tends to preserve more of the fat-free mass component than does aerobic exercise. See: Kraemer, W.J. et al. (1999). Influence of exercise training on physiological and performance changes with weight loss in men. *Medicine and Science in Sports and Exercise*, 31(9), 1320–1329.
182. Ballor, D.L. and Poehlman, E.T. (1994). Exercise-training enhances fat-free mass preservation during diet-induced weight loss: a meta-analytical finding. *International Journal of Obesity*, 18, 35–40.
183. Whenever a person exercises at a rate that exceeds the capacity of the heart and lungs to supply oxygen to the muscles, the muscles must draw more heavily on glucose (primarily in the form of muscle glycogen) because it is the *only* fuel that can metabolized to produce energy without the simultaneous utilization of oxygen. During intense exercise, a selective dependence on glucose metabolism has an additional advantage, namely, its rapidity for energy transfer compared to fats (about twice as fast).
184. Whitney, E.N. and Rolfes, S.R. (1999). *Understanding Nutrition*. Belmont, CA: West/Wadsworth.
185. Brown, G. (1999). *The Energy of Life: The Science of What Makes Our Minds and Bodies Work*. New York: Free Press.
186. McArdle, W.D., Katch, F.I., and Katch, V.L. (1996). *Exercise Physiology: Energy, Nutrition, and Human Performance*. Baltimore: Williams & Wilkins.
187. Guyton, A.C. and Hall, J.E. (1996). *Textbook of Medical Physiology*. Philadelphia: W.B. Saunders.
188. Brown, G. (1999). *The Energy of Life: The Science of What Makes Our Minds and Bodies Work*. New York: Free Press.
189. *Ibid.*
190. By conserving and even increasing the fat-free body mass (the principal metabolically active component of total body mass), exercise

contributes to total energy expenditure and weight loss both through the cost of the exercise itself and through its effect of offsetting and even reversing the depression in metabolic energy usually observed when weight loss is achieved through dietary restriction. See: 1) McArdle, W.D., Katch, F.I., and Katch, V.L. (1996). *Exercise Physiology: Energy, Nutrition, and Human Performance.* Baltimore: Williams & Wilkins; and 2) Ballor, D.L. and Poehlman, E.T. (1994). Exercise-training enhances fat-free mass preservation during diet-induced weight loss: a meta-analytical finding. *International Journal of Obesity,* 18, 35–40.

The composition of the 5.54 kg/12.2 lb loss was as follows: a 0.8 kg /1.1 lb drop in FFM combined with a 4.74 kg/10.5 lb loss of FM, inducing a drop in percent body fat to 21.44.

191. Abdel-Hamid, T.K. (2003). Exercise and diet in obesity treatment: an integrative system dynamics perspective. *Medicine and Science in Sports and Exercise*, 35(3), 400–413.

192. Brody, J.E. (2000, October 17). One-two punch for losing pounds: Exercise and careful diet. *New York Times.*

193. Pool, R. (2001). *Fat: Fighting the Obesity Epidemic.* Oxford: Oxford University Press.

194. Leermakers, E.A., Dunn, A.L., and Blair, S.N. (2000). Exercise management of obesity. *Medical Clinics of North America*, 84(2), 419–440.

195. van Baak, M.A. (1999). Exercise training and substrate utilization in obesity. *Journal of Obesity and Related Metabolic Disorders,* 23, S11–S17.

196. Brownell, K.D. and Horgen, K.B. (2004). *Food Fight.* Chicago: Contemporary Books.

197. Sterman, J. D. (1991). A skeptic's guide to computer models. In: Barney, G.O., Kreutzer, W.B., and Garrett, M.J. (Eds.) *Managing a Nation,* 2nd ed. Boulder, CO: Westview Press.

198. Sterman, J.D. (2000). *Business Dynamics: Systems Thinking and Modeling for a Complex World.* Boston: Irwin McGraw-Hill.

199. Gustafson, D.H. et al. (1999). Impact of a patient-centered, computer-based health information/support system. *American Journal of Preventive Medicine*, 16(1), 1–9.

200. Battle, E.K. and Brownell, K.D. (1996). Confronting a rising tide of eating disorders and obesity: treatment vs. prevention and policy. *Addictive Behaviors,* (21), 755–765.

201. Carey, J. (2006, May 29). Medical guesswork: from heart surgery to prostate care, the health industry knows little about which common treatments really work. *Business Week.*

Prevention and Beyond

V

Clearly if disease is man-made, then it can be man-prevented.
—*Ernst Wynder, (1975)*

The Fat Lady ... Models

Despite the growing awareness of obesity's health hazards and the wide-spread concern about its escalation, there has been a subtle but unmistakable countertrend: a societal embrace of the large man, woman, and child. In the words of Marion Nestle, author of *Food Politics*, "[W]hat used to be considered pudgy before isn't even worthy of a comment today."[1] Perhaps it is the inevitable consequence of our disappointing track record, as individuals and as a society, in treating weight gain and reversing its upward trend. Nevertheless, many health experts fear that as fat becomes mainstream, it will drive more and more people to become complacent and seriously undermine treatment and prevention efforts.[2]

There is ample evidence that weight levels to which Americans aspire have been slowly drifting upward. For example, statistical evidence can be found in the Centers for Disease Control and Prevention's Behavioral Risk Factor Surveillance Surveys (BRFSS).[3] Survey data over the last decade and a half show not only that average *actual* weights of American adults have increased, but also that the average *desired* weights among both men and women have been creeping up (by an estimated 3 pounds between 1994 and 2002).[4]

More colorful evidence of the trend can be seen on the covers of teen magazines. Instead of the stick-thin figures of the past, we are increasingly seeing more and more pictures of real teenagers in real sizes on their pages, as many of the magazines cater to "larger" readers.[5] On television, too, audiences are getting used to seeing plumper girls, and they apparently like what they see—very much. In December 2005, for example, *Libération,* a European daily newspaper, declared that a barrier was been crossed when "millions of television viewers voted and chose Magalie Bonneau, a 19-year-old student who is 5 feet 1 inch and weighs 165 pounds, as the winner of the hit talent and reality show 'Star Academy.'"[6]

But, perhaps nowhere is this acceptance more vividly illustrated than in fashion. In recent years, mainstream retailers such as Ralph Lauren and Tommy Hilfiger have begun to introduce designs for the full-figured, while

T.K.A. Hamid, *Thinking in Circles About Obesity*,
DOI 10.1007/978-0-387-09469-4_22, © Springer Science+Business Media, LLC 2009

stores popular with teenagers, such as Delia's, Gap, and Old Navy, have increasingly widened their range of sizes (some now offering clothes up to size 20) and now offer more fashionable styles in sizes 12 and up.[7] And the fashion industry did not stop there. A few years ago, the industry introduced its so-called vanity sizes, which are new cuts that are bigger but without the bigger size numbers, allowing its customers, both male and female, who have packed on the pounds to be able to wear the same sizes they wore in their trimmer days.[8] And, *quelle horreur!*, as the French are getting fatter, even French couture may be embracing the large woman. In a 2005 fashion show, designer John Galliano "stunned" the audience, as the venerable *New York Times* put it, by featuring overweight models on the runway alongside their string-bean–thin counterparts (Figure 22.1).[9]

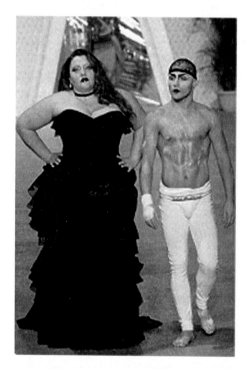

Figure 22.1 Spring 2006 ready-to-wear fashions by John Galliano, as seen in a runway review. (*Source*: http://www.style.com/fashionshows/collections/S2006RTW/complete/thumb/JNGALLNO)

To systems thinkers, none of this is surprising. The dynamic fits a familiar and recurring pattern (also referred to as an *archetype*) witnessed in a wide variety of settings and at many different levels—at the level of individuals, in organizations big and small, as well as at the macro-societal level. It is one of the nine principal systems archetypes discussed in Peter Senge's *The Fifth Discipline*, one that he calls *eroding goals*. Here is how it works.

Whenever—as individuals, as an organization, or as a society—we perceive a gap between our current state and a goal we have, we feel pressure to take action to close the gap. Two courses of action are possible. The first is to take corrective action(s) to bring our state or situation into line with the goal. For example, "when you are hungry, you eat, satisfying your hunger, when tired you sleep, restoring your energy and alertness."[10] This first path to closing the gap is termed the *fundamental solution* and is the process represented by the loop in Figure 22.2. It is the classic goal-seeking negative-feedback structure that aims to bring the state of a system in line with a goal or desired state.

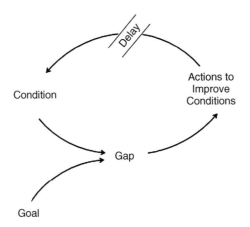

Figure 22.2 The fundamental solution

As the loop in Figure 22.2 indicates, the fundamental solution can take time and effort, which is why we are often tempted to close the gap the other way: by lowering our goals. That is the *goal erosion* path shown as the lower loop in Figure 22.3.

A critical difference between the two loops is that lowering the goal immediately closes the gap, whereas corrective actions usually take time and effort. The longer it takes or the greater the difficulty of changing our situation, the greater the temptation (and the pressure) to close the gap by lowering the goal. Whether in dealing with a personal situation, an organizational strategy, or a public policy, when failure persists and victory remains elusive, "the easiest path is to just pretend there is no bad news or better yet 'declare victory'—to redefine the bad news as not so bad by lowering the standard against which it is judged."[11]

It is no wonder that societies collude in eroding goals all the time. For example, we see it in lowered government targets for "full employment" or for

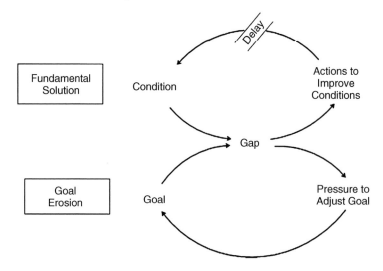

Figure 22.3 Eroding goals. If all else fails, lower your goals

balancing the federal deficit, and we have witnessed it as our targets for controlling dangerous pollutants and protecting endangered species have slid.[12] In the case of obesity, we see this erosion in the slow upward drift in our collective aspirations for desired weight and, more concretely, in the subtle but persistent "broadening of America." There are plenty of indications of this trend: All across the country, auditoriums, stadiums, and even subway cars are being fitted with new seats that are several inches wider to accommodate patrons who now cover a lot more seat than did earlier patrons.[13] Fire departments are installing gurneys that can hold patients weighing up to 600 pounds, and ambulance companies are retrofitting their vehicles with winches and plus-sized compartments to handle patients weighing up to half a ton.[14] Even the final resting place has had to accommodate our growing girth. An Indiana manufacturer of caskets now offers a double-oversize model that is 38 inches wide, compared with a standard 24 inches.[15]

While goal erosion does close the gap, it is a strategy fraught with peril, since lowering one's expectations invariably leads to poorer performance. In Senge's words, "[It is] the dynamics of compromise, the path of mediocrity." Worse yet, because the story rarely ends with a one-time reduction in the goal, the process can easily become addictive. "Sooner or later new pressures pulling reality away from the [new, lowered] goal arise, leading to still more pressures to lower the goal,"[16] and a classic downward spiral ensues of failure to meet goals, lowering the goals, temporary relief, and pressures anew to lower the goals still further.

In obesity there may be a third way, beyond tackling stubborn goals or eroding our aspirations, and that way is prevention.

The Third Path: Prevention **23**

Can't Unscramble an Egg

Since the onset of the obesity epidemic, treatment of the problem has received overwhelmingly more attention than has prevention. While this remains true today, interest in obesity prevention is slowly starting to attract increasing attention, probably because of the growing realization that it may be easier, less expensive, and more effective—at both the personal and public-policy levels—to change behavior so as to prevent weight gain, or to reverse small gains, than to treat obesity after it has fully developed.

From a public-policy perspective, there is a real and growing concern about the feasibility—economic if not medical—of treating ourselves out of this public health problem.[17] If the trends are not reversed, it is feared, the sheer number of obese individuals who will need help could very well overwhelm the already fragile health care systems in the United States and many other developed countries. Indeed, some have argued that we have already reached that point—that we no longer have sufficient health care resources to offer proper (and affordable) treatment to all who need it.[18]

Obesity prevention may also be the best way to address the health problems it causes. Many of the adverse health consequences associated with obesity result from the cumulative stress of excess weight over a long period of time and are not fully reversible by weight loss.[19] When it comes to our body, "there are real limits to what can be done to reverse the damage caused by a lifetime of unhealthy living."[20] This is true no matter how strong-willed we are.

As MIT's John Sterman so deliciously puts it: "You can't unscramble an egg (the second law of thermodynamics)."[21] Analogously, many processes in health and disease can be hard, if not impossible, to reverse. For example:

- A former smoker's risk of lung cancer is always higher than that of someone who has never smoked. "The best [one] can be is a former smoker—[one] can't be a 'never smoker.'"[22]

T.K.A. Hamid, *Thinking in Circles About Obesity*,
DOI 10.1007/978-0-387-09469-4_23, © Springer Science+Business Media, LLC 2009

- There is no way to repair the cancer-causing DNA damage that excessive exposure to the sun's ultraviolet radiation causes to our skin.[23]
- Repeated exposure to loud noise, such as from the earbuds on an iPod, a lawn mower, or a Metallica concert, can destroy the inner ear's delicate sound-conducting hair cells. Dead hair cells do not grow back, and once hearing is lost, it is gone forever.[24]

Obesity is no exception. Gaining an excessive amount of weight can induce a wide array of irreversible anatomical and physiological changes that can lead to irreparable damage. For example, obesity is often associated with damage to blood vessels and the buildup of plaque in the arteries that no amount of exercise or diet change will reverse.[25] Insulin resistance is another potentially serious and irreversible consequence of obesity, one that places people at risk for type 2 diabetes. Because the consequences of insulin resistance are often not felt for years, the effects of the elevated sugars begin to build and become irreversible, often with devastating consequences.[26] Scientific findings released within the past few years, for example, suggest that when cells do not get enough sugar as a result of insulin resistance, the lack of sugar can cause the cells to malfunction or die. When this happens in the brain, dying brain cells may set the stage for Alzheimer's disease.[27] But perhaps the one irreversibility that annoys most dieters more than any other is the one associated with the proliferation of the body's fat cells when excessive weight is gained. As was explained earlier, the increased number of fat cells that accompanies excessive weight gain is not only next to impossible to dispose of, but also acts to defend the elevation in body weight.

The implications of all this for obesity treatment and prevention are clear: It is crucial to reach the overweight patient before fat-cell proliferation sets in, weight is gained, and the irreversible damage incurred.

The Buck Starts Here

Many health care professionals believe that, while the treatment of disease needs to remain within the purview of the private health care system, prevention efforts for conditions such as obesity (and diabetes) have little chance of success without substantial government involvement and investment.[28–31] An important reason for that is *incentives*.

While America's high-tech pharmaceutical-driven health care system excels at dispensing pills and opening up bodies, it has little incentive to promote prevention. Health care is a business, and the big bucks are in the treatment of acute diseases. The goal of prevention, on the other hand, is to maintain good health and prevent disease and illness. Thus, the market and health promotion are at odds.[32]

> The market functions wonderfully when we want to sell more cereals, cosmetics, cars, computers, or any other consumer product. Unfortunately, it doesn't work in health care, where the goal should hardly be selling more [heart bypass or bariatric operations].[33]

A recent yearlong investigation by the *New York Times* provided a timely exposé of how the American health care system, due to its perverse financial incentives, is "flailing when it comes to prevention." In what is partly a fascinating piece of investigative reporting and partly a socioeconomic research study, *Times* reporter N.R. Kleinfeld successfully documents how the "undeniably biased" financial incentives in the system undermine preventive care, financially rewarding doctors and hospitals for treating complications of diseases such as obesity and diabetes, but losing them money when they try to help patients prevent them.[34]

Two sharply contrasting trajectories highlighted in the article underscore the bias in the system's economic drivers: the meteoric growth of bariatric surgery (the new high-profit, high-tech weight-loss procedure) on the one hand, and the precipitous decline in the number of prevention centers. As Kleinfeld quips, "[I]f a hospital charges, and can get reimbursed by insurance, $50,000 for a bariatric surgery that takes just 40 minutes or it can get reimbursed $20 for the same amount of time spent with a nutritionist, where do you think priorities will be?"

It is estimated that between 2001 and 2006, the number of bariatric weight-loss procedures performed in the U.S. increased by an astonishing 300 percent, from 50,000 to approximately 200,000 procedures.[35] Today, even children as young as 12 are having the surgery. Not surprisingly, the American Bariatric Society reports that its surgeons "can't keep up" with all the demand.[36] Such "healthy" growth is undoubtedly greased (if not fueled) by the fact that more and more insurers are now covering the procedure (provided that a physician determines it to be medically necessary).[37]

At the same time, the system's economic structure has hastened the closure of several diabetes prevention centers that had recently been established at a number of New York hospitals. What is particularly disturbing is that these innovative prevention centers were shut down not because they had failed their patients, but simply because they had failed to make money.

> Though regarded as medical successes, they lost money because the preventive care did not pay.... They were victims of the Byzantine world of American health care, in which the real profit is made not by controlling chronic diseases like diabetes but by treating their many complications.... Day in and day out, for example, doctors

and hospitals reap financial rewards by performing diabetes-related amputations, which are nearly always covered by insurance, experts say. But little money is available for the sort of preventive education that might have saved a foot in the first place.... It's almost as though the system encourages people to get sick and then people get paid to treat them.... In other words, our financial success in part depended on our medical failure.[38]

The prevention-unfriendly financial incentives in the system are hardly mysterious. Prevention is simply not as profitable as treatment because insurers and consumers are not willing to pay as much for care that is not a "sure thing." That is, the cost of investing in prevention is immediate and apparent, while the benefits often do not become apparent until the quite-distant future. In the case of an insurance company, there is also the added risk that the returns may accrue not to the investor, but to others, for example, when people switch jobs or insurers, sending any savings from preventive measures to competitors.[39,40]

Patients are also more inclined to pay high prices on high-tech fixes or when severe health consequences are imminent (e.g., for a bypass surgery). But when the danger is distant or when the benefits may not be apparent for a year or two, there is less willingness to make the investment (e.g., for nutrition counseling that could potentially prevent that bypass). This helps further undercut prices and profits in prevention programs.[41]

It is no wonder, then, that while the United States spent close to $2 trillion on health in 2006—or 16 percent of the gross domestic product (GDP)—less than 1 percent of that sum was spent on protecting health and preventing the illnesses and injuries that require health care services in the first place, according to Julie Gerberding, director of the Centers for Disease Control and Prevention.[42]

Obviously this needs to change. Unless we put the business of prevention on a more competitive footing with acute care, health experts warn, diseases such as obesity and diabetes are going to rage out of control. In contrast to treatment decisions and practices, the leverage here lies outside medical care and the marketplace; it lies with public policy.

Several national groups are already pressing for government intervention to restructure the health care system's financial and reimbursement structure. Such a restructuring, some experts propose, could be kick-started if government insurance programs like Medicaid began paying more for preventive efforts, a move that the private sector would be likely to follow.[43,44]

That would certainly help. However, public policy will need to look for answers beyond incentives alone. Disregarding the socioeconomic and physical environment in which the individual must live and attempt to maintain a healthy weight, even with the best incentives, would leave people struggling against an environment that is increasingly promoting overeating and sedentary behavior.[45] Thus, an important and necessary role for public policy is to create supportive macroenvironments that make healthy choices about energy intake and energy expenditure easy to make. Indeed, that is where the government may have its greatest leverage.

I explore some of these possibilities next.

Make Healthy Choices the Easy Choices

While the focus in treating disease is naturally on individuals and how to help them, success in obesity prevention will require a combination of two approaches: an individualistic orientation to help people manage their individual risk factors, in conjunction with efforts to "de-obesify" the environment in which people must live and in which they attempt to maintain their health.

> Historically, epidemics have been controlled only after environmental factors have been modified. Similarly, reductions in population levels of obesity seem unlikely until the environments which facilitate its development are modified.... If the macroenvironment [remains] obesogenic, [prevention] programs aimed at influencing individual behavior can be expected to have only a limited effect.[46]

Our physical and social environments provide us with the context in which to live our lives, such as what we eat, and how we work, play, and move around, all of which affect energy intake and expenditure. As I argued in earlier chapters, what we decide to eat is not only a matter of personal preferences, but also very much a function of what food is available in the variety of food outlets we have access to in our communities. Similarly, our choices concerning physical activity are simultaneously a function of lifestyle choices and the characteristics of our environment. These characteristics, it is important to remember, are of our own making.

Unlike nonhuman species, people are affected by more than the physical characteristics of their environment. Cultural and economic dimensions also play a role, affecting our attitudes, beliefs, and values relating to both food and physical activity. For example, in our environment of abundance, what foods people favor is a function not only of what foods are available, but also of the way food is marketed and priced and the value people place on convenience and price.[47]

That obesity was never a common health problem throughout most of human history suggests that our asymmetric energy and weight-regulating system does not ordain obesity—in the "right" environment. The challenge and opportunity for public policy on obesity prevention are to create supportive environments for making the healthy choices the *easy* choices for people, and, although this is a challenge, it is not "mission impossible." Let's not forget that communities, workplaces, schools, and many other venues are already subject to federal, state, and local government regulations that affect many of the environmental determinants of poor diets and sedentary lifestyles. Hence, the government has significant leverage and opportunity to modify government policies and programs to make the environment more conducive to healthful diet and activity patterns.[48]

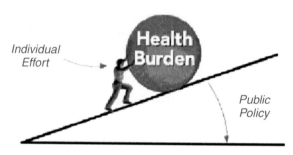

Figure 23.1 Public policy could substantially ease the burden for making health choices. (*Source:* Adapted from Milstein, B. (2008). *Hygeia's Constellation: Navigating Health Futures in a Dynamic and Democratic World.* Atlanta, GA: Syndemics Prevention Network, Centers for Disease Control and Prevention.)

Public Works to Level the Playing Field

An Ounce of Prevention is a Ton of Work.

—Paul Frame, cited in Clancey, C.M. and Kamerow, D.B. (1996). Evidence-based medicine meets cost-effectiveness (Editorial). *JAMA*, 276, 329–330

To effect broad-scale change in health behavior, government policies and programs will have to address environmental determinants of both "energy input" (link 1 in Figure 23.2) and "energy expenditure" (link 2 in Figure 23.2). That includes both the physical characteristics of the environment—matter and energy—as well as the cultural and economic dimensions (such as incentives) that shape our attitudes, beliefs, and values relating to food and physical activity (link 3 in Figure 23.2).

The good news is that obesity-prevention efforts along all these fronts have already begun nationwide. Below, I provide a sampling of the ongoing efforts (experiments) to use the levers of public policy—legislative and regulatory— to encourage broad-scale healthier lifestyles.

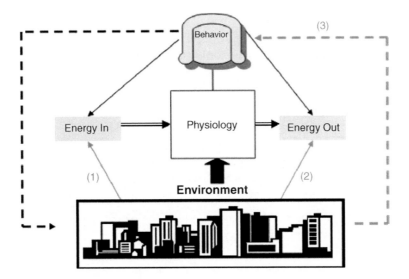

Figure 23.2 Three targets for government intervention

Energy Input

On the energy-input front, a primary target for government prevention programs has been schoolchildren. While adults certainly have the power to change their eating patterns, a growing body of evidence suggests that our childhood experiences powerfully program much of how we eat and what we like to eat.[49,50] Thus, prevention experts have long argued that children present the best window of opportunity to markedly influence lifelong eating behavior and consumption patterns.[51]

The most convenient and cost-effective setting for reaching large numbers of children and, indirectly, their families is the school, where healthy diet messages can be reinforced every day and children can practice making healthy food choices.[52] Furthermore, because most public-school students consume a large proportion of their total daily energy while at school, public schools directly, and significantly, affect the quality of food consumption for large numbers of children. Almost all public schools participate, for example, in the National School Lunch Program (NSLP), a $10 billion federally assisted meal program providing free lunches to more than 27 million public-school children each school day, and approximately seven million pupils utilize the National School Breakfast Program (NSBP).[53] It has been estimated that "meals from these programs [constitute] more than half the daily caloric intake for children who participate in both programs, particularly for those from low-income families."[54]

Children's health advocates argue that schools should not make unhealthy food available, at any time, at any place, in any amount,[55] and that all foods served in schools should meet accepted nutritional content standards.[56] Many school districts are now taking the lead to achieve just that:

> New York City, with the nation's largest school system, is using its clout to extract concessions from the food industry ... to reduce the fat and sodium content. In 2003, New York cut the fat content of lunches served at school by 30% and started offering free breakfasts to every student, ensuring they start the day right.... Los Angeles and Philadelphia have barred sales of junk food and soda in all public schools, and New Jersey is proposing a similar ban.[57]

The U.S. Congress is also moving to amend the National School Lunch Act to do on a national level what many of these school districts have been trying to do locally. In the last few years, Congress has passed several amendments requiring schools to provide only healthful food and to explicitly prohibit the sale of fatty or sugary foods such as French fries and soft drinks.[58] Starting with the 2006 school year, schools receiving federal lunch subsidies were required to create a wellness plan, a detailed strategy for how nutrition will be provided and taught.

"Thought for Food"

Legislatures are also looking at regulating the way foods are advertised to children. "Thirty years ago Congress banned cigarette ads from radio and television as a public health measure ... [and] smoking has declined ever since."[59] There is a growing belief that the advertisements for low-nutritional-value foods that target children may warrant the same restrictions.

The massive efforts by food manufacturers to encourage us to eat more food undoubtedly play a role in increasing Americans' caloric intake. In study after study, social scientists are finding that exposure to advertising messages that encourage food consumption does indeed increase food intake.[60,61] Advertising also affects food choices, especially those of children.[62,63]

It is estimated that the average American child sees 10,000 food advertisements on television each year, the overwhelming majority of them (more than 90 percent) for foods of poor nutritional quality (e.g., sugared cereals, fast food, soft drinks, and candy).[64] And these advertisements do work. There is clear evidence that repeated exposure to commercials for particular types of foods fosters children's preferences for those foods. For example, a number of investigations have revealed that "children's requests for foods were [directly] related to the frequency with which children saw the foods advertised on television."[65]

In 2006, the Institute of Medicine (IOM), an influential group of experts chartered by Congress to provide health-policy advice, issued a landmark report titled *Food Marketing to Children and Youth: Threat or Opportunity?* The report called for sweeping changes in the marketing of foods and beverages to children. Citing experiences of countries such as Sweden and Norway, which have maintained virtual bans on advertising to children since the early 1990s and have consistently shown low levels of childhood obesity, the report called on trade groups to develop and enforce marketing standards that support healthful diets.[66] If voluntary efforts fail to work, it recommends that Congress enact legislation blocking the showing of ads for high-calorie, low-nutrient foods during children's TV shows.[67] Stay tuned.

Economic Incentives

While the government can regulate school meals, it cannot aim to improve the general population's diet by seeking to control the nation's food supply. What it can do, however, is try to affect people's food preferences by manipulating relative food prices through taxes or price subsidies.[68]

Government has a long history of using taxation as a lever to discourage the consumption of products deemed to be unhealthful.[69] Excise taxes, for example, were imposed on tobacco and alcohol products and have been demonstrated to influence consumption.[70] In principle, food taxes could similarly alter the hierarchy of food prices, for example, increasing the relative cost of unhealthy foods to make them economically less attractive.[71]

In practice, however, manipulating food prices through tax policy has proven to be more problematic, much more so than taxing tobacco, for example. One major reason: "There are millions of foods and food products, and distinguishing among them [has been] terribly difficult, and politically divisive."[72] Taxation of foodstuffs also needs to be considered much more cautiously because, unlike tobacco, food is essential to life and because food consumption patterns differ by income, gender, race, and cultural background. This means that a price change may have very different effects on different population groups.[73,74]

In the 1990s, a number of states experimented with the taxation of foods deemed by policy makers to be unhealthful; there was an 8.25 percent tax on "nonessential" foods in California, a 5 percent snack food tax in Maryland, and a 7 percent tax on "nonnutritious" foods in Maine. These were all relatively hefty (some say onerous) tax rates that, not surprisingly, were largely unpopular. Eventually, all were repealed. They were widely criticized for being regressive, meaning that they affected the poor more than the rich, were arbitrary in their classification of foods, and were difficult for retailers to impose.[75,76]

More recently, a different taxation strategy has been slowly gaining traction, one deemed far more appealing and certainly politically more realistic. Rather than imposing a substantial tax burden on a commonly purchased product such as food, the new approach is to levy relatively small taxes, not to deter or penalize, but to generate revenue that could then be deployed to support health promotion efforts and to subsidize healthy foods.[77,78] The notion, in other words, is to use taxation to encourage positive changes rather than to penalize.[79]

A number of states and municipalities across the country now use this strategy. While the levied taxes, which have targeted primarily soft drinks and snack foods, are small enough (usually several cents per can or bottle) to minimize resistance, the revenues are often many millions of dollars.[80] "Arkansas, for instance, raises $40 million annually from a tax of about 2 cents per twelve-ounce can of soft drink."[81]

Because advocates of the tax-to-encourage-not-to-penalize approach propose that the bulk of the revenues be earmarked for subsidizing healthy foods, an important question is legitimately raised: Can people be influenced to consume more healthful foods if subsidies help lower their prices?[82] The answer, according to a number of controlled studies and experimental public initiatives, seems to be yes. For example, a number of studies conducted in controlled environments, such as workplace and school cafeterias, clearly show that when the prices of healthy foods, such as fruits, vegetables, and low-fat snacks, are lowered, sales of these foods increase.[83] In fact, a recent University of Minnesota study involving 12 secondary schools and 12 work sites demonstrated that it does not take that much of a drop in price to spur more sales. When the Minnesota researchers examined the effect of price reductions on sales of vending machine snacks (at both work sites and secondary schools), they found that, for some snacks, a drop of as little as a nickel spurred more sales. Not surprisingly, greater price reductions were associated with higher increases in sales—often significantly so. For example, when the price of snacks in vending machines was cut in half, sales almost doubled.[84,85]

Similar results were observed in a much larger-scale public policy experiment undertaken by the Finnish government in Karelia, a region of Finland where obesity and heart disease were serious concerns. In the early 1970s, the Finnish government started subsidizing free salads at restaurants and workplace cafeterias in Karelia to make fresh vegetables more widely available and more affordable. Again, the economic incentives worked—the intervention helped double vegetable consumption over a period of several years.[86]

Energy Output

Given the significant contribution of physical inactivity in modern society to the obesity problem, many experts believe it is imperative that the promotion of physical activity be at the heart of prevention efforts. However, with the near-ubiquity of energy-saving devices at home, at school, in the workplace, and in our neighborhoods, public policy makers will have a lot to overcome in providing Americans with opportunities for physical exertion that are both attractive and convenient.[87,88]

Obviously, the challenge here is to accomplish that without trying to force society to "go back in time." For example, it would be undesirable, as well as infeasible, to attempt to engineer physical activity back into our modern, non–labor-intensive occupations. Nor is it necessary. Increasing physical exertion can certainly be achieved without giving up the convenient modern lifestyle we have created for ourselves. A good place to start is with structured environments such as schools and workplaces, where an infrastructure already exists to provide the opportunities, means, and appropriate incentives for energy exertion.[89]

Schools are an ideal place to provide opportunities for physical activity because they reach most children and adolescents, provide a safe location, and can ensure that students receive a minimum amount of physical activity on a regular basis.[90] School programs are also important because they can build in a proclivity for regular physical activity that often persists into adulthood.[91] But the schools need the government's help. The pressure to raise academic scores in a time of shrinking education budgets has, over the last several decades, squeezed out many physical education programs. It has been estimated, for example, that at the moment, only 6 to 8 percent of America's schools provide daily physical education.[92] That is way too low. The federal government could help here by creating financial incentives for the states to expand opportunities for physical activity in schools, not only for physical education, but also for activities such as intramural and interscholastic sports programs, after-school sports, and health-related fitness programs.[93]

Similarly, for adults, the structured environments of workplaces provide many opportunities to encourage the adoption of active lifestyle behaviors.[94] With more than 100 million Americans spending the majority of their day at a worksite, the workplace is a convenient and cost-effective place at which to reach a large number of people. Furthermore, the social structure of the workplace allows people to support one another and positively reinforce behavioral change.[95] The government can help here, as well; for example, it can effectively subsidize physical activity by offering tax incentives to businesses to provide exercise opportunities for their employees.[96] An alternative tack, of course, would be to resort to penalties. Figure 23.3 provides one such example, a 2008 law enacted by the Japanese government requiring companies and local governments to meet specific health targets or else incur severe financial penalties.

Because work-site and school physical activity programs will not be an option for some adults, changes at the community level may also be necessary to further induce physical activity in the population. This can be carried out through a variety of means, but a good starting point is to encourage and support the use of walking and bicycling as alternatives to car use. Federal studies show that approximately 25 percent of all trips we make are a mile or less, and yet we make 75 percent of these trips by car.[97] The state of Minnesota provides a good model for what governmental prodding can do to change that. The state has instituted a full-time bike coordinator to oversee the state's Comprehensive State Bicycle Plan. The plan, probably the most progressive in the United States, provides robust and stable funding for education and safety programs, as well as the development of on-street and trail facilities. The result: "Minnesota adults [hike] at twice the national average . . . and almost half of the 300 million miles hiked per year are for transportation."[98]

In many cities and towns, a shift to walking and bicycling as alternatives to driving is unlikely to occur unless the cities and towns are retrofitted to facilitate that. Government initiatives and incentives are needed to promote the changes, and numerous options exist, such as zoning ordinances for the protection of open spaces, regulations that restrict inner-city centers to foot or bicycle traffic, and policy and capital investment priorities that promote the development of cycleways and walkways.[99,100] As communities are built or rebuilt, local governments could also ensure that amenities such as sidewalks and cross-walks that promote safe walking are included in any new construction or renovation. For example, "[M]uch like environmental impact assessments are required to assess the impact of building projects on natural resources, a similar 'healthy environment' impact assessment could be required to ensure that the physical environment is built to provide the opportunity to engage in healthy behaviors in that community."[101]

Demonstration projects in a variety of communities are underway:

In New York City, . . . a feasibility study [is underway] for a greenway that would extend along 5 miles of the [South Bronx] shoreline, creating a public waterfront with cycling and walking paths and recreational activities. . . .

At the other end of the spectrum, Stapleton, a planning community near Denver [is] being built from the ground up to support active living. Stapleton is located on 4700 acres of land where Denver's old airport used to be . . . [and will have 20,000–30,000 residents]. . . . Design plans call for smaller housing lots but with more parks, and open space, and with shops, restaurants, theaters, and workplaces within walking distance of homes and apartments.... [E]verything's accessible, and it's easy to walk or bike to do what you need to. About 80% of people now working in Stapleton use alternative modes of transportation.[102]

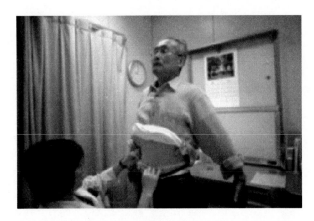

Figure 23.3 A lesson from Japan: government clout. Japan has undertaken one of the most ambitious campaigns ever by a nation to slim down its citizenry. "Under a 2008 national law ... companies and local governments must now measure the waistlines of Japanese people between the ages of 40 and 74 as part of their annual checkups. That represents more than 56 million waistlines or about 44 percent of the entire population. Companies (like Matsushita and NEC) must measure the waistlines of atleast 80 percent of their employees. Furthermore, they must get 10 percent of those deemed overweight (those exceeding government limits of 33.5 inches for men and 35.4 inches for women) to lose weight by 2012, and 25 percent of them to lose weight by 2015. If they fail to meet their targets, a company like NEC could incur as much as $19 million in penalities." (*Source:* Onishi, Norimitus. Japan Seeking Trim Waists, Measures Millions. *New York Times,* June 13, 2008. Photo credit: Ko Sasaki, *New York Times,* Redux.)

Often Preventable But Rarely Prevented

Changing our physical environment to help make healthy choices easy may be necessary for obesity prevention, but it will not be sufficient. As the next two chapters show, to succeed, we also need to change people's mental models.

Winning the "mental" prevention battle is particularly important and particularly challenging in the case of obesity because it is such a slowly building threat; for most people, weight gain typically occurs slowly, over decades. (Remember the boiling frog syndrome?) So a gradual increase in body weight might not be recognized until people are trapped in an unhealthy lifestyle, which can ultimately result in chronic obesity.[103]

The next two chapters discuss how maladaptation to slowly building threats and other mental impediments help explain one of the sad paradoxes of obesity—that it is often preventable, but rarely prevented. The next two chapters discuss how to overcome those impediments.

Location, Location, Location: Places to Intervene in Systems

24

Behavior Change Cannot Be Legislated

As we saw in the previous chapter, public policy has multiple roles to play in disease prevention. An important role is to create supportive environments in which it becomes easy to make healthy choices in both energy intake and energy expenditure. While this will be very helpful (almost necessary) in obesity prevention, reengineering our environment will not, by itself, be enough. Reducing the national waistline will require a "metanoic" jump (see Chapter 1),[104] entailing new ways of thinking and acting in managing our instincts, even as we reengineer our environment.

In public health policy, there has been a long tradition of, and a logic to, relying on so-called passive structural solutions—interventions that aim to "achieve objectives for the good of society and the people in it without requiring individual behavior change and perhaps even without the knowledge of the individual."[105] Such passive solutions, which achieve change even without the knowledge of the individual, have worked for public health interventions in sanitation, air pollution, and food fortification. But they do not work for obesity. Unlike the air we passively breath, personal energy balance is a product of deliberate lifestyle choices about how much and what to eat, and how much energy to expend and how to do it. Although human body weight regulation does reflect the outcome of interactions between people and their environment (social, economic, physical), it is human decision making (e.g., about food, work, and play) that modulates such interactions.[106]

Thus, eliminating environmental barriers to healthy food choices and active lifestyles does not, by itself, prevent obesity in the population. We must recognize that the government cannot legislate exercising more, and it cannot pass a law to force us to turn down that slice of chocolate cake.[107] No matter how many sidewalks we build or how many healthy food buffets we arrange, it will not be enough if people are not motivated to use them.[108]

T.K.A. Hamid, *Thinking in Circles About Obesity*,
DOI 10.1007/978-0-387-09469-4_24, © Springer Science+Business Media, LLC 2009

In this chapter and the next, I will argue that a significant impediment to obesity prevention has been people's persistent, widespread misconceptions about human weight and energy regulation. People's health behavior, as with all human decisions, is very much influenced by our mental models—those deeply ingrained assumptions and generalizations we form of ourselves, others, and the things with which we interact. These cognitive constructs, as was explained in earlier chapters, shape not only how people make sense of the world (looking back), but also what goals they set (looking forward) and how they act to achieve them. It is through our mental models, for example, that we define the risks we face and how we act in response—for example, whether or not to engage in prevention efforts.

Lessons from Managing America's *Other* Energy Problem

America's other energy problem is its oversized appetite for oil. Reducing oil consumption has long been an explicit and worthy goal in public policy, both to protect the environment and to reduce America's dependence on foreign oil, which many believe increases the nation's exposure to geopolitical risk.

Public policy interventions to rein in Americans' excessive oil consumption provide interesting parallels to obesity prevention as well as valuable lessons. As with public health policy, the government has had an array of options for inducing change, from regulations on car manufacturers to tax incentives for achieving efficiency in fuel consumption. In 1978, for example, Congress set minimum corporate average fuel economy (CAFE) targets for all carmakers. (These currently are set at 27.5 miles a gallon for cars and 21.6 for SUVs and other light trucks.) Over the last three decades, these CAFE targets have proven remarkably effective in prodding the industry to develop and introduce new fuel-efficient technologies. Some of the new engine innovations include designs that use four valves for each cylinder (which allows more power from a smaller, lighter engine) and computer-controlled fuel injection (which increases efficiency and cuts pollution).[109]

One of the most promising innovations has been the development of hybrid technology. With two power sources—one a gasoline-powered internal combustion engine, the other a battery-driven electric motor—the new hybrid cars are designed to run on battery power in lieu of the gas engine when driven at low speeds in local driving. As a result, these hybrids offer the potential to consume less fuel and emit fewer pollutants than most conventional automobiles.[110] Indeed, since their introduction, hybrids have, as hoped, deliver superior fuel economy. Examples of this first generation of hybrids include the two-seat Honda Insight (introduced in December 1999), which had a rating of 70 miles per gallon (mpg), and the five-seat 55-mpg Toyota Prius introduced a year later.[111]

With such impressive mpg numbers, federal, state, and local governments, not surprisingly, have been bending over backward to encourage the sale of hybrids, offering "a bewildering array of tax breaks, traffic lanes, and parking spaces dedicated to hybrid owners."[112] To many, beating the nation's oil addiction appeared tantalizingly close at hand.

The logic (or mental model) underlying this optimism and the government's initiatives to push hybrid cars is fairly straightforward. It may be captured by the simple loop in Figure 24.1 and it goes something like this: (1) Americans' average fuel consumption is higher than what the government would like it to be. → (2) To close the gap between the government's goal and the actual gasoline consumption levels, the government initiates tax breaks and other incentives to induce consumers to switch to fuel-efficient hybrids. → (3) The incentives increase the demand for hybrids. → (4) As more and more drivers switch to the smaller, more fuel-efficient hybrids, the average car size and horsepower drops, and ultimately → (5) fuel efficiency increases to the desired level.

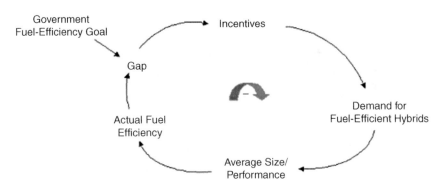

Figure 24.1 The "mental model" driving the government's intervention

The loop in Figure 24.1 represents the archetypical feedback structure of goal-seeking behavior: we compare the state of a system with our goal(s), and if a discrepancy or gap is detected, we take corrective action to close the gap and bring the system in line with the goal(s). Such a feedback process encompasses many of our conscious and subconscious decisions and underlies all goal-oriented behavior.

V. Prevention and Beyond

Initially, the results of the government's initiatives were immediate and dramatic. In four of the first five years, 2001 through 2005, hybrid sales approximately doubled, with demand for the popular models, such as the Prius, far outstripping the limited supply. In many parts of the country, for example, buyers were paying a premium to get a Prius ($1,000 to $3,000 above the advertised price), while on the used-car market, it was not unusual to pay full sticker price for a used hybrid—a practice, according to automotive experts, rarely seen outside the trade of Ferraris and other super sports cars.[113]

But while "green," environmentally conscious consumers were snapping up hybrids, the market remained quite small in absolute terms, representing about 1 percent of new vehicles sold. By 2006, reports in the media were suggesting that demand for hybrids was starting to cool off.[114]

Even more surprising, the big hoped-for improvement in fuel economy was not materializing. Indeed, fuel economy actually declined. According to the Environmental Protection Agency (EPA), overall fuel economy in the United States increased from 19.3 mpg in 2004 to 20.2 mpg in 2007 (a 5 percent increase), reversing a long trend of slowly declining fuel economy since the 1987 peak. In fact, the increases in 2005 and 2006 were the first consecutive annual increases in fuel economy since the mid-1980s. What happened? This is a perfect example of what systems scientists euphemistically call "policy resistance," which is a phenomenon frequently encountered with interventions to resolve complex social problems. The policy interventions are diluted or outright defeated because of unanticipated compensating responses—feedback effects—in the system. This tends to happen when policy makers' actions alter the state of the system so that it no longer is in sync with the goals of some of its key players, who then react to restore the balance the new policies have upset.[115]

The compensatory feedback effects that can lead to policy resistance are triggered by a gap between the state of the system and the goals of its key players. *Such a gap can occur whenever we change a system but not the goals, or the goals but not the system.* Either way, the result can be a discrepancy between the state of the system and the goals.

Compensatory feedback and policy resistance are neither new nor uncommon in public policy. The history of public policy is littered with failed efforts at change because of unanticipated compensatory feedback, from road-building programs that create suburban sprawl and actually increase traffic congestion, to flood-control efforts, such as levee and dam construction, that lead to more severe floods because they encourage people to build homes and live in flood-danger zones.[116] It happens every time we focus on the physical system but fail to change the players' goals, and it happened with the fuel-economy efforts. Interventions to improve fuel economy required one "minor" detail—American drivers had to play along. That is, they had to buy into the government's fuel-economy goals. Because hybrid technology works best in smaller vehicles, that meant that drivers had to be willing to sacrifice some pep and size in their new cars. It was a sacrifice, however, that American drivers were not willing to make. They still wanted bigger vehicles and ones that accelerate faster, and they were not willing to sacrifice any of that to go "green."

As noted above, policy resistance tends to arise when the compensating responses are *unanticipated,* and hence unplanned for. Figure 24.2 shows how the government's hybrid initiatives triggered compensatory feedback effects that were unanticipated—hence, "below the waterline"—and how they worked to undercut the push for the gas–electric hybrids.

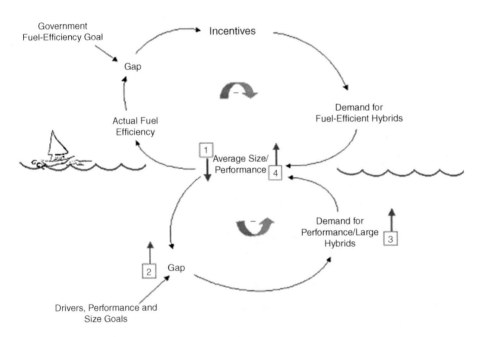

Figure 24.2 "Under the surface" compensatory feedback undercutting the government's initiatives

The lower loop in Figure 24.2 captures a chain of reactions starting in the years 2000–2001, when the hybrids were first introduced. These initial hybrids, such as the Insight, the Prius, and the hybridized Civic, were all smaller in size and lower in performance than the average American car. (The Honda Insight, for example, was a two-seater, and in the hybridized Civic, the standard 1.7-liter engine was replaced by a 1.3-liter engine.) The drop in size and performance of this first generation of hybrids, relative to the average market, is indicated in the figure with the downward-pointing arrow 1. Because people's preferences for greater acceleration and power remained largely intact, this meant that there was a gap between what most customers desired and what was being offered (upward-pointing arrow 2). The car-makers, who are fairly adept at sizing up their customers, undoubtedly recognized the gap between customer needs and actual product offerings. They could hardly have missed the fact, for example, that, while hybrids were being snapped by "green," environmentally conscious consumers, the market remained quite small in absolute terms. This created pressure on manufac-turers (upward-pointing arrow 3), who ultimately responded by increasing the average size and performance of their hybrid offerings (upward-pointing arrow 4).[117]

It was an amazing U-turn. To give customers the performance and size they wanted, carmakers started using the hybrid technology not to make cars that go farther on a gallon of gasoline, but to make a new generation of hybrid vehicles that accelerate faster.[118] To do that, they simply took the same gas–electric hybrid technology and turned the knob toward performance. Here is how that was done with the Honda Accord:

> The 2005 Honda Accord hybrid gets about the same miles per gallon as the basic four-cylinder model, . . . and it saves only about two miles a gallon compared with the V-6 model on which it is based. Thanks to the hybrid technology, though, it accelerates better. In the Accord, the mechanism was simple. Honda took the model with the 3.0-liter V-6 engine, which generates 240 horsepower, and added a 16-horsepower electric system. (That is in contrast to the Civic, in which Honda pulled out the standard 1.7-liter engine and replaced it with a 1.3-liter engine when it made a hybrid version of the car.) Combined with the electric drive, the car's horsepower remained roughly constant.. . . The main benefit is in getting from zero to 60 miles per hour in 6.9 seconds, compared with 9.0 seconds for the basic four-cylinder model. [Consumers] got what they wanted from the Accord, a hybrid with no sacrifices—not performance, amenities, or space.[119]

The Accord hybrid is not alone in using technology for power; the Toyota Highlander and the Lexus RX330, two premium vehicles, both gained horsepower when they were produced as hybrids. By using the technology for power at the expense of fuel economy, this new generation of hybrids saves hardly any fuel.[120] Rather, it represents the other face of hybrid technology, "the face that gets a big grin when the foot goes down on the accelerator."[121]

Hybrid technology, then, ended up being used in much the same way as earlier under-the-hood efficiency innovations: to satisfy the unwavering American appetite for room and zoom.[122] Greater fuel efficiency—the very thing that would reduce America's oil dependency, as well as its contribution to global warming—has taken a back seat. Again.

So, is hybrid technology ultimately a good thing or a bad thing? Has it worked, or did it fail? These are not the right questions to ask. As with any technology, it all depends on who is wielding it and for what purpose or goal. The important lesson here is that, when it comes to having an impact on oil consumption, the driver is more influential than the car. Without changing the mental models and goals of American consumers, all the fuel-efficiency inventions in the world may not make much difference.[123]

Leverage Points

Professionals who manage change in complex social systems have a great interest in "leverage points," which are places within a complex system—whether an economy, an ecosystem, a corporation, or a living body—where interventions can lead to significant and enduring improvements,[124] and where interventions produce the most bang for the "intervention buck" (see Figure 24.3).

There are usually many places to intervene in a system, but only a limited number of them are leverage points. The late Donella "Dana" H. Meadows, a pioneering American environmental scientist, teacher, and writer, was among the first to systematically classify different intervention strategies into classes and to formally describe which classes are most and least effective.

In "Leverage Points: Places to Intervene in a System,"[1] one of her best-known essays, Meadows argued that policy makers typically target intervention strategies that are relatively low-leverage, including the use of incentives (such as taxes and subsidies), regulating standards of conduct (such as the CAFE regulations for fuel economy), and regulation of information and its flows (e.g., nutritional food labeling and advertising to children). Higher-leverage interventions, which are less obvious and certainly less common, are the interventions that target the goals and shared paradigms in social systems.

By paradigms, Meadows meant the shared ideas and unstated assumptions—unstated because everyone knows them—that constitute society's deepest set of beliefs about how the world works. Her concept of paradigm, thus, constitutes a sort of meta-version of the notion of mental models I use in this book. Meadows's paradigms, in our nomenclature, are simply the aggregates of a society's widely shared mental models. Meadows offers the following examples of "shared ideas and unstated assumptions" in American culture: money measures something real and has real meaning, so people who are paid less are literally worth less; growth is good; one can "own" land; evolution stopped with the emergence of *Homo sapiens;* and the selfish actions of individual players in markets

---

[1] Meadows, D. (1999). Leverage Points: Places to Intervene in a System. The Sustainability Institute, Hartland, Vermont. http://www.sustainabilityinstitute.org/pubs/Leverage_Points.pdf

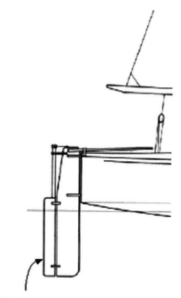

Trim tab on main rudder

Figure 24.3 The trim tab. "The principle of leverage—Where a small push can lead to a big move—is often exploited in physical systems. A wonderful mechanical illustration of that is the *trim tab*. On a large ocean-going ship, the large volume of water flowing around its large rudder makes it difficult to turn. A trim tab is a small 'rudder on the rudder' of the ship. Its function is to make it easier to turn the large rudder, which, then, turns the ship. When the trim tab is turned to one side or the other, it compresses the water flowing around the rudder and creates a small pressure differential that 'sucks the rudder' in the desired direction. The large rudder, then eventually steers the ship. The larger the ship, the more important is the trim tab." (*Source:* Senge, P.M. (1990), pp. 61–65. *The Fifth Discipline: The Art and Practice of the Learning Organization.* New York: Doubleday/Currency. Illustration courtesy of Scanmar.)

wonderfully accumulate to the common good. As was argued in earlier chapters, such cognitive constructs shape not only how people in a society make sense of the world, but also what goals they set and how they act to achieve them.

The oil-consumption case discussed above demonstrates well Meadows's point about the critical significance of goals and mental models. Consider, for example, how differently things could have transpired had the government chosen to target and had been successful in altering society's goals. Had American drivers been turned around to buy into the government's goal for better fuel economy, they could very well have taken the initiative to achieve that even without the benefit of new technological innovations by, for example, car pooling, using public transportation, or simply switching to smaller, lighter, and more efficient cars. Fuel-efficient conventional cars, we should note, were already (and still are) available with mileage ratings comparable to those of the hybrids; for example, the conventional gasoline-powered Honda Civic delivers 40 miles per gallon on the open road. (In the case of obesity prevention, we know that such cognitive strategies can work, even in the absence of macroenvironmental change. The best evidence of that comes from the many individuals in the National Weight Control Registry [NWCR] who have succeeded in losing weight and maintaining a weight loss in the current environment.[125])

As we have seen, when public policy interventions fail to address society's existing (dysfunctional) paradigms, not only are they often diluted and resisted, but they may also be twisted and mangled to serve the very behaviors they were intended to disrupt. Again, oil consumption provides a good case in point, for that is exactly what happened to the pro-hybrid laws and incentives: they ended up effectively subsidizing the *unintended* use of gas– electric hybrid technology for power and performance rather than to cut fuel consumption.

What about those generous tax incentives? They ended up rewarding the suburbanite who buys, say, a hypothetical hybrid Dodge Durango that gets 14 miles per gallon instead of 12, while the buyer of a conventional gasoline-powered Honda Civic that delivers 40 miles per gallon got no reward.[126] Even Congress's well-intentioned CAFE regulations meant that each hybrid sold became a free pass for its manufacturer to market and sell a few extra gas guzzlers because that's what their customers desired.

To get the most bang for our "intervention buck," we need to target society's mental models because that is where the the impact can be dramatic and enduring as well as immediate.

> [P]eople who have managed to intervene in systems at the level of paradigm have hit a leverage point that totally transforms systems ... whether it was Copernicus and Kepler showing that the earth is not the center of the universe, or Einstein hypothesizing that matter and energy are interchangeable.
> In a single individual it can happen in a millisecond. All it takes is a click in the mind, a falling of scales from eyes, a new way of seeing.[127]

Leveraging Paradigms . . . and Succeeding

The concept of feedback is fundamental to the processes of leverage and resistance and is key to understanding why goals play important roles in both. *Negative* feedback, for example, is often the primary driver of policy resistance in social systems. We saw that in the oil case, in which a goal-seeking negative feedback loop, driven to seek a goal that was inconsistent with the intervention, acted to resist the intention of the government policy.

But goals can also work to reinforce policy interventions. When the mental models of the players in the system are changed so that their goals are in sync with the aims of the policy, they can create a positive feedback that reinforces, rather than resists, intervention, which is what happened in Karelia, Finland.

The story began in the late 1960s, when an epidemiological study comparing the health status of residents of eastern and western Finland to other populations around the world concluded that Finnish men had the highest rates of heart-disease mortality in the world. The worst situation was found in the province of North Karelia in eastern Finland, a rural province with 180,000 inhabitants.[128,129] The major culprit was the typical Finnish diet, which is high in saturated fats and salt and low in unsaturated fats, vegetables, and fruit.[130] The results of the study were quite a shock to Karelia's residents and civic leaders, who were so alarmed that they petitioned the Finnish government for assistance in organizing some kind of intervention.[131]

In response, a massive intervention effort was launched in 1972 in the province of North Karelia, with the primary goal of transforming people's existing dietary habits. In collaboration with the World Health Organization (WHO), the North Karelia Project developed a comprehensive community-based strategy to prod and facilitate change in the public's dietary habits, specifically to reduce their intake of saturated fat, especially from dairy sources, and to increase their consumption of vegetables and fruit. All key sectors of the community were engaged, including health care organizations, schools, voluntary organizations, businesses, the food industry, and the local media.[132] It was a massive and integrated approach encompassing nutrition counseling, behavioral skill training, and social and environmental support, with sometimes subtle persuasion thrown in (by featuring role models in the local media). In addition, the government sought to nudge people in the right direction by subsidizing free salads at restaurants and workplace cafeterias.[133]

On the surface, the mental model underlying the government's effort (Figure 24.4) is not unlike that of the oil consumption case. (1) Consumption of healthy foods was lower than what the government wanted it to be. → (2) To close the gap between the government's goal and the actual consumption

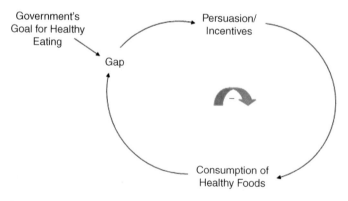

Figure 24.4 The "mental model" driving the government's intervention

levels, persuasion and incentives were deployed to induce consumers to switch to healthy diets (high in vegetable and fruit content). → (3) The persuasion and incentives increase the consumption of healthy foods. → (4) And, ultimately, health food consumption increases to the desired levels.

Unlike the oil consumption case, however, the Karelia intervention did work as intended. It took several years, but fruit consumption eventually doubled in Karelia and the consumption of vegetables almost tripled.[134] Perhaps most rewarding of all, these changes contributed to a 73 percent decline in cardiovascular disease.[135]

What happened under the waterline? Dr. Bobby Milstein of the U.S. Centers for Disease Control and Prevention (CDC) provides the following postmortem analysis of the project:

> There is no doubt that the talents and persistence of world-class health professionals were crucial to the project's success. But the engagement of ordinary citizens who felt connected to and angered by the tragedy of so many early deaths galvanized the entire effort, transforming it from an ad-hoc disease prevention project into a serious cultural movement for better health that continues even today.... Many creative innovations were devised not by experts with technical training in health care or public health, but rather by citizens who were moved to ask themselves, "What can I do to make it easier for people in North Karelia to be healthy?" To that straightforward question came an array of astonishing answers. Bakers devised lower-fat loaves, working for years to perfect breads that had less salt, more fiber, and still pleased their customers' palates. Sausage makers added mushrooms to their products to increase vegetable consumption. A food scientist at the University of Helsinki discovered a breakthrough way to lower cholesterol in margarine and immediately approached the dairy and margarine industries so that they could incorporate his discovery. No one directed the baker, sausage maker, and food scientist to pursue innovations that would make it easier for their fellow citizens to eat more healthfully, but they did. *They regarded the entire population's health as a goal worthy of their own work with themselves, their families, and their nation as beneficiaries* [emphasis added].[136]

The initial alarming revelations about the mortality rate from coronary heart disease and bleak prospects of a relatively low life expectancy, in combination with the government's massive campaign to change Karelians' hearts and minds, created enough of a one–two punch to cause a profound shift in awareness. This meant that, under the waterline, people's collective goals would now be in sync with the government's, and their behavior would now reinforce rather than resist change.

Figure 24.5 shows how the persuasion and incentive policy (the top loop) triggered reinforcing feedback effects ("below the waterline") that augmented the intended effects of government policy. By making healthy foods widely available and giving people the incentive to try them, the government

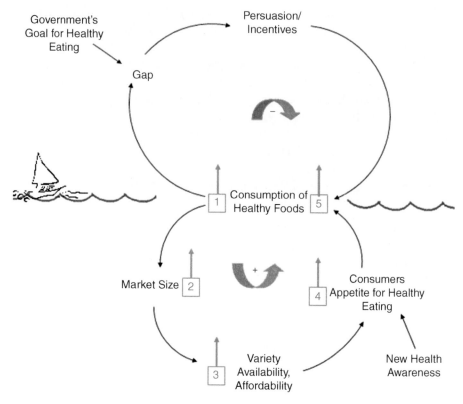

Figure 24.5 'Under the surface" feedback reinforcing government policy

encouraged people to develop a taste for them and, ultimately, increase their consumption of them. The upward-pointing arrow 1 indicates the increase in (government-induced) demand for and consumption of vegetables and fruits. To satisfy the growing demand for healthy foods, the food industry started to develop, with great creativity, a whole range of low-fat and cholesterol-reducing products. For example, "[i]n the 1980s, low-fat milks and fat spreads promoted by the Project were joined by low-fat cheeses, ice creams, sausages, etc. A specific innovation was the development of a plant-sterol-containing margarine, which was very effective in lowering blood cholesterol."[137] The increase in the variety and availability of healthy food products made it much easier for people to succeed in changing their diet and ultimately led to an increase in market size for such foods (upward-pointing arrow 3). As the demand for healthy foods picked up speed and the industry grew in size, market competition and economies of scale further spurred innovation in the development, packaging, and delivering of these foods, while also driving their relative prices lower and increasing affordability (upward-pointing arrow 4). The wider variety of choices and lower costs further increased the new demand (appetite) for healthy foods (upward-pointing arrow 4) and ultimately inducing more consumption (upward-pointing arrow 5).

With Karelians' *new* healthy-oriented diet goals now in sync with the government's intervention, a positive virtuous cycle was born, one that amplifies and reinforces, not resists or counteracts, the initial favorable change.

It is important to take note here of a significant difference between Figs 24.2 and 24.5. Notice that in the former, the last arrow that closed the loop, arrow 4, pointed up, thus opposing the initial change that was applied to the system (which was downward-pointing arrow 1). That is the telltale sign of a negative loop in action, where an initial change triggers a series of actions and responses that ultimately oppose that initial change. In Figure 24.5, by contrast, the original change (which was up for arrow 1) was reinforced as it propagated around the loop, ultimately pushing consumption further up (arrow 5).

That is the power of reinforcing feedback: a change in one direction (triggered, in this case, by government intervention) triggers reinforcing pressures that propagate around the system to produce further change in the same direction. What makes paradigm changes a particularly potent catalyst in this system is that once a shift in thinking takes hold, its implications extend way beyond a single individual. The Karelia experience provides a perfect example of that. As more and more people switched to healthy foods, their collective healthy behavior ultimately reshaped their collective environment, which, in turn, further reinforced their behavioral change. That is the power of leverage.

Back in the United States: A Challenge and an Opportunity

> The achievements in North Karelia are a source of optimism and envy in the United States, where health protection efforts ... did not yield results anywhere near as dramatic, comprehensive, nor sustained as these.[138]

In Eastern Finland, transforming the public paradigms about diet and well-being was instrumental to the government's success in inducing (and sustaining) change. By comparison, U.S. disease-prevention efforts, specifically those targeting obesity, have not yet been as successful. Mental models continue to get in the way.

A recent Harvard University study examining public attitudes toward obesity and obesity policy has shed light on the incongruence between the views and goals of public health authorities and those of the American public, and how the disconnect may be undermining obesity-prevention efforts.[139] Using unique survey data collected for the study, the Harvard researchers found that, contrary to the views of health experts, most Americans do not view obesity as a major health concern, either for the country as a whole or for themselves in particular. It was found, instead, that the general public ranked highly publicized and emotionally charged conditions, such as heart attacks and AIDS, as much bigger threats to health than obesity. (This finding is in line with numerous other public surveys in which AIDS was consistently ranked far ahead of obesity as the more serious health concern, even though obesity is a source of far more deaths than AIDS.) The researchers also found that most Americans viewed obesity as primarily the result of individual moral failure—lack of willpower to stick to a diet and exercise program—rather than environmental or physiological influences.

A public that is not seriously concerned about obesity and that still views obesity as a private matter and the result of individual failure could not be expected to tune in to the prevention message; nor would it be expected to support bold public policy initiatives to change behaviors and the environment. Not surprisingly, then, the Harvard study found that most Americans "express relatively low support for obesity-targeted policies." That is the bad news about the status of obesity prevention.

The good news for the prospects of obesity prevention, however, is that we may require only a relatively small "trim tab" to turn this ship around. The reason for this optimism is purely scientific: the energy gap that prevention efforts need to close in the population is quite small and manageable.

Obesity typically develops gradually over a relatively extended period of time. For example, research studies suggest that most people tend to put on weight at the slow rate of 2 pounds a year.[140] This suggests that, in most of us, obesity results from a strikingly small but sustained energy imbalance.[141],[142] This small energy differential is what prevention efforts need to target. (Note that, by contrast, when obesity is fully developed, the energy gap to reduce weight down to healthy levels can be substantial.) Hill et al.[143] estimate that "most of the weight gain seen in the population could be eliminated by some combination of increasing energy expenditure and reducing energy intake by 100 kcal/day." For a typical adult with an energy intake of 2,000 to 2,500 kcal/day, this is only a 4 to 5 percent change in total daily energy levels. Hence the opportunity and reason for optimism: behavior changes needed to close such a slight caloric gap are quite achievable. "For example, energy expenditure can be increased by 100 kcal/day just by walking an extra mile each day.

Similarly, it is possible to reduce energy intake by 100 kcal/day (if people could be induced to eat just a little less)."[144]

The next two chapters discuss why achieving this seemingly simple change has eluded us, and what to do to change that.

It Will Take More Than Food Pyramids

25

"Educate Them and They Will Change"

To date, the bulk of public-health interventions have relied on education to change health behaviors, by aiming to inform the public about which behaviors are good for them and which are not. The premise is that once the public "gets it," people will abandon unhealthy lifestyle behaviors and adopt those that are deemed to be good for them.[145] To take a few liberties with the famous line from the film *Field of Dreams*,[146] the belief is that "if you educate them, they will change." The primary means for accomplishing this has been reliance on population-oriented health communication campaigns that could be disseminated to a wide audience.[147,148]

Half a Century of Government Education

As early as 1952, the American Heart Association identified obesity as a cardiac risk factor modifiable through diet and exercise. This prompted a number of federal agencies and private organizations devoted to general health promotion to issue guidelines advising Americans to maintain a healthy weight by reducing energy intake, raising energy expenditure, or both.[149] Some landmark initiatives/guidelines subsequently followed:

- The Dietary Guidelines for Americans, issued in 1980 by the Department of Health and Human Services jointly with the Department of Agriculture, was among the first. Aiming to reduce the risk for major chronic diseases, it provided dietary recommendations to the public based on the current scientific knowledge. The guidelines were revised in 1985, 1990, and 1995, and now Public Law 101-445, section 3, requires publication of the dietary guidelines at least every 5 years. The sixth edition of the dietary guidelines

T.K.A. Hamid, *Thinking in Circles About Obesity*,
DOI 10.1007/978-0-387-09469-4_25, © Springer Science+Business Media, LLC 2009

was released in 2005 and continues to form the basis of federal food and nutrition education, and information programs.[150]

- In 1988, the first Surgeon General's Report on Nutrition and Health was published, declaring overweight and obesity to be one of the most prevalent diet-related problems in the United States.[151] In January 1991, the National Heart, Lung, and Blood Institute (NHLBI) of the National Institutes of Health (NIH) launched the Obesity Education Initiative (OEI) to help reduce through education the prevalence of overweight and physical inactivity.

- In 1990, the U.S. Department of Health and Human Services issued Healthy People 2000, a health-promotion and disease-prevention agenda for the nation. It was the second in a series of 10-year plans (the first was issued in 1979) and outlined specific goals to be achieved by the year 2000. Among its 10-year goals was reducing the rates of overweight among adults and adolescents (which appeared second in order only to prevention of cardiovascular disease).[152,153]

- The latest in the series, Healthy People 2010, was introduced in 2000, with a new set of health objectives to address the nation's health problems at the start of the new millennium. Healthy People 2010 places an even greater focus on overweight and obesity and outlines specific objectives to be achieved by 2010, including reducing the proportion of adults who are obese to 15 percent (from 31 percent in 2000), and reducing the proportion of children and adolescents who are overweight or obese to 5 percent (from approximately 15 percent in 2000).[154]

- And then, of course, there is the Food Pyramid. First introduced in 1991 by the U.S. Department of Agriculture (USDA), was touted as a significant step forward over the old four-basic-food-groups color wheel that it replaced. Reacting to a growing body of nutrition science and a population more sophisticated about food and health, the USDA unveiled a new and improved Food Pyramid in April 2005. The pyramid now comes in twelve versions (with new variations by activity and age) to educate Americans more precisely about their nutritional needs.[155]

The government's guidelines have also been emphasizing exercise and physical activity, in addition to nutrition. For example, in Healthy People 2010, the section on physical activity and fitness appears at the top of the list of twenty-two priority areas for behavior change. In March 2004, Health and Human Services Secretary Tommy Thompson launched a nationwide public-awareness campaign, dubbed "Small Steps," to try to educate Americans about the importance of physical activity and regular exercise.[156]

The concept of providing the public with more information seems intuitive; who would oppose it? Yet, while it seems to make perfect sense, the record does indicate that "most of these [educational] intervention programs have been disappointing in terms of obesity and weight control."[157] Why?

It Is Not Working

U.S. News & World Report published a special 11-page section warning the nation. "There is deep concern in high places over the fitness of American youth," the magazine's report began. "Parents are being warned that their children—taken to school in buses, chauffeured to activities, freed from muscle-building chores, and entertained in front of TV sets—are getting soft and flabby."

The date of that report was August 2, 1957. Nearly 50 years later, the hand-wringing continues, but now it is compounded by concerns about an obesity epidemic.[158]

The assumption (and hope) that informing the public in great detail about the potential risks of obesity, poor diet, and inactivity would automatically lead to behavior change was too optimistic. Despite the government's concerted educational efforts and a plethora of guidelines (and pyramids), the dietary and activity behaviors of Americans appear to have improved little, if at all, in the last several decades.[159] In any practical sense, the quest to control and prevent obesity cannot be considered a success.[160]

A look at the record to date reveals that the message has been loud and clear, but it has had minimal effect. On the one hand, the government's health initiatives to educate and inform the public have been quite successful in reaching large numbers of people, yet, on the other, they have not, for the most part, demonstrated the ability to modify people's behavior.[161] It is estimated, for example, that more than 80 percent of Americans recognize the Food Pyramid, and yet such recognition has not done much for the American diet. According to the USDA, only 2 to 4 percent of Americans eat according to its principles. Indeed, "[i]n the years since the pyramid was introduced, obesity rates have climbed in every state."[162] That is the irony of America's obesity epidemic: at a time when Americans arguably know more about food and nutrition than at any time in their history, they are gaining more weight.[163] The exhortations to eat right and shed pounds have not scared people away from unhealthy food.

Americans are eating hamburgers, doughnuts, French fries, and fried chicken like never before.... Apparently, all the talk about obesity causing clogged hearts, hypertension, high blood pressure, and even diabetes is falling on deaf ears.... In fact, fried chicken ... is the fastest-growing fast-food menu item in the last decade.... Yes, fried chicken: KFC has been going gangbusters. [In March 2005, KFC] introduced the Snacker, a 99-cent chicken sandwich that proved to be a runaway bestseller. The 5,525 KFC restaurant outlets in the U.S. sold 100 million Snackers in the [first] seven months, making it one of the most successful product launches in KFC history. But while Americans are digging in to the fried chicken, they're certainly not eschewing other fatty foods. Hamburger outlets served over 500 million more customers in 2004 than in the previous year. And doughnut shops served about 150 million more people [in 2004] than in 2003.... What's going on?[164]

Critics commonly attribute the failure to promote behavior change not to the government's educational approach per se, but rather to the message—both its quality and quantity. With regard to the quality of the message, it has been suggested that the government's educational initiatives over the last half-century have been notable for their "banal recommendations and lack of creativity."[165] Many of the government's guidelines, critics argue, have tended to state the obvious. "For example, the [second edition of the] otherwise landmark 1977 Senate report on diet and chronic disease prevention, *Dietary Goals for the United States*,... [advises]: 'To avoid overweight, consume only as much energy [calories] as is expended; if overweight, decrease energy intake and increase energy expenditure.'"[166]

A big part of this quality problem, critics have long argued, is that the government's health education message is all too often compromised by political pressures from the food and agriculture lobbies. As a result, Congress and federal agencies cannot muster anything but "completely uncontroversial" recommendations.[167] An illustrative example of political compromise in action is the way the Senate Select Committee led by George McGovern was pressured, in 1977, to reword its original warning to "reduce consumption of meat," ultimately turning it into "choose meats, poultry, and fish that will reduce saturated fat intake."[168]

A second critique that is often leveled at the government's message is a quantity issue—that the message (even if banal and uncreative) is being swamped by competing messages from the food industry designed to increase food consumption. The food industry is second only to the auto industry in total advertising spending—spending to the tune of $7 billion annually. No government agency seeking to promote dietary advice has the funds to compete with that. It is estimated that for every dollar the government spends on nutrition education, the food industry spends thirty to advertise its products.[169] The primary targets of the advertisements are children, the most vulnerable audience. In 2003, for example, the USDA spent $10 million on school-based nutrition education for children (on its Team Nutrition program), which was less than half the $25 million budget for the initial phase of a new campaign to sell a single brand of candy bar, the wildly popular Milky Way.[170,171]

It Is Deeper Than Just That

While both critiques raise legitimate concerns about the message, they do not provide an adequate explanation for the ineffectiveness of the government's educational initiatives. As I will argue, there is a more fundamental flaw in the strategy itself, in relying on a didactic educational approach to public health prevention and its underlying premise that knowledge alone is enough to change people's ingrained mental models and, ultimately, their behavior.

Although the notion that knowledge shapes behavior seems reasonable, the evidence to date suggests that merely providing information does not have much effect on changing health behavior.[172,173] In the words of Bill Layden, an executive at Porter Novelli, the designers of the food pyramid, "We don't expect people to learn how to drive a car by showing them an icon. . . . Changing how people eat is going to require a whole lot more than one [pyramid] image."[174]

The best evidence of the inherent weaknesses of the educational strategy is experimental evidence. A number of experiments have been conducted over the last 25 years to assess the efficacy of large-scale standardized educational interventions. These studies have consistently shown that even when the educational message was not sanitized under political pressure and was able to provide sound and objective nutritional advice, and even when it was delivered persistently over prolonged periods of time, to ensure that it registered and was not muffled by advertising, it still did not have a positive lasting effect on people's behavior.

One of the best known controlled intervention studies, aimed specifically at preventing weight gain in adults, was the Pound of Prevention (POP) study conducted in the 1990s in Minneapolis and St. Paul and two adjacent Minnesota suburbs. This was a randomized experiment designed to evaluate an educational approach to obesity prevention that focused on reducing weight gain rather than encouraging weight loss.

> Volunteers for POP were randomized to a treatment group or a no-treatment control group. . . . Intervention subjects received an educational program comprised of monthly newsletters (2-4 pages) for 3 years encouraging regular weighing, eating more fruits and vegetables (eat two servings of fruit, and three servings of vegetables each day), reducing fat intake, and increasing exercise (walk three times a week for at least 20 minutes). Additional opportunities for more intensive education, such as classes and contests, were offered twice a year. Half of the people in the intervention arm of the trial also participated in an incentive program designed to encourage them to read the newsletter (a $100 lottery drawing was held each month for members of the incentive condition who returned their monthly newsletter postcard . . . to encourage participants to open and read their newsletters and thus learn about weight gain prevention). Participation in the POP

intervention over the 3 years of the study was good ... and there was objective evidence of learning.[175]

The POP experimenters set out to demonstrate the efficacy of a cost-effective, relatively standardized, educational intervention applied to many people. Unfortunately, the educational intervention was not successful in preventing weight gain. At the end of the 3-year POP trial, there were no significant differences between the treatment groups, with all groups having gained a small amount of weight over the study period.[176]

Another experiment conducted during the same era was the California Five-A-Day for Better Health campaign. This was an intensive 5-year statewide campaign to promote increased fruit and vegetable consumption among Californians. After 5 years of an intensive statewide intervention, a careful program evaluation showed that, while there was widespread awareness among Californians of the importance of eating more fruits and vegetables, this awareness did not result in any measurable behavior change. "There was no increase in fruit and vegetable consumption in any population group."[177]

There is also ample evidence that the failure of these experiments is not a cultural issue. Similar results were obtained when comparable education-based initiatives were attempted elsewhere. The Active for Life campaign, believed to be the largest public health intervention attempted in Europe, was a 3-year intervention conducted by the former Health Education Authority (HEA) of England to promote moderate-intensity physical activity in everyday life. The multifaceted intervention, which ran from 1996 to 1999, included a variety of mass media communication components, as well as support for health care and public health professionals who developed and promoted localized, community-based physical-activity programs. Postcampaign evaluations showed that, "after three years, there was no evidence that the campaign improved physical activity, either overall or in any subgroup."[178]

These are sobering results from what were touted to be state-of-the-art communication initiatives.[179] They suggest that educational prevention strategies are unlikely by themselves to reverse the obesity epidemic, at least not in their current form.

We need to move beyond the bankrupt mass communications knowledge-accretion model of prevention, in which the aim is to stuff people's heads with nutritional guidelines and food pyramid images, to a customized knowledge-restructuring model that challenges people's deeply ingrained assumptions about health risk and well-being and that seeks to provide them with the skills and the tools needed to effectively exercise personal control over their health habits and their bodies.

Prevention requires changing our mental models about risk, our bodies, and the strategies we need to use to manage them better and prevent disease.

Prevention is, I believe, fundamentally a deep-learning issue. To many people, learning is primarily an assimilation process, as in learning a new vocabulary word or the spelling of an already known word. We call this form of learning *knowledge accretion,* or the accumulation of facts.[180] It is the easy form. The difficult form of learning is *restructuring*, in which we use new knowledge to form a new (more effective) conceptual structure of a problem or a situation. Learning in this deeper sense is discovery—discovery of mental maps and decision rules that are more appropriate to the decision task—and that can be much harder. While accretion is often relatively easy, even automatic, acquiring new conceptual understanding is neither easy nor automatic. As cognitive scientist Donald Norman[181] has argued, it often requires tools "to reflect; to explore, compare, and integrate."

Information Is Not Enough to Change Mental Models

A large part of the discussion in Part III of this book focused on the significant disparities between the widely shared (but highly simplistic) mental models of energy balance (open-loop, static, and linear) and the far more complex reality of human weight and energy regulation (with its feedback, dynamics, and nonlinearities). We also noted in Chapter 24 that recent surveys have continued to find that large segments of the population still view obesity as a private matter and a result of individual moral failure rather than as a function of a changing relationship between our physiology and the environment. Such misconceptions (among others) are important reasons why obesity prevention remains a "hard sell."

Particularly troublesome is the fundamental misconception people continue to have about the energy dynamic between humans and their environment. As I explained in Chapter 7, throughout most of history, human feeding behavior was largely done unconsciously and automatically, and obesity was never a common health problem. That long-term energy balance for our hunter-gatherer ancestors, it is important to understand, arose not out of a symmetric regulatory process or living in a stable environment, but from an asymmetric process that compensated for their unstable and food-scarce environment (akin to obtaining a positive result from multiplying two negative numbers). While our environment has now changed significantly, our "ad-libitum" mental model, like our hard-wired physiology, has not. Most of us continue to instinctively regulate our feeding behavior in accordance with the body's biological drives, but in our modern environment of constant abundance, this behavior no longer serves us well. We continue to eat to our physiological limits when food is readily available and selectively focus on foods high in energy density, and an increasing number of us are paying a big price.

It is the mismatch between our body's asymmetric system of weight-energy regulation and our modern obesifying environment that explains why we are all at risk. Understanding this is crucial if we are to alleviate a heretofore significant impediment to prevention efforts: the "it won't happen to me" illusion that instills in many people a false sense of invulnerability, that is, until they are trapped in an unhealthy lifestyle that ultimately results in chronic obesity.

Such illusions of invulnerability, as noted earlier, have been found across a wide range of diseases and hazards and are not unique to obesity. They are often an attempt to avoid the anxiety one would feel from admitting a threat to one's well-being—a form of defensive denial. In problems such as obesity or drug addiction, which many believe to be caused by behavior or personality, people may feel invulnerable not only as a result of misconceptions of disease causality (as discussed above) but also because they would like to believe that they do not have the weakness of character that allows the disease to develop in them. This mindset becomes a significant impediment to prevention. If people convince themselves that they are invulnerable to becoming obese, then they are unlikely to heed the prevention message and take the appropriate measures to reduce their risk of gaining weight. The "it won't happen to me" mindset gets in the way: Why protect yourself from an event that will not occur?

The persistence of such fundamental misconceptions, despite the drumbeat of educational campaigns and broad publicity about the obesity problem, may surprise many people and must surely frustrate policy makers, but it is no mystery to cognitive psychologists. Research in human cognition has repeatedly demonstrated that correcting mental models is rarely accomplished by new information alone. The path from acquiring information to changing one's mental models is not as direct as we tend to assume. In fact, the process often works in reverse, that is, one's mental models lead to changing the information we receive.[182]

While it may be comforting to believe that our senses reveal the world as it is, that is not how it works in reality. In sensing the world (both the physical and intellectual), we are rarely passive-objective observers; instead, our brains actively construct (model) our world, which affects what we see.[183] Literally. New research in human cognition and perception is now revealing the mechanisms by which this happens.

> [In processing sensory data, information] from the eyes, ears and body is carried to primary sensory regions in the brain. From there, it is carried to so-called higher

regions where interpretation occurs. For example, photons bouncing off a flower first reach the eye, where they are turned into a pattern that is sent to the primary visual cortex. There, the rough shape of the flower is recognized. The pattern is next sent to a higher—in terms of function—region, where color is recognized, and then to a higher region, where the flower's identity is encoded along with other knowledge about the particular bloom. . . .

The surprise is the amount of traffic the other way, from top to bottom. . . . There are 10 times as many nerve fibers carrying information down as there are carrying it up. These extensive [top-down] circuits mean that consciousness, what people see, hear, feel, and believe, is based on what neuroscientists call "top-down processing." What you see is not always what you get, because what you see depends on a framework built by experience that stands ready to interpret the raw information— as a flower or a hammer or a face. . . . If the top is convinced [that the flower you are looking at is hammer], the bottom level of data will be overruled.[184]

The above example illustrates how our expectations can (unconsciously) manipulate our visual perceptions. "Modeling of higher-level knowledge is likewise unavoidable and often equally unconscious,"[185] which sometimes gets us into trouble.

A great deal of research in behavioral decision making has revealed that our mental models do not always function as neutral, objective filters, but instead are often biased by needs and emotions.[186] For example, people often (unconsciously) seek out information that supports their existing instinct or point of view, while avoiding information that contradicts it, a behavior that psychologists call confirmation-seeking bias. This "not only affects where we go to collect evidence but also how we interpret the evidence we do receive, leading us to give too much weight to supporting information and too little to conflicting information."[187] That is why putting out more information—say, via a mass-media campaign to promote increased fruit and vegetable consumption—often fails to induce significant changes in the public's ingrained mental models.[188] Indeed, information from many different sources can prove dysfunctional because people have the tendency to retain information selectively in accordance with their prejudices and to support their preconceived notions.[189] Thus, access to more information tends to increase confidence in judgment, as people assume that their decisions are good because they can find information to support them, but it does not necessarily increase the quality of judgment. For example, "All that many people did on low-fat and fat-free products was gain weight because they figured that fat-free gave them license to eat as much as they wanted, without regard to serving size and calories per serving."[190]

Naturally, the higher the complexity of an idea or image, the more the opportunity for distortion. A pertinent example of that is in the distorted conceptions people can form of illness and disease. In a 1980 groundbreaking article titled, "The Common Sense Representation of Illness Danger," Howard Leventhal, Daniel Meyer, and David Nerenz[II] presented both reasoned argument and empirical data showing that people employ commonsense models of illness—referred to as *implicit theories of illness* or *illness schemata* in the academic literature—to define and explain illness and disease and respond to health threats.[191,192] By means of interviews with hypertensive patients, cancer patients undergoing chemotherapy, and cardiac bypass surgery patients, Leventhal and his colleagues found that lay theories of illness include four common dimensions: (1) *cause*—what factor led to the onset of the disease; (2) *consequences*—the immediate and long-term effects of the disease; (3) *time line*—the temporal course of the disease, its treatment, and whether it will reoccur; and, most fundamentally, (4) disease *identity*— what the disease is (e.g., a common cold vs. pneumonia).[193,194]

Leventhal and his colleagues also found that these multidimensional mental representations of illness play a critical role in determining how people respond to health threats—and whether they do that appropriately or inappropriately. For example:

> Kaplan[III] and Matthews et al. (1981)[IV] found that the chief factor determining heart attack victims' delay in seeking treatment (often a matter of days) was failure to label their symptoms as a heart attack (*identity*). A woman finding a lump in her breast may fail to seek medical treatment either because she does not interpret the lump as a sign of cancer, or because she does but fears the only *consequences* of the disease (death, or mastectomy) of which she has knowledge. Leventhal and Nerenz (1982)[V] report that hypertensives who believe their disease is acute rather than chronic (*time line*) are more likely to drop out of treatment. [And] several researchers have found that attributing responsibility (*cause*) for severe accidents or cervical cancer to oneself rather than to chance influences the effectiveness of coping strategies adopted by the patient.[195]

Thus, people's conceptions of disease can be distorted along all four dimensions, and such distortions have important implications on how

---

[II] Leventhal, H., Meyer, D., and Nerenz, D. (1980). The common sense representation of illness danger. In: Baum, A., Taylor, S.E., and Singer, J.E. (Eds.) *Handbook of Psychology and Health*, Vol. 4 (pp. 219–252). Hillsdale, NJ: Erlbaum.

[III] Kaplan, G.A. (1981). Understanding the understanding of heart attack: patient and physician perspectives. Paper presented at the 89th Annual Convention of the American Psychological Association, Los Angeles.

[IV] Mathews, K.A., Siegel, J.M., Kuller, L.G., Thompson, M., and Varat, M. (1981). Determinants of seeking medical care by myocardial infarction victims. Paper presented at the 89th Annual Convention of the American Psychological Association, Los Angeles.

[V] Leventhal, H. and Nerenz, D. (1982). Representations on the threat and the control of stress. In: Meichenbaum, D. and Jaremko, M. (Eds.). *Stress Prevention and Management: A Cognitive Behavioral Approach*. New York: Plenum.

people react (or *mis*-react) to disease or the threat of disease. Obesity is no exception.

Perhaps the most striking distortion is that of the identity dimension, arguably the most transparent and objective dimension. It would seem that educating people to acknowledge and accurately assess their weight status would surely rank among the most achievable prevention goals—an assured public awareness "homerun." And yet, a number of studies have demonstrated significant gaps between people's assessment of their weight status and their actual status. In one recent study, researchers sifted through data from the third National Health and Nutrition Examination Survey (NHANES III, 1988–94) to assess the degree of agreement between individuals' *actual* weight status, as measured by their body mass index (BMI), and their *perceptions* of their weight status. The researchers found that large segments of the U.S. population seriously misperceived their weight status. Interestingly, overweight men, not women, were the major culprits, with 43 percent of the overweight male subjects failing to correctly perceive that they were overweight and, instead, reporting themselves as being "about right" or underweight.[196] Significantly, for both the men and the women, the mistakes were not just at the margin (when weights were a few pounds over the overweight cut-off point); many of the mistaken perceptions were of quite large discrepancies.

Another identity-related, and potentially serious, distortion is the finding that parents of overweight children systematically underestimate their children's weight.[197] In one study, for example, "only 21% of the mothers of overweight, preschool children recognized their child as overweight."[198]

Misperceptions about weight have direct implications on people's perceptions of risk—for themselves or their children. Such misperceptions, health experts agree, are formidable roadblocks to prevention efforts.

> Information programs linking overweight and obesity with health risks might fail to induce diet and lifestyle changes if individuals fail to recognize they are overweight or obese. . . . For example, upon receiving information about the connection between weight status and health risks, a prudent individual might make diet and lifestyle changes to lose weight, hoping to reduce the health risks. However, health information programs might fail to induce this type of behavior if overweight individuals do not believe they are overweight. These individuals will assume that the message is intended for someone else. In this case, the people most in need of changing their diet and lifestyle will not do so.[199]

These findings about a dimension as basic, straightforward, and objective as identity can only serve to underscore the limitations of public education campaigns and the challenges facing prevention efforts.

It is clear from the record that the fundamental "information problem" is not too little information (i.e., *accretion*), but too little knowledge *restructuring*.

Learning from Experience: A Bad Second Option

When prevention education fails to prompt people to abandon unhealthy behavior, they often learn the consequences of unhealthy behavior the hard way: from experience.

Experience was certainly a major driver for change in Karelia, Finland. Recall that, at the time of the intervention, Finnish men were already experiencing the highest rates of heart disease mortality in the world. The alarming revelations about mortality rates and the bleak prospects of relatively low life expectancy came as a wake-up call to the citizens of North Karelia and its civic leaders, enough so that they prompted the whole community to swing into action for change.

> Looking back from our vantage point today, it is easy to see how much public strength [for change] was already present when the citizens of North Karelia ... began organizing a serious response. They were outraged, but in a constructive way.[200]

People learn many things through first-hand experience: how to walk, how to ride a bicycle, and not to touch a hot stove. "We act, observe the consequences of our action, and adjust."[201] This form of learning through direct experience has one important thing going for it: the learning experience is highly personalized. This is undeniably a big advantage when it comes to learning about health prevention, for it can help soften a heretofore-stubborn cognitive barrier to health prevention: the pervasive and enduring "it won't happen to me" illusion. By contrast, when people are lectured to in traditional mass-media–type health campaigns, what they typically hear is information about general, population-wide health risks,[202] not personalized information about their own susceptibility.

The downside to relying on first-hand experience to learn about how best to regulate our health behavior is that it is a risky, and even hazardous, proposition, because when it comes to our health, the ill effects of mistakes can be hard, if not impossible, to reverse. Thus, the price we pay for learning a good lesson can be too high in terms of morbidity and even death!

Relying on real-life experience to learn about health behavior can also be a bad deal for a second important reason. Even when the high price of misbehavior is paid in pain, suffering, and financial cost, the lessons from our experience (our payback) can be illusive.

Learning-by-doing works well as long as the consequences of our actions are rapid and unambiguous. For some conditions this is indeed the case. An example is when failure to control blood sugar levels causes a type 1 diabetic to lapse into unconsciousness. In such a case, the immediate unambiguous lesson could help those afflicted become more vigilant.

But in a system as complex as our human physiology, interventions typically induce a wide range of responses. Some are quick and immediate, while others are slow in developing, taking months or even years. The type 1 diabetic again provides a good illustration of the immediate-versus-delayed responses. Besides the immediate risk of lapsing into unconsciousness (even death), the disease also carries long-term risks that may not surface for years, including kidney failure, heart disease, and blindness. When someone smokes a cigarette, eats a piece of chocolate cream pie, or has unprotected sex, not all of the consequences are immediately evident. Yet, all of these actions can have potentially serious longer-term consequences for that person's well-being.[203] In such situations, when cause and effect do not occur close together in time, the learning process breaks down, because most of us assume that cause and effect *are* close in time and in space.[204] Experiences in everyday life deeply ingrain in us the expectation that the cause of a symptom is to be found nearby and immediately before the observed consequence.[205]

> From earliest childhood we learn that cause and effect are closely associated. If one touches a hot stove, the hand is burned here and now. When one stumbles over a threshold, the cause is immediately seen as not picking up the foot high enough, and the resulting fall is immediate. All simple feedback processes that we fully understand reinforce the same lesson of close association [in time and space] of cause and effect. However, those lessons are aggressively misleading in more complex systems.[206]

When dealing with complex systems such as our bodies, our inferences regarding causal relationships between actions and outcomes become increasingly problematic because causes may be far removed in both timing and location from their observed effects. After a long delay, consequences often are not easily traceable to the actions that produced them. As a result, we often fail to learn from our mistakes.[207] That is certainly a potential complication with obesity prevention, where the initial development of overweight comes with few major health side effects, and there is often a long lag time before its cumulative ill effects become evident.[208]

In addition to delays, the messiness of real-life experiences often causes ambiguity. Ambiguity arises whenever changes resulting from our decisions are confounded by simultaneous changes in other variables that we do not control.[209] For example, consider a newly promoted executive who starts exercising less regularly because of increased time pressures and, as a result, starts gaining weight. Ambiguity may arise because the outcome of her action (exercising less) may be confounded by a host of other changes in her situation, such as changes in the amount or quality of her diet (perhaps because time pressure also causes her to eat out more), smoking initiation or cessation, travel, increased stress on the job, and even contracting a disease or infection. The bottom line is that there are too many ways to explain why a certain outcome (say, gaining 20 pounds by the end of her first year in the new job) occurred.

Thus, in situations involving complexity, delay, and ambiguity, learning a good lesson from raw, real-life experiences can be difficult, as well as hazardous to our health.

Lessons from Business: Learning About Risky Stuff Without Experiencing the Risk

As I have argued, prevention is essentially a learning issue. The aim is to change people's mental models about risk, their bodies, and what strategies to use to better manage their health so as to avert disease. In a fundamental sense, it is not unlike learning to manage risk in business or in engineering, to maintain the long-term "health" of a complex organization or system. As with human health, changes in the business environment (whether technological, competitive, or regulatory) can cause a mismatch between an organization's environment and its current business practices or strategies. Thus, in business, as in health, the need to adapt shared mental models can also be a matter of life or (organizational) death.

How do companies learn to manage risk and avoid costly mistakes? As with health, learning from experience is always a default option. In many organizations, for example, postmortems are common business rituals, conducted after a new project or strategy has failed so as to understand why it happened and learn from the experience. However, just as in health, relying on direct experience to learn about failure is not necessarily the smartest option.

> If knowledge and skills could be developed only by direct experience, the acquisition of competencies would be greatly retarded, not to mention exceedingly tedious and hazardous.[210]

In recent years, technology-savvy organizations have become increasingly smarter at exploiting new information and modeling technologies to enhance their learning skills. In place of postmortems, for example, these companies are conducting "premortems" at the beginning of a project or new initiative to help identify the risks at the outset, which makes a lot more sense.

> A premortem is the hypothetical opposite of a postmortem. A postmortem in a medical setting allows health professionals and the family to learn what caused a patient's death. Everyone benefits except, of course, the patient. A premortem in a business setting comes at the beginning of a project rather than the end, so that the project can be improved rather than autopsied.[211]

One effective way to do this is by using "management flight simulators" (also known as virtual microworlds).[212] Analogous to the flight simulators that pilots use to learn how to fly a new aircraft, a management flight simulator is essentially a computer-based microworld of an organization and its business environment. It provides a virtual practice field for managers to imagine and rehearse the future and experience the long-term consequences of planned actions.[213]

For several decades now, pilots have been required to train for many hours on flight simulators before they are allowed to fly a new aircraft. A great deal of the training time is devoted to "experiencing" catastrophic failure, such as stalling or overshooting a landing, in order to learn how to avoid it.[214] One great advantage of these virtual flights is that "'crashing' hurts no one, and [pilots] walk away every time, better prepared for a real emergency."[215]

Managers can now do the same. Thanks to the availability of affordable, high-quality computing capabilities and increasingly user-friendly software interfaces, management flight simulators have now been acknowledged, and rightfully so, as a revolution in learning and training about complex systems. Training experts agree that simulators work because they help overcome many of the barriers to learning we face when learning from raw, real-life experiences. In a flight simulator, for example, feedback is quick and unambiguous. By compressing time and space, simulators allow us to experience more clearly the consequences of our actions, even the consequences that would normally occur months or years hence. Whether in learning to fly an aircraft, manage disease, or run an organization, a flight simulator provides a computer-based microcosm of reality in which it is safe for the learner to fail—and repeatedly if necessary. Indeed, flight simulators are the only practical (and ethical) way to "experience" disaster in advance of the real thing.[216] Furthermore, the learning experience can be highly personalized by tailoring model parameters to a specific organization or project, even to an individual.

But perhaps the flight simulator's most important learning virtue is that it makes perfectly controlled experimentation possible. In the model system, unlike in real-life experiences, the effect of changing one factor can be observed while all other factors are held unchanged. Real life offers no such control: Many variables change simultaneously, confounding the interpretation of a system's behavior and reducing the effectiveness of learning. (Controlled experimentation, it is important to note here, can be particularly useful in personal health regulation since experimentation on our bodies is often unadvisable, too slow—because consequences of lifestyle choices often take months or years to manifest—or just plain infeasible.)

The absence of adequate control in real-life experiences, where causes and effects must be disentangled through sheer subjective judgment instead of objective experimentation, leaves the question of cause and effect ambiguous and leaves us vulnerable to our own self-serving biases. That is when wishful thinking, the desirability of outcomes, and other irrational factors can easily warp our interpretations.[217,218]

No wonder, then, that flight-simulator–based learning applications are quickly catching on. Today, companies such as Cisco Systems and Canon are spending millions on virtual "practice fields" to train their employees.[219] They use this technology not only for conducting premortem-type exercises, but also to instill new business and technological skills in the organization. Management flight simulators, for example, have helped raise maintenance productivity in companies in the chemicals industry and boost service quality in the insurance industry, and they are helping top management in high-tech petrochemicals reformulate their strategies. That is why MIT's John Sterman boldly predicts that "flight simulators may someday be as integral a part of the learning process for managers as they are today for pilots."[220]

Likewise, in the military, the use of simulators is inducing a sea change in training. According to the trade publication *Military Training and Simulation News*, the U.S. Department of Defense spends about $4 billion each year on simulation and training equipment.[221] Today, U.S. troops are practicing on simulators not only how to use their ever more complex equipment, but also how to work in teams, move efficiently through a battle space, and negotiate a wide range of conflicts. At the Pentagon, military strategists increasingly rely on *military* flight simulators to test strategic options before launching a campaign in earnest. The result, according to a task force of the U.S. Defense Science Board, has been nothing less than remarkable, for example, attributing low U.S. casualties in recent conflicts such as Desert Storm to the growing use of training simulators. In its 2000 report, Training Superiority and Training Surprise, the task force concluded that "the new combat training approach ... develops, without bloodshed, individuals and units into aces."[222]

But while microworlds continue to make impressive inroads in business and the military, their use in health education remains limited. Yet, as I've argued, health is precisely the setting where complexities are the most problematic and where the stakes are the highest. So, it is hoped that this will change soon.

As I sought to demonstrate in Part IV, it is now possible to build simulation models of human physiology that faithfully mimic our bodies' functions. These types of models, which we can call *physiological* flight simulators, can serve as personal laboratories for learning about and assessing the long-term consequences of our lifestyle choices, and, just as with a pilot's flight simulator, one can do that without risking life or limb. Indeed, the interface I developed for the simulation model discussed in Part IV was designed to give the touch and feel of flight simulator software, with their dials, buttons, and graphics. The interface is shown in Figure 25.1.

The next section and Chapter 26 explain why such tools can be particularly effective in helping people see (and *believe*) the specific health risks they face, which is key to disease prevention.

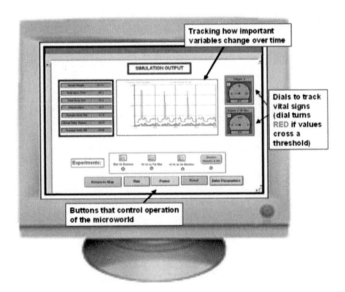

Figure 25.1 The interface of my "physiologic flight simulator"

Transforming Prevention from a Spectator Sport to a Contact Sport

People's perceptions of personal risk and their beliefs about their suscept-ibility to harm are key determinants to self-protective behavior,[223] which is precisely why the communication of health-risk information has always been a primary goal in prevention efforts. While there is little argument over the wisdom of that goal, the question of how best to communicate health-risk information remains open to debate.

The traditional approach has been to disseminate, as widely as possible, assessments of population-wide risk information about the disease or health hazard. Such assessments are impersonal by definition, providing people with population-based probabilistic indicators such as "the average person's risk of developing some disease is one in 500," rather than with personalized information indicating their own susceptibility.

This approach has not worked very well. As already noted, the record indicates that informing the public, even in great detail, about population-level potential risks has led to less behavioral change than hoped. We are starting to understand the reasons why. Studies are showing that successful communication of health-risk information "may make people aware of the risks posed by a particular pattern of behavior, but it might not change their behavior."[224] Even when people believe the message about the risk of some hazard to the population, they may not recognize the risk as personally relevant, thanks to their formidable arsenal of defensive psychological routines.[225]

Numerous studies covering a wide range of hazards and disease condi-tions have demonstrated that people systematically underestimate their personal health risks.[226] This so-called optimistic bias, also referred to as *illusion of unique invulnerability,* causes people to rate their own risk of experiencing a health problem as less than that of their peers or of the average person.[227] Though comforting, such illusions can be risky. Unrea-listic optimism in matters of health and disease often leads people to ignore legitimate risks to their health and avoid taking necessary measures to offset them.[228,229]

Such misconceptions are difficult to dispel with impersonal and general information about health risks. As long as the misconceptions persist, people will be less inclined to adopt precautionary behaviors, no matter how edu-cated they are about the risk to the population or the dire consequences of the disease.[230]

If risk information is to effect changes in people's health behavior, it must be conveyed to them in a manner they can relate to. This means providing them with risk information that applies specifically to them, that prompts them to recognize the links between the very things that they do, or do not do, and unwanted health outcomes.[231] To accomplish this, we must move from a mass-communications model of prevention to more of a "rifle shot" approach that tailors the message to fit each individual—from population-wide statistics to specific information regarding the links between a particular health problem and an individual's prior behavior or medical history.[232]

This concept is not unique to health. Mass customization, as this process is known, is taking root in a wide range of industries. In place of mass production for the increasingly elusive average customer, many businesses are already using state-of-the-art information technology to build and deliver products and services designed to fit the precise specifications of individual customers. As consumers, we have come to expect such customization, and now it needs to happen in health.

Already, a number of studies have assessed the value of customization in the domain of disease prevention. The overwhelming majority of these studies report that tailoring interventions to personal attributes does, indeed, increase the rate of behavioral change.[233] For example,

> Bull et al.[VI] found tailored health education materials to be significantly more effective for weight loss interventions than non-tailored materials. Likewise, Marcus et al.[VII] found that tailored materials were more effective than standard interventions to improve physical activity. In another randomized controlled trial [Marcus et al.] demonstrated that tailored messages improved [healthy food] intake (something that has been very hard to do with traditional media).[234]

What can transform these "rifle shot" intervention experiments from the academic realm to the realm of public policy is information technology. Computer-technology and the rapid rise of the Internet are changing the economic rules of health prevention and enabling customization and interactive communication—both technically and economically. For the first time we now have the tools to build prevention delivery systems that personalize risk information, such as customized health flight simulators, and with the Internet and the Web we have an electronic infrastructure that allows us to tailor these tools (via the facility of interactive communication) to individual users. The

---

[VI] Bull, F.C., Holt, C.L., Kreuter, M.W., Clark, E.M., and Scharff, D.(2001). Understanding the effects of printed health education materials: Which features lead to which outcomes? *Journal of Health Communication*, 6, 265–279.

[VII] Marcus, B.H., Nigg, C.R., Riebe, D., and Forsyth, L.H. (2000). Interactive communication strategies: implications for population-based physical activity promotion. *American Journal of Preventive Medicine*, 19(2), 121–126.

technology allows us to do all this efficiently and economically for large population groups.[235]

With personal computers in almost every home, it is not much of a stretch to foresee a near future where most of these home computers will have, in addition to the word processor and the Internet browser, a customized health flight simulator for each member of the family. A personal health simulator would allow each of us to have, in essence, an imaginary "virtual twin" with which to predict the state of our health under different lifestyle scenarios or health interventions. Unlike the typical population-wide statistics, this "intimate" tool would help people understand how they might develop a health problem and which behavior or personal attributes they might change to prevent it.[236] Furthermore, the specificity of individualized tools would go a long way toward breaking down people's defensive biases, such as that pervasive illusion of unique invulnerability.[237]

In contrast to the electronic medical record, which is another promising information technology that facilitates reviewing the patient's history, a microworld, such as the simulator model discussed in Part IV, is a dynamic *forward-looking* tool that contains the fourth dimension—time. Such forward-looking tools provide us with the facility to "compress time" and experience now the future results of our actions and lifestyle choices. This helps address a second trap, or illusion, that we often fall prey to: a *delay trap*. This is the tendency, often unconscious, to discount the future negative consequences of our actions.[238]

Delays between actions and their consequences tend to cast veils of uncertainty and ambiguity on the future consequences of our actions. Delays, especially long ones, as is often the case in health and disease, make it difficult to imagine the probable effects of our current actions. Obesity is a good example. It is a condition with a complex array of detrimental health consequences, but with most of the adverse effects resulting from the cumulative stress of excess weight over a long period of time.[239] That is where simulator-type tools can provide real leverage in prevention. When the consequences of our lifestyle choices take months or years to manifest, simulation becomes the main—perhaps the only—way we can foresee the long-term consequences of our decisions. With advanced graphics capabilities, these models (unlike the plain graphs in the proof-of-concept model in Part IV) can be built to illustrate vividly the severity of the consequences associated with a health problem.[240] This would help get people's attention. For example, if people could see their own arteries building deposits as they ingest high-cholesterol foods, and then visually "experience" a cataclysmic event in their cardiovascular system 20 to 40 years later, they might be more willing, experts argue, to change their behavior.[241]

It is difficult to visualize the potential, and contemplate the possibilities, of such dynamic tools using the "dynamically challenged" medium of pages of a book. So consider, for a moment, a *mirror*—not a regular mirror, but rather a hypothetical modern type of mirror, one conjured by Michael Schrage in his entertaining book *Serious Play*:

> This mirror is full-length, and you see yourself in it every time you step out of the shower. It can also instantly modify your mirror image in response to voice commands. You can see how you'd look if you lost ten pounds or gained fifteen. If you stopped exercising for two weeks. If you lifted weights three times a week for five weeks. . . . You might . . . ask the mirror to age you by three years or ten years. You could ask for best-case and worst-case versions of various aging scenarios. . . .
>
> How much time would you spend looking at the real you versus images of possible yous? Would the images of possible yous alter how you manage the real you? Would you eat less? Exercise more?. . . . In other words, would the mirror significantly change how you behave?. . . . Would such mirrors truly matter?[242]

Yes, such mirrors would matter profoundly. They would, Schrage argues, utterly transform how people see themselves and their futures (see Figure 25.2). Such a "what-if" mirror, with added simulation capabilities to make it even more dynamic and interactive, is an apt metaphor for the physiological flight simulator I am proposing here.

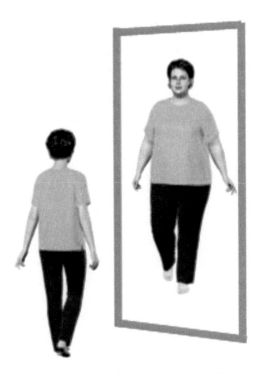

Figure 25.2 A hypothetical mirror. (*Source:* Illustration courtesy of www.mvm.com)

These technological capabilities are not a futuristic vision or wishful thinking. They are closer to becoming reality than you might think. In fact, all the technological building-blocks are available now. At Stanford's Virtual Human Interaction Lab (VHIL), for example, Professor Jeremy Bailenson and his graduate students have some exciting research underway to build such personalized simulation tools and put them into action.[243] One focus of Bailenson's research is the usefulness of virtual reality tools (a form of intimate simulators) to change human behavior, especially health behavior. For example, in a series of laboratory experiments to investigate the impact of interacting with a digital twin or altered self, he has found that the impact on health behavior is both powerful and enduring.

> Experiments in [Bailenson's] lab have shown that what you experience as your digital doppelganger ... bleeds into your real-life identity.... Seeing your altered self ... can actually change the way you behave in real life.... [I]t really does change your definition of self.[244]

In one experiment that is relevant to the obesity issue, Bailenson's team examined how interacting with a digital twin affected exercise behavior. Specifically, that experiment's goal was to assess whether seeing the long-term impacts of physical activity (or a lack of it) on their body would affect people's decisions to become more active. The researchers found not only that it did, but also that the change happened remarkably quickly. These findings, the researchers believe, are potentially highly significant. By building personalized tools that allow individuals to see how exercise benefits their digital-selves—benefits that in the real world are not immediately visible—might help people set more realistic goals and expectations and follow more carefully their health plans in the real world.[245]

"*Virtual* to Your Health"

What I am advocating, then,[246] is a new model for prevention. It is prevention by experiencing and not by being told. It is worth reemphasizing that the new model is not contingent on the development of new technologies. Rather, it is about finding new ways to use the technology we already have.

The logical place to start training people on these tools is in structured environments, such as our schools, where an infrastructure already exists to build the knowledge and the skills to apply the technology.[247] Schools are also where the leverage from starting with young bodies and minds is greatest.

Microworlds Я Us   26

[Children] have played a key role in previous social change movements such as recycling—they learned about why recycling was critical to preserving and sustaining our planet [in school] and they took the recycling mentality home with them and reminded their parents. We need to teach our children at an early age about why physical activity and healthy eating are so important. We need to provide them with the knowledge and the skills to manage energy balance in the modern environment. This would include developing basic understanding about the energy value of food and physical activity and how these work together to determine energy balance.[248]

The findings from studies on childhood obesity intervention suggest that the approach described in the above quotation would be a very wise investment. Several recent studies have found, for example, that young children respond better than adults do to obesity prevention and treatment interventions.[249,250] Particularly interesting was the finding that when children were treated *together* with their parents, "the children were successful in reducing and maintaining their weight loss, whilst over time the adults returned to their pre-study body weight."[251]

Even more encouraging, children's acquired healthy eating and exercise habits have been shown to persist into adulthood. The work of Leonard Epstein and his colleagues at Stanford University provides some of the most compelling evidence to date that positive experiences gained from prevention and treatment endure from childhood through adolescence to adulthood.[252] Following 158 children for 10 years after a treatment intervention, Epstein and his colleagues found that those who received treatment ended up markedly less overweight 10 years later than those who did not.[253,254] (At the time of the initial treatment, the children were 6 to 12 years of age and were, on average, 40 to 50 percent overweight.)

Such results should not be interpreted to mean that children have more self-control than adults. Rather, these results suggest that children's appetites

T.K.A. Hamid, *Thinking in Circles About Obesity*,
DOI 10.1007/978-0-387-09469-4_26, © Springer Science+Business Media, LLC 2009

are malleable, while those of adults may be less so.[255] Much of how we eat and what we like to eat is powerfully programmed by our experiences in childhood, especially during the first 5 years of life. This factor, according to a review by a panel of leading nutrition experts, makes us exceedingly resistant to change as adults.[256] Hence, targeting children allows us to intervene before obesity-promoting behaviors have become well ingrained.[257]

To date, successful childhood intervention studies have typically involved intensive behavior modification over extended periods and often in combination with a diet and exercise program.[258] (For example, the Epstein et al. studies involved an intensive behavior modification treatment applied over an 8- to 12-week period, followed by monthly maintenance sessions over a 6- to 12-month period, and combined with a special diet and exercise program.[259]) Such approaches are quite labor-intensive and expensive and, consequently, are infeasible to scale up—both economically and technically. On the other hand, economically scalable alternative strategies, such as traditional mass communication based approaches, have proven as ineffective with children as they have been with adults.[260–263]

Here is where information technology and computer games can be a real boon to children. As for adults, the new generation of information technology tools would allow us to build effective prevention delivery systems for children that support customization and interaction and to be able to do it efficiently and economically for large populations of children. Indeed, tools such as the health flight simulator may be a more appealing and effective medium for America's new "games generation" children, even more so than they are for the pilot, the business person, or the soldier.

More than in any preceding generation, technology (and especially digital technology) has become an important part of children's lives.[264] Outside of school, the typical American child spends more time—an average of 6.5 hours a day—in front of a screen watching videos, playing interactive games, or surfing the Internet than doing any other activity except sleeping.[265,266] This new tech-savvy generation of American children has already shown "an uncanny ability to make use of computers as routine tools for study and entertainment," and they have consistently said that they prefer them for learning instead of other print or verbal media.[267]

With technology becoming an ever-increasing part of children's lives, it is clear that computer-based health interventions are not only appropriate but also perhaps even requisite for this population. Marc Prensky,[VIII] author of *Digital Game-Based Learning*, who coined the phrase "digital native" to describe this generation, posits that children not only live in a much richer

---

[VIII] Prensky, M. (2001). *Digital Game-Based Learning*. New York: McGraw-Hill.

and distinctly different informational environment than their parents, but also that "this digital environment has helped to shape them into fundamentally different types of thinkers ... requiring a change in messaging methodologies to successfully engage and educate them."[268]

Child's Play

> We don't stop playing because we grow old; we grow old because we stop playing.
> —George Bernard Shaw

Learning by playing is natural for children. They learn some of the most difficult and complex tasks in their lives by playing, such as playing a musical instrument, shooting baskets, or riding a bicycle. By playing with so-called transitional objects, children also learn about themselves and their environment (social and physical).

> When they play with dolls, children rehearse ways of interacting with people. When they play with blocks, they teach themselves basic principles of spatial geometry and mechanics. Later in life they will learn the general properties of the pendulum through swinging on a swing and all about levers through the playground teeter-totter. The doll, the blocks, the swing, and teeter-totter are what educational theorists call "transitional objects"; the playroom or the playground is a [physical] microworld, a microcosm of reality where it is safe to play. Through experimentation with transitional objects in microworlds, children discover principles and develop skills that are relevant in reality beyond play.[269]

For the new "games generation," the doll, the block, and the teeter-totter have yielded to computers, video games, and the Internet, and the computer screen has become the new "practice field."[270] Now just over 30 years old, video games have become one of the most pervasive and influential forms of entertainment for children (and adults) in the United States and around the world. By some estimates, one out of every four American households owns a Sony Playstation, and more than 80 percent of teens (and 40 percent of adults) are video gamers.[271,272]

In recent years, a growing number of schools have started to integrate gaming technology into their instructional designs as a means to enhance student involvement, enjoyment, and commitment.[273] Teachers in disciplines as diverse as history, politics, and music theory are wrapping instructive materials in a gaming package to pique their students' interest and motivate learning.[274,275]

To educational theorists, an enticing characteristic of digital game-based instruction is the active participation it requires of the learner, who is learning by making decisions, exploring, and discovering.[276] Interestingly, this notion of active learning is not new. It was first espoused many centuries ago by the ancient Greeks, notably Socrates, who believed in education by interrogating rather than by propounding. Socrates' ideas faded, however, during the Middle Ages, when the teacher was expected to hand down the truth "from on high." It was not until the late 18th century that interest in participatory learning was revived by the French philosopher Jean Jacques Rousseau, who famously argued, "[S]tudents learn by doing rather than by having their minds stuffed with abstract principles."[277] A century or so later, and on the other side of the Atlantic, John Dewey, arguably the most influential of American philosophers and perhaps the greatest educational theorist of our time, espoused the idea of "education through personal experience."[278]

It took a while for the ideas of Socrates, Rousseau, and Dewey to take hold, but recent advances in computer technology are allowing this to finally happen.

Learning About Healthy Behavior by Playing, Not by Lecturing

> Tell me and I will forget,
> Show me and I will remember,
> Engage me and I will understand.
> —A Lakota Sioux saying

People do not want to be lectured about their bad habits. Thus, the traditional method of health preaching has not been particularly effective in promoting behavior change.[279–281] As we have seen, because children are so technologically savvy, we can create intervention programs that are wider-reaching and far more effective because they can be delivered via the channels that children and teens prefer and in the forms that they will recognize and use. In a 2007 report funded by the prestigious Robert Wood Johnson Foundation titled *Childhood Obesity Prevention and Reduction: Role of eHealth*, the authors make the technology argument specifically with regard to the childhood obesity problem:

> The ubiquity of technology in the lives of today's youth requires new pedagogical methods and paradigms for interventions to prevent and treat childhood obesity that are adapted to the learning and information-seeking styles preferred by these frequent technology users.

Digital game-based environments provide us not only with a more effective medium for reaching young people, but also with unique advantages known to be crucial to health education.[282] For example, virtual environments provide the advantage of privacy. The ability to receive personalized advice while remaining anonymous is uniquely important in health education. "If they choose to learn about [obesity, anorexia nervosa, or] birth control ... they have entree to these materials without anyone controlling what they are learning. ... Students can acquire information at their own pace, without having to ask personal questions in front of teachers or their peers."[283]

According to cognitive psychologists, controlling the action and learning by doing not only is private but also can be more empowering. Receiving "authoritarian" instruction from a teacher or a social worker, research has indicated, "stimulates 'submissive' behavior in [children]— the opposite of the empowerment required for behavior change."[284] It can also provoke negative feelings of embarrassment and guilt.[285]

Instruction can also be tailored to each child's objectives and unique style of learning. Tailored computer-based instruction allows learners to see the consequences of their choices and to recognize the links between the very things that they do—or do not do—and unwanted health outcomes.[286] This can help children "assume responsibility for their lifestyles based on personal knowledge, as opposed to following prescriptive advice based on blind trust."[287]

Finally, health educators are particularly excited about the motivating aspect of video games and the potential to harness it in facilitating behavior change. For example, the work of Stanford's Jeremy Bailenson, discussed in the previous chapter, demonstrates that the form of "pretending" in which children engage when simulating their digital selves does have significant and lingering impact on behavior. Pretending has always been a part of the way children play. In contrast to donning a costume or wearing makeup, virtual reality takes pretending to a new level. The role playing, the active hands-on involvement, and the responsibility in constructing their altered digital selves create an "intimacy" and a bond between the learners and their virtual selves. Thus, what happens (or does not happen) to them online changes the way they behave offline. For example, seeing the beneficial effects of exercise on their virtual selves—watching muscles grow or pounds melt away—can motivate "players" to become more physically active in real life.[288]

No other form of mediated or face-to-face health education offers this combination of interactivity, entertainment, challenge, decision making, feedback, repetition, and privacy,[289] and no other learning experience is as much fun.[290]

Double-Loop Playing

In Chapter 1, I discussed the distinction between single-loop learning (where a mismatch between outcomes and goals is detected and corrected, but without questioning or altering one's underlying worldview) and double-loop learning (where we use the feedback from the results of our decisions to revise and enhance our fundamental understanding of a problem or decision task). Here I propose a parallel distinction between *single-loop playing,* to polish an existing skill or for entertainment, and *double-loop playing,* to develop new thinking skills.

Just as with adults, changing children's health behavior requires changing the ingrained mental models that drive their choices about food and play. This means we will have to use our fancy new technology to do more than entertain; we need to use it to profoundly change how they think about and manage their health and well-being.

This raises obvious questions: Would this be expecting too much of children? Is it reasonable to expect that children can assimilate the knowledge and skills to manage energy balance in the modern obesifying environment (as we have been advocating for adults)? Can we expect them to develop a basic understanding about the energy value of food and physical activity and how these work together to determine energy balance? Can gaming technologies—double-loop playing—enable young children, in effect, to develop higher-order thinking skills (for example, learn to think in circles, not just in straight lines)? In short, can we expect them to become *young systems thinkers?*

On this issue we do not have to speculate. The answer to all of these questions is yes.

(Almost) Never Too Young to Think Systematically

For many years, systems thinking was considered a topic appropriate only for university-level education. That long-held assumption was first challenged in the mid-1970s, when Nancy Roberts, then a professor at Lesley College, proposed introducing the concepts of systems thinking to fifth- and sixth-grade students.[291,292] It was a bold idea, and, at the time, Roberts did not have the proper software tools to make it practical. With the accelerating advances in computer hardware and software, it was a hurdle that was quickly overcome, however. Within a decade, we had systems-thinking software with user-friendly graphic interface that would help realize Roberts's vision and make the ideas of system-thinking accessible to K-12 students.

The first significant infusion of systems thinking in K-12 education took root in the late 1980s, when Gordon S. Brown, a retired MIT dean of engineering, introduced STELLA software, one of the new-generation, truly user-friendly systems software, at the Orange Grove Middle School in

Tucson, Arizona. That initial "experiment" proved to be the original spark that ignited an explosion of interest in systems thinking—at first, within the Arizona school district and, subsequently, all over the nation.[293] Today, efforts to incorporate systems thinking into K-12 education are under way in several hundred school districts nationwide.[294]

In most of these curricular experiments, systems thinking is typically not taught as an end in itself, that is, as a separate school subject. Instead, teachers are infusing the tools and concepts of systems thinking into their traditional courses to provide their students deeper insight into and understanding of the workings of systems in disciplines such as biology, physics, chemistry, social studies, economics, and the humanities. Has it worked?

A decade or so after Orange Grove's bold experiment, several research studies were launched to objectively assess the impact and to take stock of the progress made. One such study was the STACI (Systems Thinking and Curriculum Innovation) project initiated early in the 1990s to examine the cognitive and curricular impact of using the systems thinking approach in precollege instruction in schools in Vermont, the San Francisco Bay Area, and Arizona.[295] The results from these investigations have been overwhelmingly positive.

One of the most interesting and encouraging findings was the enormous breadth of applications reported. Teachers, working with their students, in most cases, have created computer models for an enormous array of the real-life systems they teach in biology, chemistry, physics, social studies, economics, and the humanities. For example, in the physical sciences, they developed models to simulate the orbits of planets and the motion of falling objects. In the biological and health sciences, they built models to simulate the effects of alcohol consumption on the body, the spread of infectious diseases (such as the flu), and drug addition. In ecology, there is a model to look at the effects of over-fishing. In mathematics, the models range from simulating simple algebra operations (e.g., compound interest in a bank account) to high-level calculus problems (e.g., the trajectories of flying projectiles).[296]

Another particularly "bullish" finding was the palpable enthusiasm exhibited by those teachers who have experienced the impact of systems thinking on their students. That excitement is perhaps best conveyed by this sampling of teacher responses:

- Since [introducing systems thinking] our classrooms have undergone an amazing transformation. . . . [T]he students are learning more useful material than ever before. "Facts" are now anchored to meaning through the dynamic relationships they have with each other. In our classroom students shift from being passive receptacles to being active learners. They are not taught about science per se but learn how to acquire and use knowledge [scientific and otherwise].[297]

- Simulations are especially engaging, and draw out many who might not otherwise participate in more traditional discussions and activities. ... Models are extraordinarily powerful for helping to convert abstractions into concrete realities. A learner's ability to "see" a system—what goes into a stock, where feedbacks exist—and then to run a model and ascertain how the system operates under varied conditions, renders abstractions into real meaningful, concrete terms. This discovery is true for students at all levels.[298]
- Instead of hearing from a teacher or reading in a textbook that antibiotics kill bacteria, students simulated the role of a doctor discovering which minimum dose of penicillin is most effective in curing a case of strep throat. ... Instead of laboring through the immune response, with its long list of names and actions, students worked toward an operational understanding of the relation between their bodies and pathogens by changing antibiotic levels in an infected person's body.[299]

What continues to amaze educators the most, and may have even surprised Nancy Roberts herself, is how much the students can do and how early they can do it. Beginning as early as the first grade, for example, students have been taught to work with feedback loops to explain simple cycles in nature and everyday events. By fifth grade, most students have no qualms about manipulating simple computer models that have been integrated into their curriculum.[300,301] Indeed, all the advanced tools of systems thinking seem to come naturally to them.

> For example, students use *behavior over time graphs* to find patterns in historical trends, in literary plot developments, or in science experiment results. They use *[feedback] loop diagrams* to focus discussions on unintended consequences in environmental studies or patterns of escalation in social conflicts ranging from playground squabbles to the American Revolution. They use *stock/flow diagrams* to understand population dynamics in various contexts: the extinction of mammoths in social studies, the growth of yeast cells in a test tube in science, the concept of exponential growth in math. Finally, they tie all of these skills together and use (*simulation*) models, or build their own, to gain an even deeper understanding of whatever they are studying.[302]

Today, there are many advocates (including myself) for a larger infusion of systems thinking and related methods into all levels of the educational system. The systems approach not only makes education more fun and engaging for students and teachers alike—a worthy goal in itself—but, more importantly, it also helps equip children with the skills and perspective they will need to effectively address the dynamically complex problems facing them in the future, including managing their health and their bodies.[303] As John Sterman of MIT (probably the most tireless advocate for this approach) has argued: "Systems thinking techniques can enhance our [children's] intuition about complex situations, just as studying physics can improve [their] intuition about the natural world.[304]

At Home, the Real Risk Is in Expecting Too Little

Children start life with parents as caregivers in control of their food supply, as well as of their space and time environments. In addition to controlling the what, when, and where of feeding and playing, parents also shape, through their child-feeding strategies and role modeling, dietary and exercise habits and attitudes that often last a lifetime.[305] As the first teachers and mentors, parents are in the perfect position to help children acquire the knowledge and personal skills to manage their lives in a healthy manner and to assume increasing responsibility in doing so, including making their own healthy nutrition choices. Unfortunately, however, parents all too often fail to do that,[306] in large part because of lingering parental misconceptions about what children can do and how early they can do it.

In feeding, for example, many parents assume that children are fundamentally incapable of regulating their food intake—determining what, when, and how much to eat. Thus, to ensure adequate, well-balanced food intake, we see many parents, rather than empower their children with cognitive skills to make their own healthy nutrition choices, simply take over the decision-making responsibility on their children's behalf.[307] They do this with the best intentions, because they believe they can do it better or more easily, or because they do not want to saddle their children with the onerous responsibilities that personal control entails.[308] It is a common pitfall that many parents fall into—and a risky one.

Obviously, parents need to exert some control over their children's dietary options, ensuring, for example, that a variety of reasonably healthful foods and snacks are readily available on the kitchen's shelves. Naturally, if the house is stocked with cookies, cakes, candies, chips, sodas and ice cream, that is what children will want to eat. But if parents go too far in tightly controlling the what, when, and how much of feeding, they risk seriously impeding their children's abilities to build self-regulatory competence. Parents who refuse to relinquish control rob their children of the opportunity to make their own healthy nutrition choices and to acquire skills that will be crucial to their long-term health and well-being.[309,310]

Research is now starting to reveal just how unproductive the use of coercive child-feeding strategies can be and how critically they can influence long-term health behavior and well-being.[311] It has been empirically demonstrated, for example, that one of the best predictors of a child's future self-regulatory ability is the "balance of power" between child and parent in the child's early feeding experiences. Specifically, "children with the least ability to self-regulate had the most controlling mothers [and vice versa]."[312] By interfering with the development of self-regulatory skills, stringent parental control can backfire in the long term by contributing to rather than preventing dysfunctional eating patterns and, ultimately, problems such as obesity in adulthood.[313]

Shifting the responsibility and burden of accomplishing a task, such as feeding regulation, from child to parent, and in the process cause more harm than good, is a classic and common pitfall, not only in our personal lives but in our public lives as well. Systems theorists call this pitfall *shifting the burden to the intervener.*

Shifting the Burden and Its Risks

In the systems-thinking field, shifting the burden structure is one of those recurring themes or behaviors that keep popping up in all kinds of situations and settings—in family settings as well as in organizations, both large and small. The structure helps explain how well-intentioned "solutions" in a wide range of situations actually make matters worse over the long term. It comes into play when an underlying difficult problem generates symptoms that demand attention and for which quick and ready "fixes" are available that can help alleviate these symptoms. Typically, the symptomatic solution is obvious and immediately implementable, and it usually relieves the problem symptom quickly—although typically only temporarily, which is why it is considered a *symptomatic* solution. The archetypical example is giving hungry people fish rather than teaching them how to fish. In the short term, that solution helps feed the hungry; in the long term, it increases population growth without increasing people's capacity to produce more food to sustain that growth. In this case, it shifts the burden for a solution from the particular population or society to the outside relief entity (the provider of fish).

The upper loop in Figure 26.1 represents this "easy fix" route. It is a (negative) feedback loop that is intended to work as follows: problem symptom arises → apply symptomatic solution → problem symptom gone. This may sound like good news, but it really is not. Easing a problem symptom also reduces any perceived need to find more fundamental solutions. Meanwhile, the underlying problem remains unaddressed and may worsen.

The shifting-the-burden structure highlights the all-too-common human tendency to want to get rid of a nagging problem, to relieve the pressure or the pain, right away. This strong urge often leads us to resort to the quick and easy remedy rather than devote the time and thought it takes to work out a more fundamental solution. The result is that the symptoms are gone, but the underlying problem remains unresolved.[314] Peter Senge, in his book *The Fifth Discipline*, provides a simple example that illustrates this nicely:

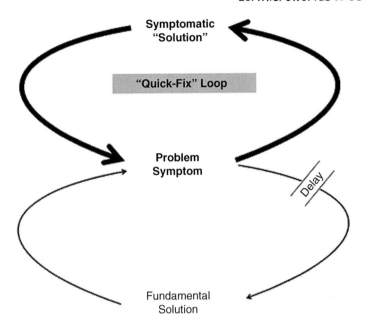

Figure 26.1 Quick-fix loop

Consider the problem of stress that comes when our personal workload increases beyond our capabilities to deal with it effectively. We juggle work, family, and community in a never-ending blur of activity. [When, eventually,] the workload increases beyond our capacity (which tends to happen for us all), the only fundamental solution is to limit the workload. This can be tough—it may mean passing up a promotion that will entail more travel or it may mean declining a position on the local school board. It means prioritizing and making choices. Instead, people are often tempted to juggle faster, relieving the stress with alcohol, drugs, or a more benign form of "stress reduction" (such as exercise or meditation). But, of course, drinking doesn't really solve the problem of overwork—it only masks the problem by temporarily relieving the stress. The problem comes back, and so does the need for drinking.[315]

The bottom loop of Figure 26.2 represents the path less traveled—the route toward a more fundamental solution to the problem (e.g., limiting the workload in Senge's example above), one that prevents the problem symptoms from recurring. Notice the delay in the fundamental solution loop. It is there to underscore the fact that most fundamental solutions (as opposed to symptomatic ones) take a lot longer to work their magic. Indeed, such delays are one reason why people tend toward the quick fix in the first place. Long term, though, the fundamental solution is the only enduring way to deal with the problem.[316]

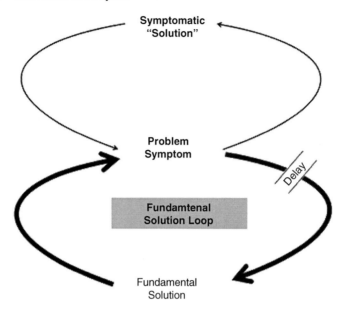

Figure 26.2 Fundamental solution loop

One common form of shifting the burden is the reliance of individuals or organizations on outside interveners to help solve their problem. Examples include parents who intervene to assume responsibility for what, when, and how their children eat, and organizations that hire consultants or other outside experts instead of training their own managers to solve problems.[317] While the outside intervener may be quite successful in relieving the problem symptoms, that success comes at a cost to the managers or the organizations, in that they never learn how to deal with the problem themselves.

In addition, symptomatic solutions often subtly erode the ability to institute the fundamental solution and, over time, reinforce dependence on the symptomatic solution (Figure 26.3). For example, turning to alcohol to relieve workload stress often leads to deterioration in health. As that happens, performance and self-confidence often deteriorate, as well. Ultimately, the person (now a stressed alcoholic with a poor performance record) becomes less and less able to fundamentally solve his or her original workload problem. That is what makes the shifting-the-burden structure so insidious: the subtle reinforcing cycle it fosters leads to increasing dependence on, and sometimes addiction to, the symptomatic solution.

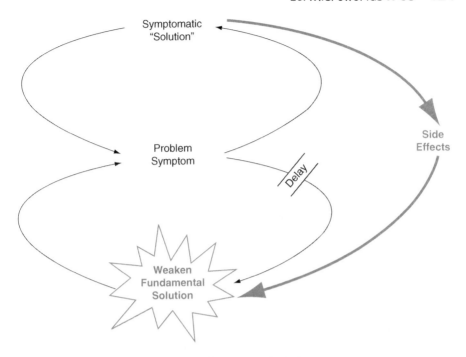

Figure 26.3 Side effects can weaken the fundamental solution

Keeping the Burden

Dealing effectively with shifting-the-burden structures requires a combination of strengthening the fundamental response and weakening the symptomatic response. To weaken the symptomatic response, we must, first and foremost, acknowledge it as such. "[For,] if symptomatic solutions are employed *as if* they are fundamental solutions, the search for fundamental solutions stops and shifting the burden sets in."[318]

One the most striking examples of the perils of shifting the burden and the wisdom of *keeping* it is the story of Helen Keller:

> [Keller was a] blind and deaf child whose parents' early attempts to protect her only made her dependent on them. Even though Helen's parents were well intentioned, they shifted the burden of responsibility for Helen's welfare to *themselves.* Helen learned that no matter what she did, her parents would accommodate her. And each incident reinforced her parents' belief that she was indeed helpless. If it had not been for the determined efforts of Helen's teacher, Ann[e] Sullivan, who refused to let Helen's handicaps prevent her from becoming self-reliant, Helen may never have achieved her real potential.[319]

Thanks to Anne Sullivan's *keeping* the burden, Keller went on to become the first deaf-blind person to graduate from college, as well as a prolific author and an activist.

The parallels between Keller's story and child-feeding practices and health prevention are unmistakable. As with Helen Keller's parents' early behavior, coercive child-feeding practices allow parents to achieve their (feeding) goals in the short term. Long term, however, these practices often prove counter-productive to the child's ability to self-regulate food intake and, thus, harmful to the child's overall well-being.[320]

As was briefly noted earlier, research studies have demonstrated empirically that exerting stringent controls over what, when, and how much children could eat tends to impede children's ability to develop self-regulatory behavior and thereby promote the very problems parents are attempting to avoid—overeating and weight gain.[321] A recent study of children aged 3 to 5 found that the more control the mother reported using over her child's eating, the less self-regulation and the more body fat the child displayed.[322] A second, longitudinal study, found that 5-year-olds with mothers who tightly controlled their food intake showed significant increases in overeating 2 to 4 years later.[323] It is ironic and, sadly, all too common that "parents who try to keep their children from getting fat may wind up producing kids who do not know how to stop eating when they have had enough."[324]

There is a silver lining in these findings, however; they demonstrate that eating is a learned behavior and one over which parental practices can exert a powerful influence.[325] To the extent that our eating patterns and preferences are learned in childhood (as they clearly seem to be), they can be modified positively.[326]

Teaching Children to Fish

Experiences with shifting-the-burden structures in many domains and different types of systems—parent–child, organizations, and societies—show that fundamental long-term solutions must strengthen the ability of the system to shoulder its own burdens.[327] This means that any intervention, whether with an individual child or an entire population, must enhance the child's ability to solve his or her problems, rather than shifting the burden to a parent or an outside relief organization.

In the case of children, the emphasis must shift from trying to coerce children into healthy eating to providing them with the tools they need to exercise personal control over their eating habits.[328] Parents, thus, should be coaches and mentors who help their children develop the necessary skills to manage their energy balance in the modern environment.[329] Like any other endeavor, effective self-regulation of feeding behavior cannot be achieved through an act of will; it requires self-regulatory skills.[330]

For example, parents need to help their children understand their bodies' built-in bias to overeat and, hence, the perils of eating in accordance with their bodies' signals, that is, eating to their physiological limits when food is readily available and overeating foods high in energy density. (In some Asian cultures, for example, children are taught not to eat until hungry, and when eating to stop before feeling full.) Parents need to help children understand that when it comes to their bodies, some of the (damaging) actions can be hard, if not impossible, to reverse, such as becoming diabetic, and to help them understand that there are trade-offs, especially between short-term gratification and long-term consequences.

The notion of transcendence—the ability to see beyond immediate stimuli—and learning to delay gratification are especially challenging, yet important, skills to emphasize because they are absolutely essential to successful self-regulation. For example, helping children understand that what begins innocently enough with a favorite dessert (or a few cigarettes) can end up many years later in obesity (or lung cancer).[331] To accomplish this, simulation-type microworlds can provide a real leverage by helping children "experience" the future status of the their bodies as a function of *their* behavior,[332,333] for example, showing sedentary teenagers a futuristic image of themselves in an obese state (Figure 26.4). This can help them see more vividly the links between the very things that they do—or do not do—and unwanted health outcomes.[334]

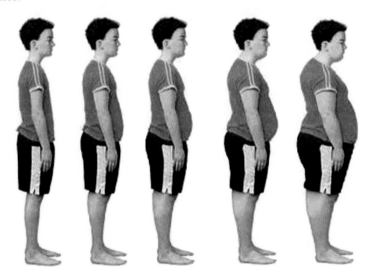

Figure 26.4 Projecting to a teenager what his body would look like if remaining sedentary

Once empowered with skills and a belief in their capabilities, children will be better able to adopt behaviors that promote health and to eliminate those that impair it.[335]

Balance of Powers and Responsibilities

In summary, parents should be encouraged to focus on the long-term goal of helping their children develop healthy self-control of feeding and to look beyond their immediate concerns regarding the composition and quantity of foods their children consume. The shift in strategy should be done smoothly and deliberately, however, not as an abrupt U-turn in which total control over food selection is suddenly handed over to children. Because children's food preferences and selection tend to be driven by familiarity (children tend to be neophobic, that is, rejecting new foods, especially those that are not sweet or salty), it has been advocated that, early on, and especially with young children, there should be a division of responsibility. Parents would be responsible for providing healthful food options, by stocking the refrigerator and kitchen cupboards with healthy foods, while keeping undesirable foods out of the house, and the children would be responsible for how much they eat (or whether they eat at all).[336]

Beyond Prevention 27

This book has discussed the historic development of the obesity epidemic and how we are dealing with it today. It also discussed how existing knowledge and technology can be deployed (and customized) to help us better manage our bodies and our health. This chapter looks forward, to ponder where we need to go from here.

Wellness Does Not Mean Only a Lack of Disease

To begin, let's explore a most fundamental question: How do we define wellness? We customarily think of health as a dichotomy—we are either sick or we are well. Such a binary viewpoint, while quite common, grossly oversimplifies the complex spectrum of human wellness and disease conditions. Human health is not merely the absence of physical impairment or disease, but a continuum in which there is a broad range of degrees of vitality and illness severity.[337]

Reducing a complex phenomenon or choice to a binary set of alternatives—in this case, health and disease—is no aberration. It is a convenient (occasionally sufficient) mental short-cut we routinely rely on, not just in thinking about our health, but in many judgmental tasks we face so as to simplify our world. Indeed, it almost seems to be part of human nature.[338]

As U.S. Supreme Court Justice Stephen Breyer observes in his book, *Breaking the Vicious Circle*:

> We simplify radically; we reason with the help of a few readily understandable examples; we categorize (events and other people) in simple ways that tend to create binary choices—yes/no, friend/foe, eat/abstain, safe/dangerous, act/don't act. The resulting categorizations do not always accurately describe another person or circumstance, but they help us make quick decisions, most of which prove helpful.[339]

Most of which! While binary thinking may help us minimize cognitive effort and make quick decisions, it dramatically oversimplifies things, which, as

Justice Breyer cautions later in his book, can seriously inhibit our understanding of a complex problem or situation. In the case of personal health and well-being, for example, it can seriously undermine our capacity to assess and manage the true health risks we face.[340]

Recent findings about the growing diabetes problem in America help underscore the pitfalls of such a binary mindset in disease diagnosis. Type 2 diabetes, which is by far the most common form of the disease, has been growing hand-in-glove with obesity and is looming as another health crisis facing the U.S. health system. Recent statistics indicate that about 20 million Americans now have type 2 diabetes. Even more ominous, more than twice as many people—45 million Americans—have impaired fasting glucose, a condition called pre-diabetes, in which a person has blood-sugar levels above normal but not high enough to be diagnosed as diabetes. What is most ominous about this condition is that most people who have it are unaware of it, and unaware that they have an increased risk of developing diabetes.[341] That risk could be significantly reduced, research is showing, with moderate weight loss and exercise. Yet, because most do not even know that they are at risk, relatively few are worrying about it, much less altering their behavior to postpone or possibly prevent the onset of diabetes.[342]

For many complex decision tasks, such as managing our health, it is essential that we make finer distinctions of the reality around us and within us. That is, it is essential that we transcend our simplistic tendency toward binary (black-and-white) thinking and embrace a more nuanced mindset, one that acknowledges reality's richer spectrum of variations (and colors).[343] This, as Fisher and Welch (1999) find, applies not only to laymen but to health professionals as well.

> Although clinicians recognize that illness severity ranges broadly (and that most chronic diseases develop over a prolonged period),... the data we have on diagnostic tests (e.g., sensitivity, specificity) assume a dichotomous model ... [and so] we often fall back on a dichotomous model when deciding to treat.[344]

Think what it would be like if managers and engineers approached business and engineering projects (whether introducing a new product or designing an aircraft or a bridge) the same way people narrowly think about and manage their health—by aiming simply to prevent failure. How far would we be from optimal performance? Quite far, no doubt. To simply focus on failure avoidance, whether in business, engineering, or health, is to effectively give up all but minimal performance. The binary mindset would necessarily blind the manager or engineer to the potential for higher levels of functioning.[345] As a consequence, the opportunity for doing better, even when utterly feasible, may never be achieved or even recognized.[346] That would not be the smartest way to run a business or design a bridge, and it should not be the way we manage our health.

Why not approach personal health management the way we manage our complex engineering and economic systems? That is, to think beyond just the absence of illness (failure avoidance) and to optimize our *health potential.* That means thinking about our wellness in terms of degrees of vitality (e.g., levels of cardiovascular robustness; immunocompetence; physical strength, stamina, and flexibility; etc.), and then seeking not merely to restore ourselves to feeling okay, but to feeling on top of the world.[347] The rest of this chapter explores why we should—and how we can—do just that.

Beyond Prevention of Disease

The idea is not entirely novel. Millennia ago, the Hippocratics and Greeks believed in the idea of "positive health," the notion that health is a state that transcends just the absence of illness (or "negative health"), and that humans should strive to attain higher and more optimal levels of functioning and well-being.[348] This was an idea far ahead of its time, and the tools needed to achieve it simply did not exist. Now, perhaps for the first time in history, we may finally have the knowledge and the technology to realize that vision.

What does "health optimization" mean, and what might an optimization health tool look like? Because no such tools exist (as far as I know), we need to venture into other domains, such as engineering, business, and professional sports, for inspiration. Many areas of engineering and business have used performance-optimization tools for years now, to help attain maximal performance of some system, product, or organization. Most of these tools are highly specialized, and tend to be rather arcane. But there is another area that is much easier for nonspecialists to relate to, and that is professional sports, in particular, Grand Prix racing, both car and sailboat racing.

On several occasions in earlier chapters, I drew on the many interesting parallels between "steering" our bodies toward health (in the current obesifying environment) and that of steering a boat (in turbulent seas). Both are complex yet delicate machines, and both are subject to personal control as well as to uncontrollable environmental forces. The analogy extends nicely to health optimization.

As a metaphor for managing our body's performance, think of sailors steering their boat on a race course. Professional sailors would not steer their boat using a simplistic *binary model,* one that simply delineates, for example, whether boat speed is nonzero or zero, whether they are ahead or behind, or whether they need to head to starboard or to port. Rather, they aim to sail their boat to its maximum potential. To do that, they rely on optimization models.

Several decades ago, naval engineers realized that simulator models could be designed to predict a specific boat's performance when it is sailed in different wind and sea conditions. Because different boats perform differently, these optimization models are "personalized" to reflect a boat's unique character-istics (such as hull shape, keel design, sizes and configuration of sails, etc.). Further, as with the human body, a boat's performance depends on environ-mental conditions, in this case, on factors such as wind strength and direction, as well as sea state. The output of these simulators, called velocity prediction programs (VPPs), is not a single number but rather a set of ear-shaped graphs, called *polar diagrams,* that predict optimal boat speed at different points of sail and wind velocities (Figure 27.1). Simply put, they tell how fast a specific boat should be able to sail in a given set of conditions.

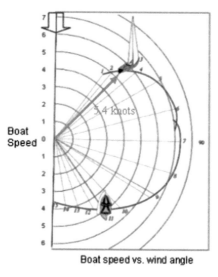

Boat speed vs. wind angle

Figure 27.1 "A polar diagram-plotted for a specific sailboat-shows the boat's theoretical maximun speed when sailed at different headings to the wind. To account for the effect of wind speed [the graph] like the one on the right (for a 7 knot wind speed) is plotted for different wind conditions.

In a *polar diagram*, the wind blows down from the top-as indicated by the arrow. The predicted boat speed at a particular heading is indicated by the length of the line from the origin to the point on the graph representing that particular heading. For example, point 3 on the graph indicates that when sailing at a 45 degree angle to the wind, this boat's theoretical maximum speed is 5.4 knots".

(*Source*: Bill Gladstone, *Performance Racing Trim,* 1983.)

Do they help? Enormously. By providing the crew with data to assess how well they are sailing the boat, whether or not the boat is sailing at its optimal speed, VPPs help the crew to maximize their boat's performance and to do it continuously throughout a race. Any time that the observed performance falls below the predicted performance, the crew can adjust the boat's trim to achieve the target performance.

Health Potential Programs for People?

> Only mediocre people are always at their best.
> —Somerset Maugham

Why not use an analogous approach to build simulators of human physiology and use them to optimize human health potential? Why not empower dieters, as we do sailors or engineers, with optimization-type tools with which they could not only avoid disease, but also "feel on top of the world"?[349]

As I will argue shortly, all the building blocks for developing such tools seem to be in place. The outstanding challenge before the medical community now is to conceptualize objective metrics for characterizing optimality in human health. To come up with the health-equivalent of *velocity* in a VPP, that would serve as optimal targets in health models—let's call the models *health potential programs* (HPPs), which ordinary people could use to optimize their health potential.

As in a VPP, optimal targets for performance would have to be personalized to account for physical differences among individuals as well as differences in goals and preferences. But unlike the VPP, a tool for optimizing health performance in humans would not be a one-dimensional affair. Rather, such tools would reflect the multiple determinants of health functioning.

Obesity provides a good case in point. A characterization of a person's optimal weight status would not, for example, be limited to a single number, such as body weight in pounds or body mass index (BMI), but would need to encompass other dimensions, such as measures of body composition (how much of one's weight is fat) and fat distribution (where in the body the fat is located). On each of these dimensions—BMI, body composition, or fat distribution—what constitutes "optimal" would not be the same for everyone. For example, the optimal BMI might depend on whether the primary concern is mortality (life-and-death or longevity issues), morbidity (disease conditions or risks), or the ability to function.[350] Body composition targets may also depend on whether a person already has weight-related medical problems or a family history of such problems.[351] The bottom line is that performance metrics in health must be defined, as with a VPP, to fit the precise specifications and preferences of each person.

Beyond optimal weight and body composition, there is much more to what would constitute optimal health. To reflect the multiple determinants of health functioning, without simultaneously overwhelming people, HPPs could reflect a *manageable* set of about five critical health factors. The set of possible factors is quite large and may include optimal cholesterol level, cardiorespiratory endurance, levels of immunocompetence, cardiovascular robustness, flexibility, and so on.[352] Again, the set of factors would be personalized to fit the individual needs and circumstances of each person (e.g., gender, age, preferences, medical history, etc.).

Is all this far-fetched? Not at all. In fact, the process has already begun—sort of. Not surprisingly, the largest strides toward optimization of human performance have been taken where we find the keenest competition—in sports. Over the last few years, a number of commercial tools—from companies such as Garmin, Nike, and Polar—that help athletes achieve higher levels of performance have become popular. Analogous to sailing's VPP, these electronic taskmasters (some call them "butt-kickers") are designed to continually push athletes to do their personal best by helping them find their potential maximum power output and then train to achieve it. (Interestingly, several of these products have also been called "polars.")[353]

Garmin, for example, offers a range of wrist gadgets called Forerunners (Figure 27.2) that lets runners, bikers, or walkers map out their workouts and then track pace, heart rate, calories burned, and other performance data as they train. A big selling point for the Forerunner is its built-in workout buddy, or virtual partner, that the user can program to perform (for example, run or bike) at a certain target level and then train against it.[354]

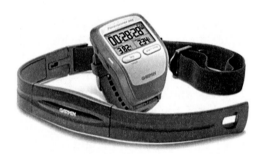

Figure 27.2 Garmin's Forerunner

Adopting such sophisticated models of performance allows athletes to set higher standards while training, which can help energize them to work harder to enhance their capacities. That is the obvious benefit. But there is also a second, perhaps less apparent, beneficial effect. In the process of learning how to tweak one's body to squeeze out maximum performance, one invariably learns a great deal about oneself. It is no coincidence, for example, that athletes, as a group, tend to have the most sophisticated understanding (second only to medical professionals) of how the body works. In the course of optimizing their speed, endurance, or stamina, they learn a lot about metabolism, nutrition, maximal oxygen uptake, muscle fiber types, maximum heart rate and stroke volume, and so on.

For now, the models are still relatively crude and narrowly focused. For example, this current generation of devices allows users to set their own performance targets, as opposed to relying (as does a VPP) on a computational model of an individual's physiological characteristics to derive truly optimal performance targets. Also, these fitness tools are limited to optimizing athletic performance rather than overall health. But we may not be far from taking the obvious next step toward full-fledged HPPs that aim to enhance overall wellness for everybody. There are two reasons to think so. First, as I argue in the next section, all the building blocks for developing such tools are in place. Second, we are starting to see more and more prognostications about such future capabilities, as in the quotation below, not in academic journals like *The Futurist* or *Science*, but in popular magazines like *Business Week,* which is usually a good indicator that a technology or innovation is getting close to realization.

> [O]ver the coming decade, each of us will give birth to far more fleshed out simulations of ourselves [and] ... will use them ... to predict how to ... steer us clear of diseases, and ramp up our productivity.... This mathematical modeling of humanity promises to be one of the great undertakings of the 21st century.[355]

The Second Flowering

Historians have called the late 19th century the time of the "great flowering of medicine." It was then that, thanks to advances in microscopy and a deeper understanding of germs and human physiology, scientists were able to identify the cause of one infectious disease after another.[356] Today, we may be on the verge of a second flowering, one in which medicine seeks not just to overcome disease, but to develop our capacities so that our human potential finds its optimal expression. It would signal a shift in which health care becomes more personalized, more preventive, and ultimately more predictive.[357,358]

What may be driving this second flowering? From history, we have learned that technology-based transformative leaps, whether in engineering, business, or medicine, rarely arise from the budding of a single great idea or invention. Rather, such advances typically arise from the synergetic convergence of diverse sets of component technologies. Often, these components lie dormant for years or even decades, waiting for the right circumstances to be pulled into full development and widespread use. Taken separately, the components may offer only marginal improvement, but when they are integrated to form an ensemble of technologies, they induce revolutionary change. This innovation dynamic has recurred many times in diverse industries and for a wide variety of technologies. One of the classic examples is the aircraft industry of the 1930s, when five key technologies first converged and led to the development of the revolutionary DC-3 aircraft, often said to be the first airplane able to support itself both economically and aerodynamically (Figure 27.3).[359]

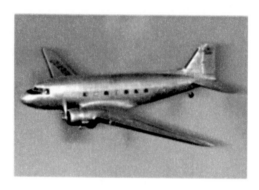

Figure 27.3 Innovation in the aircraft industry: an example case study.

"The DC-3 was the first airplane able to support itself economically as well as aerodynamically.

By the 1930s, innovations such as radial air-cooled engines, retractable landing gear, monocoque bodies wing flaps, and variable-pitch propellers had been developed separately and independently. Individually these innovations offered only minor improvements. For example, the radial-air-cooled engines offered substantial increases in power-to-weight ratio over earlier designs, but installing them only had marginal effect because older airplane designs with canvas-covered wings braced with struts and landing wheels protruding below were not streamlined. When they were all finally *integrated* for the first time in the DC-3, they made the modern air-transport business possible.

To succeed, the DC-3 needed all five, four were not enough. One year earlier, the Boeing 247 was introduced with all of them except wing flaps. Lacking wing flaps, Boeing's engineers found that the plane was unstable on take-off and landing and had to downsize the engine.' (*Source:* Senge, P.M. (1990). *The Fifth Discipline: The Art and Practice of the Learning Organization* (p. 6). New York: Doubleday/Currency.)

Similarly, the second flowering in medicine is being driven not by one thing but by the synergetic convergence of four component technologies that, together, represent the growing entwinement of the healing and information sciences: (1) Advances in molecular biology, which are expanding our understanding of the fundamental processes that underlie how the body works. (2) Advances in systems and computational sciences, which are allowing us to mathematically model and predict these processes. (3) Ubiquitous computing systems and intelligent sensors that can sense, analyze, and communicate the physiological data needed to personalize these models. (4) The Internet, which provides the infrastructure to efficiently and economically deliver these capabilities to large numbers of people.

As with the aircraft industry of 80 years ago, the integration of these component technologies will, I believe, induce revolutionary change in health care in the coming decade.

Advances in Molecular Biology: The Know-How

As demonstrated by the recent deciphering of the human genome, advances in molecular biology are expanding our understanding of the biological processes underlying health and disease and allowing us to close in on the genetic variations that define individual differences. Understanding why some people are prone to particular diseases or why one person responds to a drug and another does not is yielding more accurate diagnoses and development of more personalized treatments and is energizing the field of personalized medicine.[360]

Philosophically, one of the most profound insights stemming from our growing understanding of the molecular underpinnings of biological processes is the emerging conceptualization of biology as an information science. In the words of Leroy Hood, a member of the Caltech team that developed the DNA sequencer used in the successful mapping of the human genome: "If you think about biology, it differs from all of the other scientific disciplines in one striking sense; that is, at its core it has a digital code—the genome."[361]

The successful mapping of the human genome is likely to fundamentally change how we practice medicine, and it is already happening. More and more, we are seeing biological processes, such as protein production, being described and handled as algorithms. As we shift to the age of "personalized" medicine, physicians can be expected to become increasingly dependent on the digitization of information from the human body.[362]

Computational Modeling of Physiological Processes: The Models

Researchers in biology, biochemistry, mathematics, and computer science, among other fields, have been working for decades on the development of computer models of human physiology. Thanks to exponential leaps in available computer power, rapid progress in describing the precise and complex details of how human physiology actually works, and the development of mathematical tools to represent those details, increasingly lifelike models of human physiology are now feasible to build and are beginning to yield real health dividends.[363]

In one of the two primary research thrusts in this area, researchers are building simulations of specific body organs or physiological subsystems. Examples include models to simulate the lungs, the pancreas, the gut, and the heart.[364] The virtual-heart (or cardiome) project is probably the most ambitious, and is among the most advanced, of these organ-oriented modeling efforts. Insights gleaned from the virtual-heart modeling project are already making significant contributions to medicine, and one of its biggest may be as a tool to help researchers discover better heart drugs.[365] Ultimately, researchers aim to develop personalized virtual hearts to incorporate unique characteristics of individual patients, to find out, for example, what some new drug will do to a particular heart.[366]

The second major research thrust involves the development of integrative models of the entire human body. The organs and subsystems in the human body are not isolated islands, but are highly interrelated. Integrated models complement the organ-oriented work and allow scientists to better understand these interdependencies, such as how an experimental heart drug affects the kidneys or another physiological subsystem in the body.[367] (Note that the obesity-related simulation model discussed in Part IV, which captures a multitude of subsystems involved in the regulation of body composition, energy intake, and expenditure, lies between these two diametric model classes.) An example of a whole-body modeling effort is the *Archimedes* model, a comprehensive simulation model of human physiology that was originally developed to study diabetes and the myriad complications it can cause throughout the entire body.[368]

As with the organ-oriented programs, most researchers working on whole-body models ultimately aim to exploit advances in molecular biology and genetics to build personalized models that would help doctors assess treatments tailored to individual patients.[369] The development of such intimate models is now closer to realization because of the component technology discussed in the next subsection.

Ubiquitous Computing and Intelligent Sensors: The Personal Specs

The key to developing tailored models is personalized and timely data that capture the specificity of different individuals. Ubiquitous information technologies provide that capability.

Ubiquitous computing is the so-called third wave in computing—after the mainframe and the personal computing eras—in which information-processing technologies diffuse into our everyday objects and activities. "As opposed to the desktop paradigm, in which a single user consciously engages a single device for a specialized purpose, someone 'using' ubiquitous computing engages many computational devices and systems simultaneously, in the course of ordinary activities, and may not necessarily even be aware that [he or she is] doing so."[370]

This new paradigm was first articulated almost two decades ago in "The Computer for the 21st Century," a seminal article by the late Mark Weiser and his colleagues at the famed Xerox Park.[371] At the time, the exotic hardware technologies needed to achieve their vision were not yet available. But today, after a decade and a half of hardware progress, all the critical elements, such as mobile and wearable computers, intelligent noninvasive sensors, and wireless networks that tie them all together, are available, as are viable commercial products that continue to shrink in size and soar in IQ.[372]

The home provided the first obvious target for creating ubiquitous computing environments, and personal health provided a compelling "killer" application.[373] Several researchers and commercial labs around the world are already building experimental prototypes to test a range of specific functionalities. For example, the Japanese electronics giant Matsushita is working on a prototype house of the future that is chock-full of ubiquitous computing elements to keep track of the owner's health. "The bedroom, for instance, has an electrocardiometer, a blood-sugar meter and a thermometer, among other gadgets, [that can take measurements as we lie down or sleep], and links that can transfer [the] data ... to the home computer or doctor's office."[374]

Another room in the house that is undergoing a major transformation is the bathroom. Intelligent sensors and microchips embedded in the toilet and the plumbing are transforming the bathroom, at least in this vision of the future, into a full-blown online health-monitoring system. By measuring variables such as weight, fat content, and urine sugar levels, these prototype bathrooms can effectively provide users with a "morning checkup" together with their first flush.[375]

Such home-based applications are all examples of so-called infrastructure systems, where ubiquitous computing elements are embedded within a particular physical locale—in this case, the home. A second major category of ubiquitous computing technologies is mobile and wearable systems, also called *body area networks* (Figure 27.4). Body area networks are particularly attractive in health because they provide all the computing functionality wherever the user might be.[376]

Body area networks rely on sensors embedded into "smart" fabrics and materials (researchers at MIT, for example, have built electronic circuits entirely from textiles). These sensors will eventually appear in a range of consumer products—from shoes to keyboards to jewelry and even makeup. They will monitor changes in

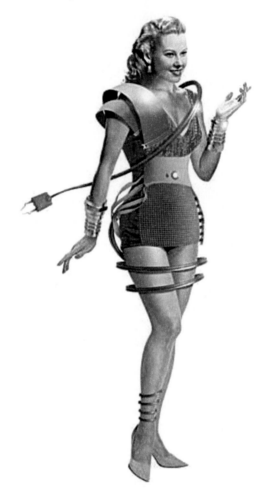

Figure 27.4 Body area network. (*Source:* Illustration by Viktor Koén.)

our temperature and other vital signs.... [And] they will transmit the results to interfaces that are already integral parts of our lives, such as cell phones, video screens, and appliances.[377]

While many of the early experimental applications have targeted patients with special needs for transmitting data to family or health practitioners, the overarching future goal is to build wellness-management and preventive tools. Such mobile-wearable systems would be designed not to alert others (e.g., about some medical emergency), but to enhance the way our bodies communicate their needs to us so that we can respond promptly to our shifting interior landscapes and ultimately decrease the risk of disease.[378]

The Internet: The Information Infrastructure

Like earlier communication technologies (e.g., the telephone and the radio), the Internet is expected to have far-reaching transformative consequences in many fields, particularly in health care, because health care is an information-intensive domain, one that depends on the development and interpretation of highly specialized knowledge.[379]

According to Internet World Stats, approximately 75 percent of the U.S. population now uses the Internet either at home or at work. This dramatic penetration, attained in a little over a decade, since the invention of the Web browser, is almost as fast as that of the telephone. This is quite remarkable, considering that the computer is far more complicated to use.[380]

The Internet provides an efficient electronic infrastructure for delivering the new generation of information-based tools for personal health management, and for doing it economically for large numbers of people. And because it facilitates interactivity and active participation, it provides the ideal vehicle for customization.

And the timing may be just right. The explosive growth of computer-based electronic communication is converging with another powerful trend: the increase in people's initiative in taking greater responsibility for their well-being.[381] This is opening enormous possibilities for empowering people with the tools they need to more effectively manage their well-being with potentially far-reaching transformative consequences.[382]

Not Automating, . . . Obliterating

> Every now and then, humanity wakes up, looks at itself in the mirror and realizes that it's been wasting a lot of effort doing things the old way just for the sake of tradition.
>
> —David Pogue, 2005[383]

Although, as the above overview suggests, an impressive collection of prototypes and experimental applications already exists, we have yet to take the bold "disruptive" steps that pull the multiple component technologies into widespread applications that induce revolutionary advances in personal health management. I believe that is largely because, in practice, we have done little more than use the new technologies to mechanize old ways of doing business and, in some cases, to simply substitute one medium (electronics) for another.

The Internet provides a good case in point: while millions of people now search it regularly for health and medical information—according to a Harris poll, more than 50 percent of U.S. adults did in 2007[384]—for most people, e-health is limited to using the Internet as a vast medical encyclopedia for health information (e.g., to search for information about diseases, diets, drugs, and doctors).[385] While many of the recently developed health-oriented sites brandish computerized tools for personal health management, most of these are electronic reincarnations of "legacy" tools from the pre-Internet era (Figure 27.5). For example, de rigueur fixtures on most of the weight-loss web sites are BMI and caloric balance calculators. Both, as we have learned, are highly simplistic models. Because their inputs are easy to measure and their computations can be performed manually, they were a necessary compromise in earlier times when we were computationally poor. That accessibility had its price. As we saw in Part III, the energy balance equation is a static, backward-looking instrument that is a poor predictor of changes in body weight. Similarly, the BMI has proven to be a poor indicator of healthy weight status because it fails to capture important predictors such as body composition and fat distribution.[386]

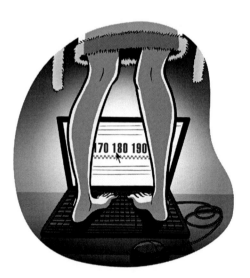

Figure 27.5 To date, most applications of information technology to personal health management have been rather pedestrian. (*Source:* Illustration courtesy of Christoph Hitz.)

The implicit assumption underlying such applications, and one that seems to be widely shared, is that mere automation of whatever manual processes people do automatically helps somehow. But it does not, and it has not. Helping people calculate their BMI faster and more accurately cannot address its fundamental performance deficiencies.

The propensity to use our new capabilities in medical informatics to mechanize old ways of doing business (rather than to enable new ones) is starkly reminiscent of the early uses of computer technology in business operations. In the 1960s and 1970s, when many organizations started adopting information technology to streamline their operations, most took the path of least resistance: replacing their inefficient manual data-processing operations with automated ones. Archaic administrative processes were often left largely intact; they were simply performed faster and more efficiently with the fancy new technology. But making inherently inefficient processes faster did not address their fundamental deficiencies. As a result, many of these early investments in information technology did not yield the anticipated dramatic improvements.[387]

The inclination to cling to our traditional routines of doing things, even as we attempt to modernize our tools, is not peculiar to information technology. It has been a recurring theme that has hampered many efforts at change, across many industries and technologies. The story below, from the military domain, is a classic tale from the colorful literature on organizational change:

> In the early days of [World War II] when armaments of all kinds were in short supply, the British, I am told, made use of a venerable field piece that had come down to them from previous generations. The honorable past of this light artillery stretched back, in fact to the Boer War. In the day of uncertainty after the fall of France, these guns, [now] hitched to trucks [rather than to horses as during the Boer War], served as useful mobile units in the coast defense. But it was felt that the rapidity of fire could be increased. A time-motion expert was, therefore, called in to suggest ways to simplify the firing procedures. He watched one of the gun crews of five men at practice in the field for some time. Puzzled by certain aspects of the procedures, he took some slow-motion pictures of the soldiers performing the loading, aiming, and firing routines. When he ran these pictures over once or twice, he noticed something that appeared odd to him. A moment before the firing, two members of the gun crew ceased all activity and came to attention for a three-second interval extending throughout the discharge of the gun. He summoned an old colonel of artillery, showed him the pictures, and pointed out this strange behavior. What, he asked the colonel, did it mean. The colonel, too, was puzzled. He asked to see the pictures again. "Ah," he said when the performance was over, "I have it. They are holding the horses." This story, true or not, and I am told it is true, suggests nicely the pain with which the human being accommodates himself to changing conditions. The tendency is apparently involuntary and immediate to protect oneself against the shock of change by continuing in the presence of altered situations the familiar habits, however incongruous, of the past.[388]

In business, the breakthrough came when companies stopped thinking about using information technology to automate existing practices and started leveraging the power of the computer to reengineer their business processes. In the words of Michael Hammer, the man who literally wrote the book on process reengineering,

> At the heart of reengineering is the notion of discontinuous thinking—of recognizing and breaking away from the outdated rules and fundamental assumptions that underlie operations. Unless we change these rules, we are merely rearranging the deck chairs on the Titanic. We cannot achieve breakthroughs in performance by cutting fat or automating existing processes. Rather, we must challenge old assumptions and shed the old rules that made the business under-perform in the first place.[389]

It is time to do the same in health; it is time to stop "holding the horses."

The shift from "industrial" to "information-age health care" will involve much more than just putting our current health education pamphlets up on the Web and using information technology to simply automate old ways of doing business. Instead of embedding outdated processes (like the ubiquitous BMI and caloric calculators) in silicon and software, we should obliterate them and start over.[390] It is time to use the technology not to automate existing processes but to enable new ones.

In this book, I argued for and, I hope, have demonstrated the feasibility and utility of a new generation of dynamic tools that support interaction and customization for personal health and wellness management. With the great advances in systems sciences, medicine, and computer technology over the last few decades, we are now in a position to put such tools into full development and widespread use. It is truly a new age in health care.

Notes

1. Mitchell, D. (2005, November 12). (Super-size comeback for fast food. *New York Times*.
2. Arnst, C. (2006, January 9). Helping your kid slim down. *Business Week*.
3. While the BRFSS data are not longitudinal, observations from different survey years can point to overall trends in the population.
4. Burke, M.A. and Heiland F. (2005). Social Dynamics of Obesity. CSED Working Paper No. 40, Center on Social and Economic Dynamics, The Brookings Institution, John Hopkins University.
5. Haskell, K. (2002, October 13). Sizing up teenagers. *New York Times*.
6. Sciolino, E. (2006, January 25). France battles a problem that grows and grows: fat. *New York Times*.
7. Haskell, K. (2002, October 13). Sizing up teenagers. *New York Times*.
8. Brody, J. (2004, January 20). The widening of America, or how size 4 became a size 0. *New York Times*.
9. Sciolino, E. (2006, January 25). France battles a problem that grows and grows: fat. *New York Times*.
10. Sterman, J.D. (2000). *Business Dynamics: Systems Thinking and Modeling for a Complex World*. Boston: Irwin McGraw-Hill.
11. Senge, P.M. (1990). *The Fifth Discipline: The Art and Practice of the Learning Organization*. New York: Doubleday/Currency.
12. *Ibid.*
13. Fountain, H. (2002, October 13). Living large: our just (burp!) desserts. *New York Times*.
14. Zezima, K. (2008, April 8). Increasing obesity requires new ambulance equipment. *New York Times*.
15. Nielsen, S.J. and Popkin, B.M. (2004). Changes in beverage intake between 1977 and 2001. *American Journal of Preventive Medicine*, 27(3), 205–210.
16. Senge, P.M. (1990). *The Fifth Discipline: The Art and Practice of the Learning Organization*. New York: Doubleday/Currency.

17. Brownell, K.D. and Horgen, K.B. (2004). *Food Fight*. Chicago: Contemporary Books.
18. Gill, T.P. (1997). Key issues in the prevention of obesity. *British Medical Bulletin*, 53(2), 359–388.
19. Jeffery, R.W. (1998). Prevention of obesity. In: Bray, G.A., Bouchard, C., and James, W.P.T. (Eds.). *Handbook of Obesity*. New York: Marcel Dekker.
20. Kalota, G. (2005, April 17). The body heretic: it scorns our efforts. *New York Times*.
21. Sterman, J.D. (2000). *Business Dynamics: Systems Thinking and Modeling for a Complex World*. Boston: Irwin McGraw-Hill.
22. Kalota, G. (2005, April 17). The body heretic: it scorns our efforts. *New York Times*.
23. Szabo, L. (2005, December 19). Will the sins of your past catch up with you? *USA Today*, p. 5d.
24. *Ibid*.
25. Kalota, G. (2005, April 17). The body heretic: it scorns our efforts. *New York Times*.
26. Urbina, I. (2006, January 11). In the treatment of diabetes, success often does not pay. *New York Times*.
27. Fackelmann, K. (2005, August 25). Does diabetes lurk behind Alzheimer's? *USA Today*.
28. Critser, G. (2003). *Fat Land: How Americans Became the Fattest People in the World*. Boston: Mariner Books.
29. Larkin, M. (2003). Can cities be designed to fight obesity? *Lancet*, 362, 1046–1047.
30. Koplan, J.P., Liverman, C.T., and Kraak, V.I. (Eds.). (2005). Preventing childhood obesity: health in the balance (executive summary). *Journal of the American Dietetic Association*, 105(1), 131–138.
31. Nestle, M. and Jacobson, M.F. (2000). Halting the obesity epidemic: a public health policy approach. *Publitc Health Reports*, 115, 12–24.
32. Kleinfeld, N.R. (2006, January 9). Diabetes and its awful toll quietly emerge as a crisis. *New York Times*.
33. Barlett, D. and Steele, J. (2004, October 24). The health of nations (op-ed piece). *New York Times*.
34. Kleinfeld, N.R. (2006, January 9). Diabetes and its awful toll quietly emerge as a crisis. *New York Times*.
35. Pear, R. (2006, July 24). Obesity surgery often leads to complications, study says. *New York Times*.
36. Santora, M. (2004, November 26). Shedding baby fat through surgery. *New York Times*.
37. Mitka, M. (2003). Surgery for obesity: demand soars amid scientific, ethical questions. *JAMA*, 289(14), 1761–2.

38. Urbina, I. (2006, January 11). In the treatment of diabetes, success often does not pay. *New York Times*.
39. *Ibid.*
40. McGinnis, J.M. (2001), Does proof matter? Why strong evidence sometimes yields weak action. *American Journal of Health Promotion*, 15(5), 391–396.
41. Urbina, I. (2006, January 11). In the treatment of diabetes, success often does not pay. *New York Times*.
42. Gerberding, J.L. (2005). Protecting health—the new research imperative. *JAMA*, 294(11), 1403–1406.
43. "In one of the boldest moves yet by an insurer to bring the rising cost of obesity under control, Blue Cross and Blue Shield of North Carolina [has reportedly started] to cover the cost of helping its members tackle their weight problems. The not-for-profit insurer, based in Chapel Hill, N.C., said more than 1.1 million members of its commercial health plans will be eligible for the program, one of the first in the U.S. to cover preventive weight management as well as medical treatments for obesity. Starting [in 2005], qualifying Blue Cross members [became] covered for four doctors' visits per year, along with needed diagnostic tests and counseling by dieticians" (McKay, B. [2004, Oct 13]. Blue Cross of North Carolina to cover cost of treating obesity. *Wall Street Journal*.).
44. Urbina, I. (2006, January 11). In the treatment of diabetes, success often does not pay. *New York Times*.
45. Swinburn, B., Egger, G., and Raza, F. (1999). Dissecting obesogenic environments: the development and application of a framework for identifying and prioritizing environmental interventions for obesity. *Preventive Medicine*, 29, 563–570.
46. Egger, G. and Swinburn, B. (1997). An "ecological" approach to the obesity pandemic. *BMJ*, 315, 477–480.
47. Brownell, K.D. and Fairburn, C.G. (Eds.). (1995). *Eating Disorders and Obesity: A Comprehensive Handbook*. New York: Guilford Press.
48. Nestle, M. and Jacobson, M.F. (2000). Halting the obesity epidemic: a public health policy approach. *Public Health Reports*, 115, 12–24.
49. Parker-Pope, T. (2003, December 9). How to give your child a longer life. *Wall Street Journal*.
50. Hodges, E.A. (2003). A Primer on early childhood obesity and parental influence. *Pediatric Nursing*, 29(1), 13–16.
51. U.S. Department of Health and Human Services. (2000, November). *Healthy People 2010: Understanding and Improving Health*, 2nd ed. Washington, DC: U.S. Government Printing Office.
52. Foreyt, J.P. and Cousins, J.H. (1993). Primary prevention of obesity in Mexican-American children. *Annals of the New York Academy of Sciences*, 699, 137–146.

53. Mercer, S.L., et al. (2003). Possible lessons from the tobacco experience for obesity control. *American Journal of Clinical Nutrition*, 77(suppl), 1073S–82S.

54. Carter, R.C. (2002). The impact of public schools on childhood obesity. *msJAMA Online*, 288, 2180.

55. Brownell, K.D. and Horgen, K.B. (2004). *Food Fight*. Chicago: Contemporary Books.

56. Koplan, J.P., Liverman, C.T., and Kraak, V.I. (Eds.). (2005). Preventing childhood obesity: health in the balance (executive summary). *Journal of the American Dietetic Association*, 105(1), 131–138.

57. Arnst, C. and Kiley, D. (2004, October 11). The kids are not all right. *Business Week*.

58. Burros, M. (2006, April 6). Bill strikes at low-nutrition foods in school. *New York Times*.

59. Schlosser, E. (2002). *Fast Food Nation: The Dark Side of the All-American Meal*. New York: Perennial.

60. Buckley, N. (2003, February 18). Unhealthy food is everywhere, 24 hours a day, and inexpensive. *Financial Times*, p. 13.

61. Goode, E. (2003, July 22). The gorge-yourself environment. *New York Times*, p. F1.

62. Nestle, M. and Jacobson, M.F. (2000). Halting the obesity epidemic: a public health policy approach. *Public Health Reports*, 115, 12–24.

63. French, S.A., Story, M., and Jeffery, R.W. (2001). Environmental influences on eating and physical activity. *Annual Review of Public Health*, 22, 309–335.

64. Wadden, T.A., Brownell, K.D., and Foster, G.D. (2002). Obesity: responding to the global epidemic. *Journal of Consulting and Clinical Psychology*, 70(3), 510–525.

65. Birch, L.L. and Fisher, J.O. (1998). Development of eating behaviors among children and adolescents. *Pediatrics*, 101(3 Suppl), 539–549.

66. Shell, E.R. (2002). *The Hungry Gene: The Inside Story of the Obesity Industry*. New York: Grove Press.

67. Hellmich, N. (2005, December 7). Drastic changes urged in marketing food to kids. *USA Today*.

68. Frazao, E. and Allshouse, J. (2003). Strategies for Intervention: commentary and debate. *Journal of Nutrition*, 133, 844S-847S.

69. Bray, G.A, Bouchard, C., and James, W.P.T. (Eds.). (1998). *Handbook of Obesity*. New York: Marcel Dekker.

70. Brownell, K.D. and Horgen, K.B. (2004). *Food Fight*. Chicago: Contemporary Books.

71. Bray, G.A, Bouchard, C., and James, W.P.T. (Eds.). (1998). *Handbook of Obesity*. New York: Marcel Dekker.

72. Shell, E.R. (2002). *The Hungry Gene: The Inside Story of the Obesity Industry.* New York: Grove Press.
73. Mercer, S.L., et al. (2003). Possible lessons from the tobacco experience for obesity control. *American Journal of Clinical Nutrition,* 77(suppl), 1073S–1082S.
74. Frazao, E. and Allshouse, J. (2003). Strategies for Intervention: commentary and debate. *Journal of Nutrition,* 133, 844S–847S.
75. Mitka, M. (2003). Economist takes aim at "big fat" US lifestyle. *JAMA,* 289(1), 33–34.
76. Wadden, T.A. and Stunkard, A.J. (Eds.). (2002). *Handbook of Obesity Treatment.* New York: Guilford Press.
77. *Ibid.*
78. Wadden, T.A., Brownell, K.D., and Foster, G.D. (2002). Obesity: responding to the global epidemic. *Journal of Consulting and Clinical Psychology,* 70(3), 510–525.
79. Brownell, K.D. and Horgen, K.B. (2004). *Food Fight.* Chicago: Contemporary Books.
80. Wadden, T.A., Brownell, K.D., and Foster, G.D. (2002). Obesity: responding to the global epidemic. *Journal of Consulting and Clinical Psychology,* 70(3), 510–525.
81. Brownell, K.D. and Horgen, K.B. (2004). *Food Fight.* Chicago: Contemporary Books.
82. French, S.A. (2003). Pricing effects on food choices. *Journal of Nutrition,* 133, 841S–843S.
83. Wadden, T.A., Brownell, K.D., and Foster, G.D. (2002). Obesity: responding to the global epidemic. *Journal of Consulting and Clinical Psychology,* 70(3), 510–525.
84. French, S.A. (2003). Pricing effects on food choices. *Journal of Nutrition,* 133, 841S–843S.
85. Glanz, K., Rimer, B.K., Lewis, F.M. (Eds.). (2002). *Health Behavior and Health Education: Theory, Research, and Practice.* San Francisco: Jossey-Bass.
86. Brownell, K.D. and Horgen, K.B. (2004). *Food Fight.* Chicago: Contemporary Books.
87. Wadden, T.A. and Stunkard, A.J. (Eds.). (2002). *Handbook of Obesity Treatment.* New York: Guilford Press.
88. Wadden, T.A., Brownell, K.D., and Foster, G.D. (2002). Obesity: responding to the global epidemic. *Journal of Consulting and Clinical Psychology,* 70(3), 510–525.
89. Peters, J.C., Wyatt, H.R., Donahoo, W.T., and Hill, J.O. (2002). From instinct to intellect: the challenge of maintaining healthy weight in the modern world. *Obesity Reviews,* 3, 69–74.

90. Partnership for Prevention. (2000). *Nine High-Impact Actions Congress Can Take to Protect and Promote the Nation's Health.* Washington, DC: Partnership for Prevention.

91. Carter, R.C. (2002). The impact of public schools on childhood obesity. *msJAMA Online,* 288, 2180.

92. Arnst, C. and Kiley, D. (2004, October 11). The kids are not all right. *Business Week.*

93. Carter, R.C. (2002). The impact of public schools on childhood obesity. *msJAMA Online,* 288, 2180.

94. U.S. Department of Health and Human Services. (2001). *The Surgeon General's Call to Action to Prevent and Decrease Overweight and Obesity.* Rockville, MD: U.S. Dept. of Health and Human Services, Public Health Service, Office of the Surgeon General.

95. Hennrikus, D.J. and Jeffery, R.W. (1996). Worksite intervention for weight control: a review of the literature. *American Journal of Health Promotion,* 10(6), 471–498.

96. Mitka, M. (2003). Economist takes aim at "big fat" US lifestyle. *JAMA,* 289(1), 33–34.

97. Koplan, J.P. and Dietz, W.H. (1999). Caloric imbalance and public health policy. *JAMA,* 282(16), 1579–1581.

98. French, S.A., Story, M., and Jeffery, R.W. (2001). Environmental influences on eating and physical activity. *Annual Review of Public Health,* 22, 309–335.

99. Koplan, J.P., Liverman, C.T., and Kraak, V.I. (Eds.). (2005). Preventing childhood obesity: health in the balance (executive summary). *Journal of the American Dietetic Association,* 105(1), 131–138.

100. Swinburn, B., Egger, G., and Raza, F. (1999). Dissecting obesogenic environments: the development and application of a framework for identifying and prioritizing environmental interventions for obesity. *Preventive Medicine,* 29, 563–570.

101. Peters, J.C., Wyatt, H.R., Donahoo, W.T., and Hill, J.O. (2002). From instinct to intellect: the challenge of maintaining healthy weight in the modern world. *Obesity Reviews,* 3, 69–74.

102. Larkin, M. (2003). Can cities be designed to fight obesity? *Lancet,* 362, 1046–1047.

103. Bjorntorp, P. (2001). Thrifty genes and human obesity. Are we chasing ghosts? *Lancet,* 358, 1006–1008.

104. "Metanoia" means a fundamental shift of mind or, more literally, transcendence *("meta"*—above or beyond, as in "metaphysics") of mind ("noia," from the root *"nous,"* of mind). See: Senge, P.M. (1990). *The Fifth Discipline: The Art and Practice of the Learning Organization.* New York: Doubleday/Currency.

105. Kumanyika, S.K. (2001). Minisymposium on obesity: overview and some strategic considerations. *Annual Review of Public Health*, 22, 293–308.

106. Blundell, J.E. and King, N.A. (1996). Overconsumption as a cause of weight gain: behavioral-physiological interactions in the control of food intake (appetite). In: Ciba Foundation Symposium (Ed.). *The Origins and Consequences of Obesity* (pp. 138–154). Hoboken, NJ: John Wiley.

107. Zernike, K. (2003, November 9). Food fight; is obesity the responsibility of the body politic? *New York Times*.

108. Glanz, K., Rimer, B.K., Lewis, F.M. (Eds.). (2002). *Health Behavior and Health Education: Theory, Research, and Practice.* San Francisco: Jossey-Bass.

109. Wald, M.L. (2006, March 30). Automakers use new technology to beef up muscle not mileage. *New York Times*.

110. Wald, M.L. (2005, July 17). Hybrid cars burning gas in the drive for power. *New York Times*.

111. Leonhardt, D. (2006, February 8). Buy a hybrid, and save a guzzler. *New York Times*.

112. Kitman, J.L. (2006, April 16). Life in the green lane. *New York Times*.

113. Brooke, L. (2006, April 30). Challenging Toyota's hybrid hegemony. *New York Times*.

114. *Ibid.*

115. Sterman, J.D. (2000). *Business Dynamics: Systems Thinking and Modeling for a Complex World.* Boston: Irwin McGraw-Hill.

116. Sterman, J.D. (2006). Learning from evidence in a complex world. *American Journal of Public Health*, 96(3), 505–514.

117. White, J.B. (2006, May 2). Can Americans kick their V-8 power addiction. *Wall Street Journal*, p. D6.

118. Wald, M.L. (2006, March 30). Automakers use new technology to beef up muscle not mileage. *New York Times*.

119. Wald, M.L. (2005, July 17). Hybrid cars burning gas in the drive for power. *New York Times*.

120. *Ibid.*

121. White, J.B. (2006, May 2). Can Americans kick their V-8 power addiction. *Wall Street Journal*, p. D6.

122. Wald, M.L. (2005, July 17). Hybrid cars burning gas in the drive for power. *New York Times*.

123. It will be interesting to see whether the recent steep surge in oil prices—increasing from around $60/barrel in the early part of 2007 to close to $150/barrel in mid- 2008—will be painful enough to help recalibrate Americans' priorities.

124. Senge, P.M. (1990). *The Fifth Discipline: The Art and Practice of the Learning Organization.* New York: Doubleday/Currency.

125. Peters, J.C., Wyatt, H.R., Donahoo, W.T., and Hill, J.O. (2002). From instinct to intellect: the challenge of maintaining healthy weight in the modern world. *Obesity Reviews*, 3, 69–74.

126. Kitman, J.L. (2006, April 16). Life in the green lane. *New York Times*.

127. Meadows, D. (1999). Leverage Points: Places to Intervene in a System. The Sustainability Institute, Hartland, Vermont.

128. Pekka, P., Pirjo, P., and Ulla, U. (2002). Influencing public nutrition for non-communicable disease prevention: from community intervention to national programme experiences from Finland. *Public Health Nutrition*, 5(1A), 245–251.

129. Milstein, B. (2008). *Hygeia's Constellation: Navigating Health Futures in a Dynamic and Democratic World*. Atlanta, GA: Syndemics Prevention Network, Centers for Disease Control and Prevention.

130. Puska, P., Vartiainen, E., Tuomilehto, J., Salomaa, V., and Nissinen, A. (1998). Changes in premature deaths in Finland: successful long-term prevention of cardiovascular diseases. *Bulletin of the World Health Organization*, 76(4), 419–425.

131. Milstein, B. (2008). *Hygeia's Constellation: Navigating Health Futures in a Dynamic and Democratic World*. Atlanta, GA: Syndemics Prevention Network, Centers for Disease Control and Prevention.

132. Puska, P., Vartiainen, E., Tuomilehto, J., Salomaa, V., and Nissinen, A. (1998). Changes in premature deaths in Finland: successful long-term prevention of cardiovascular diseases. *Bulletin of the World Health Organization*, 76(4), 419–425.

133. Shell, E.R. (2002). *The Hungry Gene: The Inside Story of the Obesity Industry*. New York: Grove Press.

134. Pietinen, P., Vartiainen, E., Seppänen, R., Aro, A., and Puska, P. (1996). Changes in diet in Finland from 1972 to 1992: impact on coronary heart disease risk. *Preventive Medicine*, 25, 243–250.

135. Shell, E.R. (2002). *The Hungry Gene: The Inside Story of the Obesity Industry*. New York: Grove Press.

136. Milstein, B. (2008). *Hygeia's Constellation: Navigating Health Futures in a Dynamic and Democratic World*. Atlanta, GA: Syndemics Prevention Network, Centers for Disease Control and Prevention.

137. Pekka, P., Pirjo, P., and Ulla, U. (2002). Influencing public nutrition for non-communicable disease prevention: from community intervention to national programme experiences from Finland. *Public Health Nutrition*, 5(1A), 245–251.

138. Milstein, B. (2008). *Hygeia's Constellation: Navigating Health Futures in a Dynamic and Democratic World*. Atlanta, GA: Syndemics Prevention Network, Centers for Disease Control and Prevention.

139. Lee, T. and Oliver, E. (2002). *Public Opinion and the Politics of America's Obesity Epidemic.* John F. Kennedy School of Government, Harvard University, Faculty Research Working Papers Series (RWP02–017).

140. Larkin, M. (2003). Can cities be designed to fight obesity? *Lancet, 362,* 1046–1047.

141. Cutler, D.M., Glaeser, E.L. and Shapiro, J.M. (2003). Why have Americans become more obese? *Journal of Economic Perspectives,* 17(3), 93–118.

142. Nielsen, S.J. and Popkin, B.M. (2004). Changes in beverage intake between 1977 and 2001. *American Journal of Preventive Medicine,* 27(3), 205–210.

143. Hill, J.O. et al. (2003). Obesity and the environment: where do we go from here? *Science,* 299, 853–855.

144. *Ibid.*

145. Nestle, M. et al. (1998). Behavioral and social influences on food choice. *Nutrition Reviews,* 56(5), S50–S74.

146. Glanz, K., Rimer, B.K., Lewis, F.M. (Eds.). (2002). *Health Behavior and Health Education: Theory, Research, and Practice.* San Francisco: Jossey-Bass.

147. Gill, T.P. (1997). Key issues in the prevention of obesity. *British Medical Bulletin,* 53(2), 359–388.

148. Bray, G.A, Bouchard, C., and James, W.P.T. (Eds.). (1998). *Handbook of Obesity.* New York: Marcel Dekker.

149. Nestle, M. and Jacobson, M.F. (2000). Halting the obesity epidemic: a public health policy approach. *Public Health Reports,* 115, 12–24.

150. *Ibid.*

151. *Ibid.*

152. *Ibid.*

153. Nestle, M. (2002). *Food Politics: How the Food Industry Influences Nutrition and Health.* Berkeley, CA: University of California Press.

154. Racette, S.B., Deusinger, S.S., and Deusinger, R.H. (2003). Obesity: overview of prevalence, etiology, and treatment. *Physical Therapy,* 83(3), 276–288.

155. Severson, K. (2005, April 24). The government's pyramid scheme. *New York Times.*

156. Butler, D. (2004). Health experts find obesity measures too lightweight. *Nature,* 428, 244.

157. Gill, T.P. (1997). Key issues in the prevention of obesity. *British Medical Bulletin,* 53(2), 359–388.

158. Kolata, G. (2002, September 10). 5 decades of warnings fail to get Americans moving. *New York Times.*

159. Nestle, M. and Jacobson, M.F. (2000). Halting the obesity epidemic: a public health policy approach. *Public Health Reports,* 115, 12–24.

160. Pool, R. (2001). *Fat: Fighting the Obesity Epidemic*. Oxford: Oxford University Press.

161. Bray, G.A, Bouchard, C., and James, W.P.T. (Eds.). (1998). *Handbook of Obesity*. New York: Marcel Dekker.

162. Severson, K. (2005, April 24). The government's pyramid scheme. *New York Times*.

163. Oliver, J.E. and Lee, T. (2005). Public opinion and the politics of obesity in America. *Journal of Health Politics, Policy and Law*, 30(5), 923–954.

164. Gogoi, P. (2005, November 11). Fat times for fast food: Americans back to eating giant burgers, fried chicken. *Business Week*.

165. Nestle, M. and Jacobson, M.F. (2000). Halting the obesity epidemic: a public health policy approach. *Public Health Reports*, 115, 12–24.

166. *Ibid*.

167. Elliott, A. (2003). US Food industry ensures that consumers are not told to eat less. *BMJ*, 327(7423), 1067.

168. Pollan, M. (2008). *In Defense of Food: An Eater's Manifesto*. New York: Penguin Press.

169. Philipson, T. (2001). The world-wide growth in obesity: an economic research agenda. *Health Economics*, 10, 1–7.

170. Shell, E.R. (2002). *The Hungry Gene: The Inside Story of the Obesity Industry*. New York: Grove Press.

171. CSPI. (2003). *Pestering Parents: How Food Companies Market Obesity to Children*. Center for Science in the Public Interest (CSPI), Washington, DC.

172. Nestle, M., et al. (1998). Behavioral and social influences on food choice. *Nutrition Reviews*, 56(5), S50–S74.

173. Skelton, J.A. and Croyle, R.T. (Eds.). (1991). *Mental Representation in Health and Illness*. New York: Springer-Verlag.

174. Severson, K. (2005, April 24). The government's pyramid scheme. *New York Times*.

175. Winett, R.A., et al. (2005). Long-term weight gain prevention: a theoretically based Internet approach. *Preventive Medicine*, 41, 629–641.

176. *Ibid*.

177. Neuhauser, L. and Kreps, G.L. (2003). Rethinking communication in the E-health era. *Journal of Health Psychology*, 8(1), 7–23.

178. Tufano, J.T. and Tarras, B.T. (2005). Mobile eHealth interventions for obesity: a timely opportunity to leverage convergence trends. *Journal of Medicine and Internet Research*, 7(5), e58.

179. Neuhauser, L. and Kreps, G.L. (2003). Rethinking communication in the E-health era. *Journal of Health Psychology*, 8(1), 7–23.

180. Norman, D.A. (1993). *Things that Make Us Smart: Defending Human Attributes in the Age of the Machine*. Reading, MA: Addison-Wesley.

181. *Ibid.*
182. Sterman, J.D. (2000). *Business Dynamics: Systems Thinking and Modeling for a Complex World.* Boston: Irwin McGraw-Hill.
183. *Ibid.*
184. Blakeskee, S. (2005, November 22). This is your brain under hypnosis. *New York Times.*
185. Sterman, J.D. (2000). *Business Dynamics: Systems Thinking and Modeling for a Complex World.* Boston: Irwin McGraw-Hill.
186. Peterson, C. and Stunkard, A.J. (1989). Personal control and health promotion. *Social Science and Medicine,* 28, 819–828.
187. Hammond, J.S, Keeney, R.L., and Raiffa, H. (1998). The hidden traps in decision making. *Harvard Business Review,* 76(5), 47–58.
188. Senge, P.M. (1985). System dynamics, mental models, and the development of management intuition. *Proceedings of the 1985 International Conference of the System Dynamics Society,* P. 788, Keystone, Colorado.
189. Hogarth, R.M. and Makridakis, S. (1981). Forecasting and planning: an evaluation. *Management Science,* 27(2), 115–138.
190. Brody, J. (2004, March 23). Sane weight loss in a carb-obsessed world: high fiber and low fat. *New York Times.*
191. Skelton, J.A. and Croyle, R.T. (Eds.). (1991). *Mental Representation in Health and Illness.* New York: Springer-Verlag.
192. Goldman, S.L., Whitney-Saltiel, D., Granger, J., and Rodin, J. (1991). Children's representations of "everyday" aspects of health and illness. *Journal of Pediatric Psychology,* 16(6), 747–766.
193. *Ibid.*
194. Lau, R.R. and Hartman, K.A. (1983). Common sense representations of common illnesses. *Health Psychology,* 2(2), 167–185.
195. *Ibid.*
196. Kuchler, F. and Variyam, J.N. (2003). Mistakes were made: misperception as a barrier to reducing weight. *International Journal of Obesity,* 27, 856–861.
197. Etelson, D., Brand, D.A., Patrick, P.A., and Shirali, A. (2003). Childhood obesity: do parents recognize this health risk? *Obesity Research,* 11(11), 1362–1368.
198. Eckstein, K.C. et al. (2006). Parents' perceptions of their child's weight and health. *Pediatrics,* 117(3), 681–690.
199. Kuchler, F. and Variyam, J.N. (2003). Mistakes were made: misperception as a barrier to reducing weight. *International Journal of Obesity,* 27, 856–861.
200. Milstein, B. (2008). *Hygeia's Constellation: Navigating Health Futures in a Dynamic and Democratic World.* Atlanta, GA: Syndemics Prevention Network, Centers for Disease Control and Prevention.

201. Senge, P.M. (1990). *The Fifth Discipline: The Art and Practice of the Learning Organization.* New York: Doubleday/Currency.
202. Weinstein, N.D. (1987). Unrealistic optimism about susceptibility to health problems: conclusions from a community-wide sample. *Journal of Behavioral Medicine,* 10(5), 481–500.
203. High Performance Systems. (2001). *An Introduction to Systems Thinking.* Hanover, NH: High Performance Systems.
204. Senge, P.M. (1990). *The Fifth Discipline: The Art and Practice of the Learning Organization.* New York: Doubleday/Currency.
205. Forrester, J.W. (1996). System Dynamics and K-12 Teachers: A lecture at the University of Virginia School of Education. System Dynamics Group report number D-4665-4, Sloan School of Management, MIT. System Dynamics Group report number D-4224-1, Sloan School of Management, MIT.
206. Forrester, J.W. (1994). Learning through System Dynamics as Preparation for the 21st Century. System Dynamics Group report D-4434-1, Sloan School of Management, MIT.
207. Dörner, D. (1989). *The Logic of Failure.* New York: Metropolitan Books.
208. Pi-Sunyer, X. (2003). A clinical view of the obesity problem. *Science,* 299, 859–860.
209. Sterman, J.D. (2000). *Business Dynamics: Systems Thinking and Modeling for a Complex World.* Boston: Irwin McGraw-Hill.
210. Bandura, A. (1997). *Self-Efficacy: The Exercise of Control.* New York: W.H. Freeman.
211. Klein, G. (2007, September). Performing a project premortem. *Harvard Business Review.*
212. The term "microworld" was coined by educator and computer scientist Seymour Papert (developer of "Logo"), to refer to microcosms of reality that serve as laboratories for learning. See: Papert, S. (1980). *Mindstorms: Children, Computers, and Powerful Ideas.* New York: Basic Books.
213. Sterman, J. D. (1992). Teaching takes off: flight simulators for management education. *OR/MS Today,* 40–44.
214. Prensky, M. (2001). *Digital Game-Based Learning.* New York: McGraw-Hill.
215. Sterman, J.D. (2006). Learning from evidence in a complex world. *American Journal of Public Health,* 96(3), 505–514.
216. Sterman, J.D. (2000). *Business Dynamics: Systems Thinking and Modeling for a Complex World.* Boston: Irwin McGraw-Hill.
217. *Ibid.*
218. Einhorn, H.J. and Hogarth, R.M. (1978). Confidence in judgment: persistence of the illusion of validity. *Psychological Review,* 85(5), 395–416.

219. Jana, R. (2006, March 27). On-the-job video gaming: interactive training tools are captivating employees and saving companies money. *Business Week*.

220. Sterman, J.D. (1992). Teaching takes off: flight simulators for management education. *OR/MS Today*, 40–44.

221. Macedonia, M. (2002, March). Games soldiers play. *IEEE Spectrum*, pp. 32–37.

222. *Ibid.*

223. Weinstein, N.D. (1987). Unrealistic optimism about susceptibility to health problems: conclusions from a community-wide sample. *Journal of Behavioral Medicine*, 10(5), 481–500.

224. Rothman, A.J. and Kiviniemi, M.C. (1999). Treating people with information: an analysis and review of approaches to communicating health risk information. *Journal of the National Cancer Institute Monographs*, No. 25, 44–51.

225. *Ibid.*

226. *Ibid.*

227. Weinstein, N.D. (1987). Unrealistic optimism about susceptibility to health problems: conclusions from a community-wide sample. *Journal of Behavioral Medicine*, 10(5), 481–500.

228. Taylor, S.E. and Brown, J.D. (1988). Illusion and well-being: a social psychological perspective on mental health. *Psychological Bulletin*, 103, 193–210.

229. Weinstein, N.D. (1987). Unrealistic optimism about susceptibility to health problems: conclusions from a community-wide sample. *Journal of Behavioral Medicine*, 10(5), 481–500.

230. Harris, L.M. (Ed.) (1995). *Health and the New Media: Technologies Transforming Personal and Public Health*. Mahwah, NJ: Lawrence Erlbaum.

231. Bandura, A. (1997). *Self-Efficacy: The Exercise of Control*. New York: W.H. Freeman.

232. Rothman, A.J. and Kiviniemi, M.C. (1999). Treating people with information: an analysis and review of approaches to communicating health risk information. *Journal of the National Cancer Institute Monographs*, No. 25, 44–51.

233. Revere, D., Dunbar, P.J. (2001). Review of computer-generated outpatient health behavior interventions. *Journal of the American Medical Information Association*, 8, 62–79.

234. Neuhauser, L. and Kreps, G.L. (2003). Rethinking communication in the E-health era. *Journal of Health Psychology*, 8(1), 7–23.

235. Harris, L.M. (Ed.) (1995). *Health and the New Media: Technologies Transforming Personal and Public Health*. Mahwah, NJ: Lawrence Erlbaum.

236. Rothman, A.J. and Kiviniemi, M.C. (1999). Treating people with information: an analysis and review of approaches to communicating health risk information. *Journal of the National Cancer Institute Monographs*, No. 25, 44–51.
237. Taylor, S.E. and Brown, J.D. (1988). Illusion and well-being: a social psychological perspective on mental health. *Psychological Bulletin*, 103, 193–210.
238. Plous, S. (1993). *The Psychology of Judgment and Decision Making*. New York: McGraw Hill.
239. Jeffery, R.W. (1998). Prevention of Obesity. In: Bray, G.A., Bouchard, C., and James, W.P.T. (Eds.). *Handbook of Obesity*. New York: Marcel Dekker.
240. Rothman, A.J. and Kiviniemi, M.C. (1999). Treating people with information: an analysis and review of approaches to communicating health risk information. *Journal of the National Cancer Institute Monographs*, No. 25, 44–51.
241. De Kler, R. (1998). Clinical simulations: a pedagogical and chronological perspective. In: Anderson, J.G. and Katzper, M. (Eds.). *Proceedings of the 1998 Medical Sciences Simulation Conference* (pp. 181–6). San Diego, CA: Society for Computer Simulation International.
242. Schrage, M. (2000). *Serious Play: How the World's Best Companies Simulate to Innovate*. Cambridge, MA: Harvard Business School Press.
243. Platoni, K. (2008, January/February). Seeing is believing. *Stanford Magazine*, pp. 48–55.
244. *Ibid.*
245. *Ibid.*
246. I am certainly not the first to do so.
247. Peters, J.C., Wyatt, H.R., Donahoo, W.T., and Hill, J.O. (2002). From instinct to intellect: the challenge of maintaining healthy weight in the modern world. *Obesity Reviews*, 3, 69–74.
248. *Ibid.*
249. Wadden, T.A., Brownell, K.D., and Foster, G.D. (2002). Obesity: responding to the global epidemic. *Journal of Consulting and Clinical Psychology*, 70(3), 510–525.
250. Critser, G. (2003). *Fat Land: How Americans Became the Fattest People in the World*. Boston: Mariner.
251. Gill, T.P. (1997). Key issues in the prevention of obesity. *British Medical Bulletin*, 53(2), 359–388.
252. Bray, G.A, Bouchard, C., and James, W.P.T. (Eds.). (1998). *Handbook of Obesity*. New York: Marcel Dekker.
253. Gawande, A. (2002). *Complications: A Surgeon's Notes on an Imperfect Science*. New York: Metropolitan Books.

254. Gill, T.P. (1997). Key issues in the prevention of obesity. *British Medical Bulletin*, 53(2), 359–388.

255. Gawande, A. (2002). *Complications: A Surgeon's Notes on an Imperfect Science*. New York: Metropolitan Books.

256. Nestle, M., et al. (1998). Behavioral and social influences on food choice. *Nutrition Reviews*, 56(5), S50–S74.

257. Wadden, T.A., Brownell, K.D., and Foster, G.D. (2002). Obesity: responding to the global epidemic. *Journal of Consulting and Clinical Psychology*, 70(3), 510–525.

258. Gill, T.P. (1997). Key issues in the prevention of obesity. *British Medical Bulletin*, 53(2), 359–388.

259. Bray, G.A, Bouchard, C., and James, W.P.T. (Eds.). (1998). *Handbook of Obesity*. New York: Marcel Dekker.

260. Tufano, J.T. and Tarras, B.T. (2005). Mobile eHealth interventions for obesity: a timely opportunity to leverage convergence trends. *Journal of Medicine and Internet Research*, 7(5), e58.

261. Belkin, L. (2006, August 20). The school-lunch test. *New York Times Magazine*, p. 30.

262. Bray, G.A, Bouchard, C., and James, W.P.T. (Eds.). (1998). *Handbook of Obesity*. New York: Marcel Dekker.

263. Stice, E., Shaw, H., and Marti, C.N. (2006). A meta-analytic review of obesity prevention programs for children and adolescents: the skinny on interventions that work. *Psychological Bulletin*, 132(5), 667–691.

264. Ahern, D.K., Phalen, J.M., Le, L.X., and Goldman, R.E. (2007). *Childhood Obesity Prevention and Reduction: Role of eHealth*. Boston: Health e-Technologies Initiative.

265. Schlosser, E. (2002). *Fast Food Nation: The Dark Side of the All-American Meal*. New York: Perennial.

266. Nestle, M. (2002). *Food Politics: How the Food Industry Influences Nutrition and Health*. Berkeley, CA: University of California Press.

267. Shortliffe, E.H. (1997). How will the information revolution change the practice of medicine? *Presented at the ABIM Summer Conference on Societal Forces Reshaping American Medicine-Implications for Internal Medicine*, Durango, Colorado.

268. Ahern, D.K., Phalen, J.M., Le, L.X., and Goldman, R.E. (2007). *Childhood Obesity Prevention and Reduction: Role of eHealth*. Boston: Health e-Technologies Initiative.

269. Senge, P.M. (1990). *The Fifth Discipline: The Art and Practice of the Learning Organization*. New York: Doubleday/Currency.

270. Gould-Kreutzer, J. M. (2006). Foreword: system dynamics in education. *System Dynamics Review*. 9(2), 101–112.

271. Ahern, D.K., Phalen, J.M., Le, L.X., and Goldman, R.E. (2007). *Childhood Obesity Prevention and Reduction: Role of eHealth*. Boston, MA: Health e-Technologies Initiative.

272. Squire, K. (2003). Video games in education. *International Journal of Intelligent Simulations and Gaming*, 2(1).

273. *Ibid.*

274. Sawyer, B. (2002). Serious games: improving public policy through game-based learning and simulation. *Woodrow Wilson International Center for Scholars*: 31, http://wwics.si.edu/subsites/game/index.htm.

275. Edwards, C. (2006, February 20). Class, take out your games: how teachers are using computer games to pique the interest of tech-savvy kids. *Business Week*.

276. De Kler, R. (1998). Clinical simulations: a pedagogical and chronological perspective. In: Anderson, J.G. and Katzper, M. (Eds.). *Proceedings of the 1998 Medical Sciences Simulation Conference* (pp. 181–186). San Diego, CA: Society for Computer Simulation International.

277. Honan, W.H. (2002, August 14). The college lecture, long derided, may be fading. *New York Times*.

278. Dewey, J. (1963). *Experience and Education*. New York: Macmillan. (Original work published 1938).

279. Tufano, J.T. and Tarras, B.T. (2005). Mobile eHealth interventions for obesity: a timely opportunity to leverage convergence trends. *Journal of Medicine and Internet Research*, 7(5), e58.

280. Nestle, M. et al. (1998). Behavioral and social influences on food choice. *Nutrition Reviews*, 56(5), S50–S74.

281. Fairburn, C.G. (1995). The prevention of eating disorders. In: Brownell, K.D. and Fairburn, C.G. (Eds.). *Eating Disorders and Obesity. A Comprehensive Handbook* (pp. 289–293). New York: Guilford Press.

282. Lieberman, D.A. (1998). Health education video games for children and adolescents: theory, design, and research findings. Paper presented at the Annual Meeting of the International Communication Association (48th, Jerusalem, Israel, July 20–24).

283. Harris, L.M. (Ed.) (1995). *Health and the New Media: Technologies Transforming Personal and Public Health*. Mahwah, NJ: Lawrence Erlbaum.

284. Neuhauser, L. and Kreps, G.L. (2003). Rethinking communication in the E-health era. *Journal of Health Psychology*, 8(1), 7–23.

285. Kline, K.N. (1999). Reading and reforming breast self-examination discourse: claiming missed opportunities for empowerment. *Journal of Health Communication*, 4, 119–141.

286. Lieberman, D.A. (1998). Health education video games for children and adolescents: theory, design, and research findings. Paper presented at

the Annual Meeting of the International Communication Association (48th, Jerusalem, Israel, July 20–24).

287. Harris, L.M. (Ed.) (1995). *Health and the New Media: Technologies Transforming Personal and Public Health.* Mahwah, NJ: Lawrence Erlbaum.

288. Platoni, K. (2008, January/February). Seeing is believing. *Stanford Magazine*, pp. 48–55.

289. Lieberman, D.A. (1998). Health education video games for children and adolescents: theory, design, and research findings. Paper presented at the Annual Meeting of the International Communication Association (48th, Jerusalem, Israel, July 20–24).

290. Sawyer, B. (2002). Serious games: improving public policy through game-based learning and simulation. *Woodrow Wilson International Center for Scholars*: 31, http://wwics.si.edu/subsites/game/index.htm.

291. Roberts, N. (1975). A Dynamic Feedback Approach to Elementary Social Studies: A Prototype Gaming Unit. Ph.D. dissertation, Boston University.

292. Roberts, N. (1978). Teaching dynamic feedback systems thinking: an elementary view. *Management Science*, 24(8), 836–843.

293. Lyneis D. A. (2000). Bringing system dynamics to a school near you suggestions for introducing and sustaining system dynamics in K-12 Education. International System Dynamics Society Conference, Bergen, Norway.

294. Forrester, J.W. (1991). System Dynamics and the Lessons of 35 years. Working paper No. D-4224-4, System Dynamics Group, Sloan School of Management, Massachusetts Institute of Technology Cambridge, MA.

295. Mandinach, E.B. and Cline, H.F. (1993). Systems, science, and schools. *System Dynamics Review*, 9(2), 195–206.

296. Alessi, S. (2000). The application of system dynamics in elementary and secondary school curricular. http://www.c5.cl/ieinvestiga/actas/ribie2000/charlas/alessi.htm.

297. Forrester, J.W. (1993). System dynamics as an organizing framework for pre-college education. *System Dynamics Review*, 9(20), 183–194.

298. Forrester, J. W. (1999). System Dynamics: the Foundation Under Systems Thinking. Sloan School of Management, Massachusetts Institute of Technology Cambridge, MA.

299. Hight, J. (1995). System dynamics for kids. *Technology Review*, Vol. 98, No.2, section on MITnews, from the Association of Alumni and Alumnae of MIT.

300. Forrester, J. W. (1999). System Dynamics: the Foundation Under Systems Thinking. Sloan School of Management, Massachusetts Institute of Technology Cambridge, MA.

301. Forrester, J.W. (1996). System Dynamics and K-12 Teachers: A lecture at the University of Virginia School of Education. System Dynamics Group report number D-4665-4, Sloan School of Management, MIT. System Dynamics Group report number D-4224-1, Sloan School of Management, MIT.

302. Lyneis D. A. (2000). Bringing system dynamics to a school near you suggestions for introducing and sustaining system dynamics in K-12 education. International System Dynamics Society Conference, Bergen, Norway.

303. *Ibid.*

304. Sterman, J.D. (1994). Learning in and about complex systems. *System Dynamics Review*, 10, 291–330.

305. Story, M., Neumark-Sztainer, D., and French, S. (2002). Individual and environmental influences on adolescent eating behaviors. *Supplement to the Journal of the American Dietetic Association*, 102(3), S40–S51.

306. Brown, P.J. and Bentley-Condit, V. (1998). Culture, evolution, and obesity. In: Bray, G.A., Bouchard, C., and James, W.P.T. (Eds.). *Handbook of Obesity*. New York: Marcel Dekker.

307. Johnson, S.L. and Birch, L.L. (1994). Parents' and children's adiposity and eating style. *Pediatrics*, 94(5), 653–661.

308. Bandura, A. (1997). *Self-Efficacy: The Exercise of Control*. New York: W.H. Freeman.

309. Hodges, E.A. (2003). A primer on early childhood obesity and parental influence. *Pediatric Nursing*, 29(1), 13–16.

310. Johnson, S.L. and Birch, L.L. (1994). Parents' and children's adiposity and eating style. *Pediatrics*, 94(5), 653–661.

311. *Ibid.*

312. Hodges, E.A. (2003). A primer on early childhood obesity and parental influence. *Pediatric Nursing*, 29(1), 13–16.

313. *Ibid.*

314. Senge, P.M. (1990). *The Fifth Discipline: The Art and Practice of the Learning Organization*. New York: Doubleday/Currency.

315. *Ibid.*

316. *Ibid.*

317. *Ibid.*

318. *Ibid.*

319. Kim, D. and Anderson, V. (1998). *Systems Archetype Basics*. Waltham, MA: Pegasus Communications.

320. Capaldi, E.D. ed. (1996). *Why We Eat What We Eat: The Psychology of Eating*. Washington, DC: American Psychological Association.

321. Birch, L.L. and Fisher, J.O. (1998). Development of eating behaviors among children and adolescents. *Pediatrics*, 101(3 Suppl), 539–549.

322. Johnson, S.L. and Birch, L.L. (1994). Parents' and children's adiposity and eating style. *Pediatrics*, 94(5), 653–661.

323. Parker-Pope, T. (2003, December 9). How to give your child a longer life. *Wall Street Journal*.

324. New York Times. (1994, November 10). Over-control of eating leads to fat children, study warns. *New York Times*.

325. Birch, L.L. and Fisher, J.O. (1998). Development of eating behaviors among children and adolescents. *Pediatrics*, 101(3 Suppl), 539–549.

326. Capaldi, E.D. ed. (1996). *Why We Eat What We Eat: The Psychology of Eating*. Washington, DC: American Psychological Association.

327. Senge, P.M. (1990). *The Fifth Discipline: The Art and Practice of the Learning Organization*. New York: Doubleday/Currency.

328. Bandura, A. (1997). *Self-Efficacy: The Exercise of Control*. New York: W.H. Freeman.

329. Peters, J.C., Wyatt, H.R., Donahoo, W.T., and Hill, J.O. (2002). From instinct to intellect: the challenge of maintaining healthy weight in the modern world. *Obesity Reviews*, 3, 69–74.

330. Bandura, A. (1997). *Self-Efficacy: The Exercise of Control*. New York: W.H. Freeman.

331. Baumeister, R.F., Heatherton, T.F., and Tice, D.M. (1994). *Losing Control: How and Why People Fail at Self-Regulation*. San Diego: Academic Press.

332. *Ibid.*

333. Lerch, F.J. and Harter, D.E. (2001). Cognitive support for real-time dynamic decision making. *Information Systems Research*, 12(1), 63–82.

334. Bandura, A. (1997). *Self-Efficacy: The Exercise of Control*. New York: W.H. Freeman.

335. *Ibid.*

336. Capaldi, E.D. ed. (1996). *Why We Eat What We Eat: The Psychology of Eating*. Washington, DC: American Psychological Association.

337. Fisher, E.S. and Welch, H.G. (1999). Avoiding the unintended consequences of growth in medical care. *JAMA*, 281(5), 446–453.

338. Wood, D. J. and Petriglieri, G. (2005). Transcending polarization: beyond binary thinking. *Transactional Analysis Journal*, 35(1), 31–39.

339. Breyer, S. (1993). *Breaking the Vicious Circle: Toward Effective Risk Regulation*. Cambridge, MA: Harvard University Press.

340. *Ibid.*

341. Kaufman, F.R. (2005). *Diabesity: The Obesity-Diabetes Epidemic that Threatens America—And What We Must Do to Stop It*. New York: Bantam Books.

342. Manning, A. (2006, May 30). Study: 73 M have diabetes or are at risk in U.S. *USA Today*.

343. Wood, D. J. and Petriglieri, G. (2005). Transcending polarization: beyond binary thinking. *Transactional Analysis Journal*, 35(1), 31–39.

344. Fisher, E.S. and Welch, H.G. (1999). Avoiding the unintended consequences of growth in medical care. *JAMA*, 281(5), 446–453.

345. Collins, M.D. (2005). Transcending dualistic thinking in conflict resolution. *Negotiation Journal*, 21(2), 263–280.

346. Brehmer, B. (1990). Strategies in real-time, dynamic decision making. In: Hogarth, R. (Ed.). *Insights in Decision Making: A Tribute to Hillel J. Einhorn*. Chicago: University of Chicago Press.

347. Brown, G. (1999). *The Energy of Life: The Science of What Makes Our Minds and Bodies Work*. New York: Free Press.

348. *Ibid*.

349. *Ibid*.

350. Dalton, S. (Ed.). (1997). *Overweight and Weight Management: The Health Professional's Guide to Understanding and Practice*. Gaithersburg, MD: Aspen.

351. Flegal, K.M., Troiano, R.P. and Ballard-Barbash, R. (2001). Aim for a healthy weight: what is the target? *Journal of Nutrition*, 131, 440S–450S.

352. Bandura, A. (1997). *Self-Efficacy: The Exercise of Control*. New York: W.H. Freeman.

353. For example, the Polar M52 developed by the Polar Company.

354. Gutner, T. (2005, August 15). A workout pro close at hand. *Business Week*.

355. Baker, S. and Leak, B. (2006, January 23). Math will rock your world. *Business Week*.

356. Capell, K., Arndt, M. and Carey, J. (2005, September 5). Drugs get smart. *Business Week*.

357. Millenson, M.L. (2006, February 14). The promise of personalized medicine: a conversation with Michael Svinte. *Health Affairs*, published online, pp. w54–w60.

358. Baker, S. and Leak, B. (2006, January 23). Math will rock your world. *Business Week*.

359. Senge, P.M. (1990). *The Fifth Discipline: The Art and Practice of the Learning Organization*. New York: Doubleday/Currency.

360. Capell, K., Arndt, M. and Carey, J. (2005, September 5). Drugs get smart. *Business Week*.

361. Hood, L. (2003). System biology: integrating technology, biology, and computation. *Mechanisms of Ageing and Development*, 124, 9–16.

362. Millenson, M.L. (2006, February 14). The promise of personalized medicine: a conversation with Michael Svinte. *Health Affairs*, published online, pp. w54–w60.
363. Freedman, D.H. (2004, March). The virtual heart. *Technology Review*, pp. 62–68.
364. Economist. (1998, July 18). Model behavior. *The Economist*, pp. 69–70.
365. Freedman, D.H. (2004, March). The virtual heart. *Technology Review*, pp. 62–68.
366. Economist. (1998, July 18). Model behavior. *The Economist*, pp. 69–70.
367. Freedman, D.H. (2004, March). The virtual heart. *Technology Review*, pp. 62–68.
368. Carey, J. (2006, May 29). Medical guesswork: from heart surgery to prostate care, the health industry knows little about which common treatments really work. *Business Week*.
369. Casti, J.L. (1997). *Would-be Worlds: How Simulation Is Changing the Frontiers of Science*. New York: John Wiley .
370. Wikipedia.(2007). Ubiquitous Computing. http://en.wikipedia.org/wiki/Ubiquitous_computing.
371. Weiser, M. (1991). The computer of the 21st century. *Scientific American*, 265(3), 66–75.
372. Abowd, G.D., Mynatt, E.D., and Rodden, T. (2002). The human experience. *Pervasive Computing*, 1(1), 48–57.
373. Want, R., Pering, T., Borriello, G., and Farkas, K.I. (2002, January–March). Disappearing hardware. *Pervasive Computing*, pp. 36–47.
374. O'Neil, J. (1999, May 18). "Smart toilet" keeps track of health. *New York Times*.
375. Brooke, J. (2002, October 8). Japanese masters get closer to the toilet nirvana. *New York Times*.
376. Want, R., Pering, T., Borriello, G., and Farkas, K.I. (2002, January–March). Disappearing hardware. *Pervasive Computing*, pp. 36–47.
377. Williams, D. (2006, February). Can I hear me now? *Harvard Business Review*, pp. 37–38.
378. *Ibid*.
379. D'Andrea Tyson, L. (2000, July 24). A startling medical breakthrough: The Internet. *Business Week*.
380. Markoff, J. (2004, December 30). Internet use said to cut into TV viewing and socializing. *New York Times*.
381. Kassirer, J.P. (1995). The next transformation in the delivery of health care. *New England Journal of Medicine*, 332(1), 52–53.
382. U.S. Congress, Office of Technology Assessment. (1995). *Bringing Health Care Online: The Role of Information Technologies*, OTA-ITC-624. Washington, DC: U.S. Government Printing Office.

383. Pogue, D. (2005, September 22). Aha! Video straight to a computer. *New York Times*.

384. Lohr, S. (2007, August 14). Dr. Google and Dr. Microsoft. *New York Times*.

385. Neuhauser, L. and Kreps, G.L. (2003). Rethinking communication in the E-health era. *Journal of Health Psychology*, 8(1), 7–23.

386. Ebbeling, C.B. and Ludwig, D.S. (2008). Tracking pediatric obesity: an index of uncertainty? *JAMA*, 299(20), 2442–2443.

387. Hammer, M. (1990, July/August). Reengineering work: don't automate, obliterate. *Harvard Business Review*, pp. 104–112.

388. Morison, E. (2004). Gunfire at sea: a case study of innovation. In: Tushman, M.L. and Anderson, P. (Eds.). *Managing Strategic Innovation and Change: A Collection of Readings*, 2nd ed. Oxford: Oxford University Press.

389. Hammer, M., (1990). Reengineering work: don't automate, obliterate. *Harvard Business Review*, July/August, pp. 104–112.

390. Phrase first coined by Michael Hammer.

Subject Index

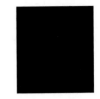

A

Active Living Program, of San Diego State
  University, 117
Active overconsumption, 93
Adipocyte proliferation, 66
Adipocytes, 66
"Ad-libitum" mental model, 137
Adrenaline, 297
Advertisements, food, 108, 364
Alzheimer's disease, 9
America's eating habits, 80–86
Amino acids, significance, 296
Amish communities, 115
Anthropological perspective, 56–58
Appetite regulation
  short-term and long-term, 208
Asymmetries in human energy regulation,
  208–210
Archetype, 353
Arthritis, 9
Automatic feeding control, 137

B

Ballistic behavior, 311
Bariatric surgery, 358
Bathtub exercise, 268–275, 279–280
Behavioral Risk Factor Surveillance Surveys
  (BRFSS), 353
Beta cells, 292
Binary thinking, 425
Bioenergetics system, human, 28, 278
Biology–environment interactions, 55–56
Biopsychosocial perspective, 55
Blood glucose, 294
Blood's glucose concentration, in normal
  individual, 292
Body area networks, 435
Body composition, 298–301
  Forbes's experiments, 301

Body fat topology, 8
Body mass index (BMI), 5–6, 89, 128–129
Body weight, 78
Boiled-frog parable, 3–39
"Bonking", 298
Boom–bust cycles, in food availability, 135
Bounded rationality, 266

C

Carbohydrate-based fuel, 66
Carbohydrate diet, high, impacts, 332
Chlorofluorocarbons (CFCs), 17
Chubby children, 122
Coercive feeding, 417, 422
Cognitive control, 138–140, 215, 216
Cognitive processes, 175
Compensatory feedback effects, 373
Complex nonlinear feedback systems, 279
Computer modeling tools, 281
  of complex systems, 283
  as personal health decision support systems,
    335–336
Computer models, use, 37
Computer simulation, 282, 284
Confirming-evidence bias, 21
Continuing Surveys of Food Intake by
  Individuals (CSFII), 78–79
Conventional wisdom, 171
Customization, 39, 243, 323, 336, 405, 410,
  437, 440

D

Deep/double-loop learning, 22–26
  barriers, 27
Deep-freezing technology, 82
De novo lipogenesis, 295
Diabetes, 3, 8, 131, 143, 209, 358, 359, 360, 389,
  426, 434

T.K.A. Hamid, *Thinking in Circles About Obesity*,
DOI 10.1007/978-0-387-09469-4, © Springer Science+Business Media, LLC 2009

Diet and exercise regimens, comparison
    experiment, 326
    integration physical activity and dieting, 334
    manipulation of diet composition, 332–334
    time aspect in excercising, 330–332
Dietary fat, 94
Dietary protein, importance, 296
Diet books, 171
Dieting, 13
Diffusion of innovations, 172
Discrimination, against obese people, 11
Double-loop learning, 22–26, 414
Double-loop playing, 414
Drive-through window restaurants, 91

E
Eating out, 90–91
Eating pattern, trends, *see* Feeding behavior,
    human
Economic incentives, 114, 365–366
Economic Research Service (ERS), of the U.S.
    Department of Agriculture (USDA), 79
Economic value of time, 81
Energy balance equation, 32–36, 325
    in academic literature, 171–172
    plumbing analogy, 180–182
    principles, 172
Energy-balance model, of body weight
    regulation, 18–19, 184
    complexities, 277–279
Energy conservation measures, 19–20
Energy deficiency and basal metabolism, 65
Energy deficit, 305
Energy expenditure
    bathtub analogy, 197–199
    determinants, 186–191
    implications for treatment, 193–196
    and responses to imbalances, 191–193
    at workplace, 113–115
    See also Energy balance equation
Energy expenditure (EE) subsystem, 278–279
Energy intake
    American eating habits, 80–86
    due to poor quality of food, 78–79
    food abundance and overconsumption, 80
    See also Energy balance equation
Energy intake (EI) subsystem, 287
Energy metabolism and regulation, 291–298
Energy regulation, asymmetrical
    in energy expenditure, 64–65
    in energy intake, 60–64
    in energy storage, 65–67
Energy regulation, management, 267
Environmental Protection Agency (EPA), 373

Epinephrine, 297
Eroding goals, 354–355
Essential fat, 298
Esterification, 300
Exercise intensity, 330–332
Exercise metabolism, 297–298
Exercising, 122–123
Expectancy-valence theory, 265

F
Fast-food restaurants, 91–92
    demand-pull, 103–105
    food quality, 92–93
    health impacts of fast foods, 94–95
    impact of advertising and promotion,
        107–108
    portions of, 95–100
    portions sizes of fast food, 95–100
        children's food habit, 98–99
    supply force, 105–108
    U.S. market, 97
Fat-analysis scales, 299
Fat cells, 62, 63, 66, 67, 127, 143, 204, 207,
    209–213
Fat cell theory, 212, 227
Fat-enriched foods, 93
Fat-Free Mass (FFM), 301
Fat Mass (FM), 299–300, 326–328
Fatty foods, 58
Feedback processes, 31–32, 36–37
    multiple possible scenarios, 242
    use of computer simulations, 243
Feeding behavior, human, 69–70
    amnestic patients, 71
    drive to overeat, 106–107
    of free-living adult Americans, 106
    socioeconomic-technological factors,
        changing, 80–86
    time and space dimensions, 86–100
Feeding regulation, assymetrical, 60–63
Fidgeting, 127–128
Finland, health status of residents, 379–380
Flows, 219–221
Food pyramid, 387–408
Forerunners, 430
Free fatty acid metabolism, 292–296
French portion sizes, 96

G
Game-based learning, 410
Genetics, 14, 58, 126, 128, 434
Glucagon, 296
Gluconeogenesis, 296

Glucose and free fatty acid metabolism, 292–296
Glucose regulation, in human body, 292–296
Glycogenesis, 295
Glycogenolysis, 296
Goal erosion path, 355
Goals, 215, 223, 224–230
Goal- seeking negative-feedback structure, 354, 373
Government initiatives and incentives, for exercising, 367

H

Health care, as business industry, 357–358
Health potential programs (HPPs), 429–431
Health risks, with obesity, 8–9
Healthy people 2010, 388
Homeostatic mechanism, 65–66
Homeostatic processes, 19
Homeostatic system, 210–213
Homo sedentarius, 120
Hormone-sensitive lipase, 295
Human–environment interactions
    feeding behavior, 69–70
    and function of lifestyle choices and preferences, 72
    with physical environment, 76
    role of physical characteristics, 72–74
    socioeconomic factors, 73–74
    See also Feeding behavior, human
Human genome mapping, 433
Hybrid technology, 371–373, 375–376
Hysteresis, 318

I

Illusion of control, 174
Illusion of unique-invulnerability, 20, 404, 406
Individual-centered "theory", 54
Individual differences, in weight regulation experiment
    dieting, 304
    overfeeding, 318–320
    static and dynamic aspects, 318
Information technologies, in health management, 38, 438, 440
Insulin resistance, 357
Insulin secretion, 293
Internet, 433, 437, 438
Involuntary energy expenditure, 304

K

Kitchen appliances, advanced, 83
    and cost savings, 86–87
Kung San tribe, of Kalahari Desert, 58

L

Learning deficiency, 23
Leptin, 63, 127, 207
Leverage points, 127, 377–379
Lifestyle changes and obesity, 4
Linear thinking, 177–180

M

Macronutrients, 65, 94, 95, 190, 206, 278, 289
Maladaptation, 4
Mass customization, 323
Mental maps, discovery, 23
Mental models, 16–18, 169
    autopilot's "mental model", 25–26
    health education, 390–392
Metabolism, defined, 291–292
Metanoia, 28
Microworlds, 38
    as operational models, 284–287
    subsystems, 287–288
        body composition, 298–301
        energy expenditure (EE), 290–291
        energy intake (EI), 289–290
        energy metabolism and regulation, 291–298
Military flight simulators, 402
Molecular biology, 433
Multiloop nonlinear feedback systems, 240
Muscle glycogen depletion, impact, 298

N

National School Breakfast Program (NSBP), 362
National School Lunch Act, 364
National School Lunch Program (NSLP), 363
National Weight Control Registry (NWCR), 140
Natural Selection, Principle of, model, 176
Negative energy balance, 240–241
Negative feedback loops, 102–103, 197, 379
    glucose metabolism, 297
Nonlinearity, 179
Nonsmokers and obesity, 7–8
North Karelia Project, 380
Nutritional excess, impacts, 300

O

Obesity
    associated health risks, 8–9, 357–358
        disabilities among older adults, 9
    causes, 3–5
    deaths, 7
    global impact, 11–12
    impacts, 7–9

Obesity (cont.)
  health care costs, 11
  management
    analysis of different dimensions, 28–31
    body management, 14–16
    role of emotions, 20–22
    strategies, 12–13
  people perception, 6–7, 393
    about weight-loss programs, 13–14
  prevention, *see* Prevention
  sociocultural impact, 10–11
  trends, 3, 5–7
ob gene, 127
Oil consumption, 371, 379–380
  public regulation policy, 371–372
One-size-fits-all model, 322–323
Optimism, unrealistic, 20–21
Optimistic bias, 404
Outcome feedback, 280
Overweight children, 6
"Owning one's disability" method, 10

P
Passive entertainment, 118
Passive overconsumption, 94
Personal control, 53
Personal differences and obesity
  body weight and body mass index (BMI), 126
  genetic factor, 126–130
Personalized health decision support systems,
    335–336
Phenotype, 130
Physiologic asymmetries, 60, 67
Physiological drives, control
  dieting and self-control, 215–216
  laboratory experiments, 221–222
  management of stock-and-flow system,
    219–220
  and resource management, 221–222
Physiological flight simulators, 403
Pima Indians, 130–131
Plaque in arteries, 358
Polar diagrams, 428
Policy resistance phenomenon, 374
Positive feedback loops, 102–103
Positive feedback processes, 102, 141
Positive health, idea, 427
Predictive judgment, 265
Prevention
  approaches, 335–336
  childhood obesity intervention
    child-feeding strategies and role
      modeling, 422–423
    concepts of systems thinking, 418–420

    digital method of teaching, 422–424
    double-loop playing, 414
    play therapy, 414–415
    shifting-the-burden structure, 421–422
    teaching of healthy eating habits, 422–423
  energy-input aspects, 362–363
  goal of, 357–358
  health care costs, 359
  health education
    clearing misconceptions, 393–394
    development of technologies, 412–413
    failure of, 426–427
    Government efforts, 386–388
    informing the public, 388–389
    learning from experience, 398–400
    for mental models, 392–398
    weaknesses of the educational strategy,
      391–393
  intervention strategies with low leverage
    points, 376–377
  prevention-unfriendly financial
    incentives, 360
  private health care system, 357
  promotion of physical activity, 366–367
  public legislative and regulatory policy, 361,
    363–364
  taxation of foods, 364–365
  U.S. disease-prevention efforts, 382–384
Processed foods, 83
Prostate cancer, 9
Protein/amino acid metabolism, 296
Proteins, obligatory loss, 296

R
Recidivism, 192
Resting energy expenditure (REE), 64, 290, 304
Resting metabolic rate (RMR), 127
Risk assessment, 397, 404

S
Satiation, 60, 71, 204, 205, 206
Satiety, 62, 70, 71, 93, 94, 99, 204, 205, 206, 208
Self-efficacy, 235, 237
Self-help books, 18, 170
Self-regulation skills, 144
Self-reinforcing process, 101–102
Shifting the burden, 418–420, 422–423
Silver-bullet, 26, 142–144
Simulation models, *see* Microworlds
Single-loop learning, 23, 24
Single-loop playing, 414
Smokers and obesity, 8
Snacking habit, 87
Societal maladaptation, 4

Soft-drink consumption, 88–90
Stable equilibrium, 112
STACI (Systems Thinking and Curriculum Innovation) project, 415
Stocks, 219–221, 232, 233, 234
STELLA software, 415
Strength model of human self-regulation, 217–218
Storage fat, 298
Sugar-sweetened drinks, 89
Super-sizing foods, 96, 97, 99
Surface/single-loop learning, 22–26

T
Taxation, 365, 366
Television viewing, 118–119, 122
Theory of illness, 395–396
Thermic effect of activity (TEA), 278
Thermic effect of feeding (TEF), 304, 308
Thermic effect of food (TEF), 278
Time delay, in obesity management, 15
Tipping-point phenomena, 100–101
Transcendence, notion, 423
Trial and error learning, 22
Triglycerides, 295, 299
Type 2 diabetes, 426

U
Ubiquitous information technologies, 434
Unrealistic goals, 224–230
    and dieter's personal agendas, 230–231
Unrealistic optimism, 20, 21, 404

V
Vanity sizes, 354
Variety of foods, 58, 71, 106, 107, 361
Video games, 118, 119, 411
Virtual-heart (or cardiome) project, 434

W
Weight-cycling, risk factors, 235
Weight cycling ("yo-yo dieting") phenomenon, 26, 234
Weight gain, trend in United States, 3, 5–7, 135–137
Weight loss, assessment
    caloric deficit to achieve desired weight loss
        experiment, 312–314
        failure to achieve, 314–315
    diet regimen, overview, 303–305
Weight-loss programs, 14
Weight regulation, individual differences
    experiment
        dieting, 320–322
        one-size-fits-all model, 322–323
        overfeeding, 318–320
        static and dynamic aspects, 318
Wellness and disease conditions, 425
Wellness movement, 53
Women and obesity
    labor-force participation, 81, 84, 103–104
    technological innovations, role, 81–84

Y
Years of life lost (YLL), due to obesity, 7–8